SUPPLY CHAIN MANAGEMENT IN THE DRUG INDUSTRY

SUPPLY CHAIN MANAGEMENT IN THE DRUG INDUSTRY

Delivering Patient Value for Pharmaceuticals and Biologics

Hedley Rees

WILEY

A JOHN WILEY & SONS, INC., PUBLICATION

Published by John Wiley & Sons, Inc., Hoboken, New Jersey.
Published simultaneously in Canada.

For general information on our other products and services or for technical support, please contact our Customer Care Department within the United States at (800) 762-2974, outside the United States at (317) 572-3993 or fax (317) 572-4002.

Wiley publishes in a variety of print and electronic formats and by print-on-demand. Some material included with standard print versions of this book may not be included in e-books or in print-on-demand. If this book refers to media such as a CD or DVD that is not included in the version you purchased, you may download this material at http://booksupport.wiley.com. For more information about Wiley products, visit www.wiley.com.

Library of Congress Cataloging-in-Publication Data:

Rees, Hedley.
  Supply chain management in the drug industry : delivering patient value for pharmaceuticals and biologics / Hedley Rees.
       p.   ;   cm.
  Includes index.
     ISBN 978-0-470-55517-0 (cloth)
  1. Pharmaceuticals industry–Materials management.   I. Title.
  [DNLM: 1. Drug Industry–organization & administration. QV   736   R328s   2011]
  HD9665.5.R44 2011
  615.1068′5–dc22   2010023288

Printed in Singapore

10 9 8 7 6 5 4 3 2

To

Carol, my wife and North Star in life

Morfydd, my mother and first mentor

Jack, my father and biggest fan
(his eyes told me, *he* never could)

CONTENTS

CONTRIBUTORS

Jo-anna Allen

Jo-anna is currently associate director of sales at Shire Human Genetics Therapy Team. Previously, she ran her own consultancy, JOST Consulting, was field sales manager at Sanofi Pasteur MSD, national sales manager at Cephalon, and senior regional business manager at Elan Pharmaceuticals.

Dan Barreto

Dan is staff vice president for quality assurance at C. R. Bard. From 1978 to 1996, Dan held various positions at the FDA as investigator, manager of investigators, and member of the FDA management development team. Previously, Dan was manager of compliance for medeva and vice president for international compliance at Janssen Pharmaceutica.

Joshua Bashford

For the past ten years, Josh has been a researcher studying the basic science of metabolic disorders and cardiovascular disease at the Metabolic Diseases Institute at the University of Cincinnati. In addition to research responsibilities, he has enjoyed involvement with project management, program development, and consulting across multiple disciplines.

Owen Berkeley-Hill

Owen has a degree in engineering from Salford. He worked at Ford Europe and spent time in North America on Ford's first BPR project before returning to England to become an internal process-improvement consultant and was assigned to the Ford production system, Ford's lean journey. He graduated with a Master's degree in lean operations in 2003 and retired from Ford in 2005.

Jill Bunyan

A registered pharmacist and experienced regulatory consultant, Jill gained a Ph.D. in pharmaceutics from the University of Strathclyde in 1992. With experience in hospital, retail, and industrial pharmacy, Jill then joined a regulatory affairs consultancy in 1995, before setting up independently in 2009.

Sarah Callens

Sarah is a process development specialist at eXmoor Pharma Concepts Ltd. Previously, she developed characterization assays for regulatory submission and is developing a second-generation manufacturing process for stem cell therapies at ReNeuron. Her prior experience includes working at Onyvax and Stryker Biotech. She has a B.Sc. degree from the Evergreen State College.

Dee Carri

Dee established her own company, Torque Management, in 2002. During her career, Dee has held a number of senior management positions: at Gartner UK as consulting director, at PA Consulting Group in Ireland as e-business development director, and at Elan Corporation as vice president of information technology.

Javaid M. Cheema

Javaid started with Toyota in Nagoya in 1984, serving until 1996. Following this, he held senior roles at Molex Interconnect and Benteler Automotive. He holds an M.S. degree in industrial and systems engineering from the University of Michigan, an MBA from the University of Central Oklahoma, and a graduate diploma in manufacturing management from Tokyo Poly-Technique University, Hashimoto City.

Emil W. Ciurczak

Emil, currently at Doramaxx Consulting, has experience at Ciba-Geigy, Sandoz, Berlex, Merck, and Purdue Pharma. Emil consults widely, including with the FDA. He was a member of the PAT subcommittee (validation) for the FDA and is a member of the PAT expert committee for the USP. Emil has advanced degrees in chemistry from Rutgers and Seton Hall universities.

Andrew Cox

Andrew, until recently professor and director of the Centre for Business Strategy and Procurement at Birmingham University Business School, is a graduate of Lancaster and Michigan Universities and holds a Ph.D. degree from Essex University. He was awarded the Swinbank Medal for outstanding services by the Chartered Institute for Purchasing and Supply, and is a Fellow of the RSA. He is a visiting professor at Birmingham, San Diego, and Nyenrode Business Universities, as well as president and chairman of the Advisory Board of the International Institute for Advanced Purchasing and Supply.

Patrick Crowley

Pat was vice president for pharmaceutical development at GlaxoSmithKline R&D until 2008. His work has been in dosage form design (formulation), initially at Wyeth and then at Beecham Pharmaceuticals, SmithKlineBeecham, and GlaxoSmithKline (U.S.) as these organizations consolidated. He holds a pharmacy degree from University College Dublin.

Peter Evans

Peter is a top consultant in procurement and supply management. He started PEEP Consulting in 2007 after being a partner at ADR Int'l. His clients include Eli Lilly, Wyeth, and Alcan. Before joining ADR in 1992, he held senior positions at Philips, Thorn EMI, GEC, and GKN Group. He holds a Ph.D. degree in chemistry from the University of Wales and is a Fellow of the Chartered Institute of Purchasing and Supply.

Ian Glenday

Ian started his lean journey running a fermentation plant producing enzymes. He completed an MBA at Bradford Business School, then joined Reckitt & Colman, where he became head of policy deployment at Colman's. Ian currently divides his time between working with Dan Jones at the Lean Enterprise Academy and helping businesses to make their own lean transformations.

Elisabeth Goodman

Elisabeth is owner and principal consultant of RiverRhee Consulting. She has 25 years' experience in pharmaceutical R&D, most recently at GlaxoSmithKline, in management and consultancy roles supporting global business teams. Elisabeth has a B.Sc. degree in biochemistry and an M.Sc. in information science.

Nicki Haggan

Nicki is an experienced consultant specializing in bridging the divide between business and IT functions. A graduate of UMIST, she has more recently been awarded an M.Sc. degree in IT and management from Sheffield Hallam University. Nicki has undertaken a number of different roles within the pharmaceutical industry and is currently employed as a process improvement analyst for the contract research Organization PPD.

Adrian Hampshire

Adrian is managing director for the newly formed EMEA region of BioPharm Systems, where he is responsible for the European Practice's delivery of business change and process optimization. Prior to joining BioPharm Systems, he enjoyed an extensive career in information technology in the pharmaceutical industry. He has degrees in animal physiology and computer sciences.

Richard Harrison (contributing on behalf of S. A. Partners)

Richard has extensive senior sales and marketing experience at the board level with global premium branded consumer businesses. An alumni of London Business School, he joined S. A. Partners in 2002, and formed the Sales Transformation Partnership in 2010. He is an advanced master practitioner in neuro-linguistic programming and a Shingo Prize winner.

Peter Hines

Peter is former chairman and honorary professor at the Lean Enterprise Research Centre, Cardiff Business School. He has written or cowritten several books, including *Staying Lean*, which won a Shingo Prize in 2009. Peter is chairman of S. A. Partners, a specialist consultancy applying lean thinking. He holds a B.A. degree from Cambridge University and an M.B.A. and Ph.D. from the University of Cardiff.

Robert Ireland

From 1971 to 1980 Bob worked for Burroughs Wellcome (now GSK) as a commercial apprentice and in international marketing, and from 1980 to 1997 Bob was director and managing director of a number of medical device companies. Bob currently serves as vice president of Kowa Pharmaceuticals Europe Company.

Daniel T. Jones

Daniel is a management thought leader and advisor in applying lean process thinking pioneered by Toyota to all kinds of businesses around the world. He is the founding chairman of the Lean Enterprise Academy in the UK. He is the author with James P. Womack of several best-selling management books: *The Machine That Changed the World*, *Lean Thinking*, and *Lean Solutions*.

Niels C. Kaarsholm

Niels joined Fertin Pharma as vice president and head of research and development in 2007, before joining MC2 Biotek, Denmark in 2010. During his previous tenure with Novo Nordisk, he held positions as principal scientist, department head, project director, and vice president of protein engineering. He holds a Ph.D. degree.

Ron Krawczyk

Ron is a managing partner with Blue Fin Group, a healthcare consulting company. He is known as one of the innovative designers in our industry, due in part to his broad experience and ability to intuitively understand the uniqueness of each healthcare product, patient, provider, payer, channel, and manufacturer. His industry experience has been with companies such as Johnson & Johnson, Rhône Poulenc Rorer, Arcola, and Centocor, Eli Lilly, Pharmacia, and Schering Plough.

Donna Ladkin

Donna is professor in leadership and ethics at the Cranfield School of Management, where she is also director of the masters in management research program, leading to a Ph.D. degree. She is the author of numerous articles on leadership as well as the book *Rethinking Leadership: A New Look at Old Leadership Questions*, published by Edward Elgar. She hold a Ph.D. degree.

Martin Lush

Martin is a senior partner at David Begg Associates, having held senior management positions in manufacturing and quality assurance. He has provided consultancy and training support in over 23 countries. He has helped many companies dramatically improve the effectiveness of their quality control systems, believing that quality systems *must* add value.

Malcolm McDonald

Malcolm, until recently professor of marketing and deputy director at the Cranfield School of Management, is a graduate of Oxford University and the Bradford University Management Centre, and holds a Ph.D. degree from Cranfield University. He works with operating boards of big multinationals, such as IBM, Xerox, and BP. He has written forty-three books and is a professor at Cranfield, Henley, Warwick, Aston, and Bradford business schools.

Matt McGrath

Matt is the managing partner of Barnes/Richardson's Washington, DC office, where he has practiced international trade and customs law for 30 years. He counsels a wide range of domestic and foreign clients in trade matters before federal agencies, U.S. courts, and multilateral panels.

Jennifer Miller

Jennifer created and led business operations within the pharmaceutical sciences group for Pfizer's Global R&D Division. She is currently working on a global program to enhance Pfizer's ability to bring innovative health care solutions to patients. Previously, Jennifer held roles within finance at Pfizer. Before joining Pfizer, she spent five years with KPMG in New York and served as an officer in the U.S. military.

Edward Narke

Ed has experience in regulatory affairs, process development, and quality assurance gained at companies such as Lonza and Wyeth. In 2006, he cofounded Design Space InPharmatics, a CMC consultancy. He has authored and submitted more than 100 regulatory submissions and holds a B.A. degree from the University of Pittsburgh and an M.A. in chemistry sciences and chemical engineering from Villanova University.

Chris Oldenhof

Chris is currently manager of external regulatory affairs at DSM. Within the European Chemical Industry Council he is the president of the Active Pharmaceutical Ingredients Committee (APIC) and a board member of the European Fine Chemicals Group. He holds a Ph.D. in organic chemistry.

Ranjana Pathak

Ranjana is currently vice president of quality assurance at Endo Pharmaceuticals. She has vast experience in quality and compliance gained at Endo and as principal quality scientist at DuPont Pharmaceuticals. She holds a D.H.A. degree from the University of Phoenix, an M.B.A. from Dowling College, and a B.Sc. in chemistry from the University of Mumbai.

Marla Phillips

Marla is the director of pharma and device initiatives at Xavier University. She began working for Merck in 1996 as a project chemist. After four years, Marla took over as head of quality for the Merck North Carolina facility. In 2005 she began consulting with former FDA inspectors conducting global mock inspections. She received a B.S. degree in chemistry from Xavier University, and a Ph.D. in organic chemistry from the University of North Carolina.

Nick Rich

Nick is managing director of Montalt Enrich Limited, a provider of Lean TPM Consultancy. He is honorary associate professor at Warwick Medical School and honorary Fellow at Cardiff Business School. He was an original founding member of the Lean Enterprise Research Centre, an adviser to government, and a Shingo Prize examiner of organizational excellence for the UK (Utah State University/ Manufacturing Institute).

Ruth Rowe

Ruth is an English studies graduate with subsequent experience in two major charities before moving into retail. Ruth became a business adviser in 2004 and her passion for making a difference to small businesses has led to her current role as business support manager for flexible support for business.

James Ryan (contributing on behalf of Morrison & Foerster)

By background James is a research scientist, having completed an honors degree in experimental pathology at the University of St. Andrews before undertaking a Ph.D. degree in epigenetics. Subsequently, James has trained and qualified as a solicitor and is now an associate in the technology transactions group at the London office of Morrison & Foerster.

Jack Shapiro

Since 1988, Jack has been president of JM Shapiro Healthcare Marketing Research and Management Consulting in Maywood, New Jersey. His clients include the pharmaceutical industry, hospitals, insurance companies, and other industry stakeholders. In prior roles, Jack was at Upjohn, Squibb, Lederle Laboratories, Pfizer International, and Ayerst Laboratories.

David Stokes

David is global head of life sciences and principal consultant for *Business & Decision*. He is a reviewer of a number of GAMP good practice guides, including *A Risk-Based Approach to Electronic Records & Signatures*, *Global Information Systems: Control and Compliance*, and most recently, *Data Archiving*. David authored *Successfully Validating ERP Systems*, published by the Parenteral Drug Association.

Steve Waite

Steve is the chief administrative officer for Bayer HealthCare UK/Ireland. He is responsible for providing and managing all business services to the Bayer Group of companies in the UK and Ireland, including finance and control, information technology, procurement, product supply, property and site services, legal, and human resources and pensions.

Stephen Ward

Stephen is development director at Stabilitech. Prior to that he was director of development at Onyvax and also worked on the hepatitis immunotherapy and antigen delivery platform at Medeva. His Ph.D. degree from Imperial College London focused on recombinant vaccine design and the use of attenuated bacterial delivery systems to protect against mucosal pathogens.

Brian Williams

Brian's early career was with the Wellcome Foundation, Cyanamid, Warner Lambert–Parke Davis, and Merck Sharp and Dohme. For 20 years he worked for Bayer as both production and quality assurance director. Brian is a qualified person, a chartered engineer, and a member of the Institute of Chemical Engineers and the Royal Pharmaceutical Society. He is a practicing retail pharmacist.

Tim Williams

Tim is managing director of I Balloon, a project management consulting firm. Previously, he was business director for Japanese accounts at Autoliv. From 2002 to 2006 he was based in Nagoya and managed the global Camry passenger airbag project. Tim has an Honour's degree in mechanical and manufacturing engineering and an M.B.A. from the University of Manchester's Business School.

Katie Wood

Katie currently works as a clinical science specialist for Genentech Inc., where she oversees the development and initiation of early phase studies in the United States, the European Union, and the Asia-Pacific. She has worked in multiple therapeutic areas and has experience in initiating, managing, and closing out phase I to III studies in global locations.

Janet Woodcock

Janet is the director of the Center for Drug Evaluation and Research of the FDA. She has served the FDA as deputy commissioner and chief medical officer and as deputy commissioner for operations and chief operating officer. In these roles, she oversaw scientific and medical regulatory operations. Dr. Woodcock served as director of the Center for Drug Evaluation and Research from 1994 to 2005. She previously held other positions at the FDA, including director of the Office of Therapeutics Research and Review and acting deputy director of the Center for Biologics Evaluation and Research. Dr. Woodcock received her M.D. degree from Northwestern Medical School and completed further training and held teaching appointments at the Pennsylvania State University and the University of California in San Francisco. She joined the FDA in 1986.

PREFACE

I was staying at a budget hotel on the outskirts of London when I checked my Blackberry for email. It was probably around 3.00 a.m., so my sight was less than perfect. Squinting allowed me to make out the opening: "My name is Jonathan Rose, the Wiley editor for pharmaceutical science books." Jonathan went on to say: "With interest, I note that you are leading the coming workshop 'Supply Chain Management in Pharma/Biotech.' Given the importance of managing supply chain procedures and costs during drug production and manufacture, I believe that a book explaining the concepts, methods, and applications of supply chain management to the pharmaceutical industry would make a timely and well-received text. Such a book would be an important reference and resource for professionals involved in drug development and manufacturing, quality assurance and control, chemical and biological engineering, and regulatory personnel."

That is what I hope to have achieved with this book. I have attempted, of course, to contribute the maximum possible from my own personal databanks; along with this is supplementary commentary from what I can best describe as "expert witnesses." The contributors have been hand picked by me to reinforce, support, and move forward the sentiments in the book. Their powerful contributions are of varying length and depth.

I hope that you enjoy what we present here. The style is meant to entertain as well as to inform; and by informing, the hope is that the overall theme of the book will strike home—the pharmaceutical industry must change in radical ways if supply chains of the future are to meet stakeholder expectations.

Acknowledgments

The learning that goes into a book is so varied and random, how can anyone credit all who have contributed? To those forgotten, I apologize, and if you will contact me, it will be rectified in my next book.

First, of course, I owe the contributors a huge debt of thanks, as I do John O'Neill, former director of operations at Bayer Manufacturing in Bridgend, South Wales (Chapter 16), currently VP of manufacturing operations at Bayer Healthcare, Consumer Care, who taught me, by demonstration, what strategic thinking was about and how it should be executed, as well as for sponsoring my executive M.B.A. This leads me to the Cranfield University School of Management, for providing the faculty and environment for that life-changing program. Leo Murray, who headed the school in those days (1994–1995), seemed to know every pupil personally and certainly made me feel part of things. They worked on the whole person, not just the business boffin in us.

Next is Michael Carroll in his time as director of manufacturing at British Biotech (later to become head of technical operations at Novartis, Horsham, UK), whose incisive approach to pharmaceutical manufacturing strategy pushed me to incorporate new ways of thinking about supply chains; also Malcolm Hughes, formerly at Roche, who I worked with at British Biotech, for reviewing Chapter 4 and staying connected all these years.

The people at Vanguard Medica, one of the pioneers of virtual drug development, comprised a special team of high-caliber drug developers and business folks with a deep sense of pride in their work. Nick Heightman was a perfect boss, and special thanks to Sally Waterman, then VP of nonclinical development, now COO at Poly-Therics, whose training notes in drug development I still use; and Michael Gamlen, owner of Pharma Training Services and Pharma Development Services, the company that commissioned the workshop cited earlier by Jonathan Rose; and Peter Worrall, then CFO, now CEO of Pharminox, who provided a "spot on" quote for my newsletter on the value of procurement, which is included in the book—I still owe him a pint!

At Ortho-Clinical Diagnostics, John Gethin, general manager of the Cardiff site, demonstrated true understanding of the lean methodology as he unleashed improvement potential that the tool-heads had failed to unearth. He helped me move on to better things, which may be the subject of another book one day.

From OSI Pharmaceuticals, I must thank Bob Simon, executive director of regulatory affairs and manufacturing, who had the patience of a saint with me and others around him. Without his sponsorship and forbearing, my experience at OSI could have been very different; also to Geraldine Chapman, human resources director, for being so supportive on the UK side of the pond.

As an independent, those contributing to my learning opportunities for the book are almost too many to mention. Frank Wheeler, of the now defunct "Entrepreneur Action," planted many of the business idea seeds; Chris Barnett, expert consultant in pharmaceutical quality and compliance, who reviewed Chapter 4 and made some excellent comments; Judy Callanan, who organizes training courses (including mine) for Pharma Training Services and does a difficult job with aplomb; and David Cotterell, managing director of Apex Healthcare Consulting, who was my first client and paid his invoices on time, which is so vitally important to an independent consultant.

Recently I have joined Alacrita Consulting. My skills sets are not in much demand for Alacrita, since they are experts in drug development, and as you will see throughout the book, supply chain management competencies are little sought after in this territory. They have been brilliant to network with, though, and my thanks go to Anthony Walker and Rob Johnson for inviting me to join them; also, thanks again to Anthony for reviewing some chapters (he did not agree with all of it!) and hooking me up with Pat Crowley, who did such an excellent job in Chapter 3.

Ram Balani, CEO of FDASmart, has been incredibly interested in what I am doing, and I thank him for that and also for introducing me to Jennifer Miller of Pfizer (Chapter 17) and to Michelle Hoffman, editor of *Pharmaceutical Technology*.

A final thank you goes to my colleagues on the UK Bio-Industry Association's Manufacturing Advisory Committee (BIA MAC), especially the following people, who have been massive advocates of quality by design and modernization: Brendan Fish, our chairman, formerly of Medimune, now at GSK; Rob Winder, communications manager at BIA; Jim Mills, formerly at Xenova, now CEO of Cantab Biopharmaceuticals; Mike Hoare, professor of biochemical engineering and co-director of the Advanced Centre for Biochemical Engineering (Mike is the godfather of bioprocessing in the UK); and Dean Chespy (another member of the Welsh contingent, along with Mike Hoare, Steven Ward, and myself), development manager for life sciences at Siemens; also thanks to Robert Mansfield, former CEO of Vanguard Medica and Neuropharm, who proposed me for membership in the committee, and Tony Bradshaw, previous head of bioProcessUK and now co-director of the HealthTech and Medicines Knowledge Transfer Network, who accepted me; and Mark Bustard, head of bioProcessUK, for maintaining such an important link with BIA MAC.

HEDLEY REES

April 2010

PART I
Surveying and Mapping the Territory

1 Setting a Transformational Agenda

1.1 AIMS AND ASPIRATIONS OF THE BOOK

The skill and coordination required of scientific, technical, and business experts in bringing new medicines to market is immense. There is, however, the potential to make those efforts significantly more productive by thinking in supply chain management (SCM) terms from the earliest stage of drug development. Our intention in this book is to help readers to reach that potential by working on a number of levels.

1.1.1 A Practical Guide for the Industry

First, the book aims to be a practical guide to the application of SCM processes and practices in a pharmaceutical setting. The objective is to provide information to those in the industry wishing to contribute to improved supply chains. The key aim, therefore, is to help individuals and teams appreciate the impact they have on working supply chains; experience shows that this is a far broader spectrum of involvement than may initially be appreciated. Then, armed with that appreciation, readers can identify specific ways in which they can make a vital contribution to an organization's success in supporting patient needs for pharmaceutical products and services. With enhanced understanding among all the stakeholders, there is a real opportunity to help reduce the astonishingly high attrition rates with which this industry lives on a daily basis.

1.1.2 Understanding Constraints for SCM Practitioners

The second aim of the book is to provide SCM professionals, both inside and outside the sector, with a deeper understanding of the special constraints that operate in this industry. The regulations that apply are designed specifically to protect the health and well-being of patients. There is often confusion, however, as to what is or is not acceptable to industry regulators. The default position often becomes "change nothing." The message must be that although change is not straightforward and can be time consuming, it is necessary in order to continue to provide patients with products that are "fit for purpose" and meet their requirements as to quality, cost, and delivery lead time. To date, many talented supply chain professionals have avoided this sector or are not able to fully exercise their skills within the sector. This needs to change—and by providing more insight into the constraints, it is hoped that innovative ways of working can be adopted in a fashion similar to that of other safety-critical sectors. All the evidence suggests that industry regulators are now positively encouraging this approach through modernization initiatives, which we discuss in detail throughout.

The basis for achieving the two goals above is my own work, founded on everyday experiences of bringing drugs to clinical trial sites and markets. These experiences are based on work from early-stage drug development through to large-scale phase III and postmarket (phase IV) trials and commercial sale in global territories. The emphasis is on understanding and utilizing *simple* and *effective* ways to build, manage, and improve the performance of the supply chain. The simple approach is essential in that complexity abounds in both pharmaceuticals and SCM. Simplicity, in combination with effective working methods that focus on meaningful outcomes rather than on tools and techniques, can be extremely powerful.

I believe that these goals are achievable. There are, as well, several more ambitious goals that *could* be a by-product. The first of these is to help inspire and catalyze a step change in culture and attitude that must take place in the pharmaceutical industry.

1.1.3   Catalyzing Change of Culture

The manufacturing and distribution supply base of this sector has many issues before it, but this has always taken second place to the search for new blockbuster products and markets. The world is now changing its attitude to prescription medicines, with issues of cost, integrity (adulteration and counterfeiting), quality, efficacy, and safety all moving the supply chain center stage. The changes required are at the roots of the industry, and in this book we dig down deep.

The scientific community of pharmaceuticals has historically held innovation in manufacturing at arm's length, focusing attention on discovery research. Jon Clark, associate director of policy at the U.S. Food and Drug Administration's (FDA's) Center for Drug Evaluation and Research, observed at the Marcus Evans Summit Manupharma conference held in 2005: "The pharmaceutical industry has one of the most technically advanced discovery organizations, but remains more conservative when it comes to using 'cutting edge' technology in manufacturing." This quotation from Clark's presentation at that summit is a suggestion of ways in which the pharmaceutical industry could improve by adopting process analytical technology and quality by design approaches. There will be more on those subjects later in the book, specifically in Chapter 14, but for now, readers should simply understand them to be methods of introducing improvements into the supply chain using principles founded in best manufacturing practices.

1.1.4   Engaging Pharmaceuticals in Supply Chain Management

My last aim or aspiration, call it what you will, is to encourage engagement of the huge intellectual resource within pharmaceuticals and SCM in a search for increasingly effective processes to manage complex supply chains. That scientific attention in discovery research has resulted in rapidly developing technologies in the modeling and analysis of complex biological systems. As will become clear throughout the book, supply chains are less complex subjects than humans but have the added complication of the more unpredictable "person" component. The discipline of SCM could benefit significantly from the intellectual rigor of the pharmaceutical sector. As readers new to the discipline will begin to understand, SCM is by no means well defined or fully understood, even by the many "experts" operating in the territory. There is a dire need for continuing research and discovery of ways that are sustainably better, rather than chasing tools, techniques, and "information system" gimmicks that add little or no value, yet still attract the attention of many.

1.1.5   Examining the Two Worlds

To stand a chance of achieving these goals, it will be necessary to examine the two very different worlds of pharmaceuticals and SCM in some detail. I do not apologize to experts in either or both fields for striking a baseline at fundamentals. When visiting these settings, the level is pitched at first principles to provide a foundation for further research or investigation. It will be for the reader to follow an interest or curiosity into further depth beyond the needs of understanding SCM in pharmaceuticals.

1.2   BOOK FORMAT

The focus of the book is on factual information about the pharmaceutical industry and SCM. To aid readers' understanding of some of the less straightforward concepts or issues, the presentation is supplemented by three distinct types of auxiliary material.

1.2.1   Guest Contributor Slot

The guest slots are inputs of varying length that aim to inform and underscore the messages in the text. There is no particular pattern to the inclusion of these speakers other than the fact that I encountered them at some point and recognized that they had valuable tales to tell in relation to the book's content (as an aside, see Section 16.4). The speaking panel includes long-term colleagues and friends of the author, eminent professors, industry colleagues, and contacts made in the course of doing business, where a particular shared view or interest has prompted dialogue. They are taken from a broad spectrum of industrial, academic, and consultancy backgrounds. The unifying theme is that they have particular insights or expert knowledge that is of direct importance to the aims of this book. The style is particular to each speaker, but the messages are clear and consistent. After each slot, I emphasize an important point or points for reinforcement, but each slot stands alone as a learning opportunity. It should also be noted that the contributors do not necessarily subscribe to all the views that I express throughout the book.

1.2.2   Observations, Views, and Experiences of the Author

In these sections I include particular findings, experiences, and insights of mine during many years of operating in pharmaceutical supply chains and through personal and professional development. This is not to suggest that these views are any better or worse than anyone else's. We all have a tale to tell and valuable knowledge to impart. The perspective that I bring is from one who rather than entering academia or career consultancy has remained a practitioner. This means that I have been "doing" throughout my working life, aside from the time taken to study. I have been able to apply that valuable study and use it to determine what works and what does not work in practice. The doing has kept me grounded in the gray mists of ambiguity that pervade all modern organizations.

Some of these sections are recountings of actual events in the form of practical case studies. In the main, they are anonymous, so that, as a colleague used to say, we may "protect the innocent." The serious aspect of this is that searching for guilty parties can be a major inhibitor to organizational learning, as people fear for their jobs or career prospects. This circumstance is studied further in chapters on improvement and exemplar thinking, but it is important here to note that the vast majority of participants in organizational "mistakes" are innocent parties trying to do their best under difficult circumstances.

This is the spirit in which the case studies are examined. They aim to get at the fundamental lessons from situations where things did not appear to turn out well, were handled less than effectively, or did not involve the correct course of action or involvement; and specifically, to extract every last ounce of understanding from examples that demonstrate exemplar ways of working.

1.2.3   A Helpful Metaphor

The aim of using metaphors is to draw out the reader's identification with unfamiliar concepts. Sometimes, the only way to really identify with another person's pain or pleasure is to imagine an analogous situation that has similar implications. As with all metaphors, they are not perfect analogies, and the reader could spend time picking out differences that distinguish them from the case in point. They will, though, be close enough to convey a sense of identity with the essence of the concept. Although at first glance it may seem patronizing toward the many highly educated and scientifically gifted people reading the book, it is not, of course, my intention and hopefully, will not be taken that way.

1.3   INTENDED READERSHIP

Most readers will be in one or more of the broad categories described below.

1.3.1   Operating in Pharmaceuticals or Biopharmaceuticals Outside SCM

The responsibility areas involved include the following:

- Research chemistry and biochemistry
- Chemical and biochemical engineering

- Chemistry, manufacturing, and controls
- Preclinical development
- Clinical development
- Regulatory affairs
- Quality assurance
- Finance
- Marketing
- Informatics and information systems
- Business development
- Licensing
- Pharmacovigilance
- General management

See Chapter 3 for a definition of some of the technical terms.

1.3.2 Working in SCM Outside Pharmaceuticals or Biopharmaceuticals

Areas of responsibility include the following:

- Purchasing
- Procurement
- Supply management
- Operations
- Production management
- Inventory management and control
- Production and material planning
- Demand planning
- Logistics
- Warehouse management
- Import/export
- SCM
- General management

1.3.3 Occupying a SCM Role in Pharmaceuticals or Biopharmaceuticals

For example, readers may have the responsibility for planning and management of inventory in a clinical trial supply environment. Their background may be technical, such as in pharmaceutical sciences, and they may have moved into clinical supplies as a career development step. There may well, therefore, be gaps both in aspects of the drug development process and in common practices in SCM.

1.3.4 Off-Label Use

In pharmaceuticals, there is the well-known concept of off-label use, where a medicine is prescribed by a physician for conditions that were not part of the original approval to market and sell the drug. Possibly, there will be an analogous element of off-label use for this book, as prospective readers become aware that some of the principles apply in a complementary sense to their specific interests. This may include some additional categories:

- Academia outside SCM, such as marketing, finance, and human resources
- Venture capitalists (someone suggested that they would lose interest after the first page!)
- Industrial, non-supply chain responsibility areas outside pharmaceuticals (e.g., product design, marketing, finance)
- People looking to discover sound principles of SCM, not the surrounding baggage
- Others of a curious nature with regard to all things organizational

1.4 A BOOK ABOUT TWO WORLDS IN CONTRAST

It is time to look more closely at these different worlds. The world of pharmaceuticals is complex even on the simplest plane. It is a world populated with some of the most intellectually gifted people on the planet. It is a place of ethics, scientific rigor, personal challenge, human caring, and highly professional standards, but also a world of blockbuster drugs, huge gross profit margins, captive markets, and patent protection—a place where business and science often collide.

The other world, that of supply chains and SCM, is equally complex, although perhaps not immediately obvious to the uninitiated. It is a relatively young discipline, challenged by risk and uncertainty, constant need for innovation, quality improvements, customer choice, cost containment, and delivery deadlines; also often a place of wild demand fluctuations, dysfunctional relationships, problematic defect rates, departmental silos, and customer complaints. Ironically, in many respects, it too is populated by equally talented and intellectually bright and committed people.

So begins a voyage through these worlds in the hope that each can learn from the other to leverage better outcomes for the central character of this book: a patient—the ultimate consumer of pharmaceutical medicines.

1.5 THE PHARMACEUTICAL LOTTERY

1.5.1 Failure Is Never Far Away

Probably the number one preoccupation of anyone working in the world of pharmaceuticals is the risk of failure, and it is this aspect that differentiates it from other industry sectors. Figure 1.1 tells the story of the lottery that is pharmaceutical

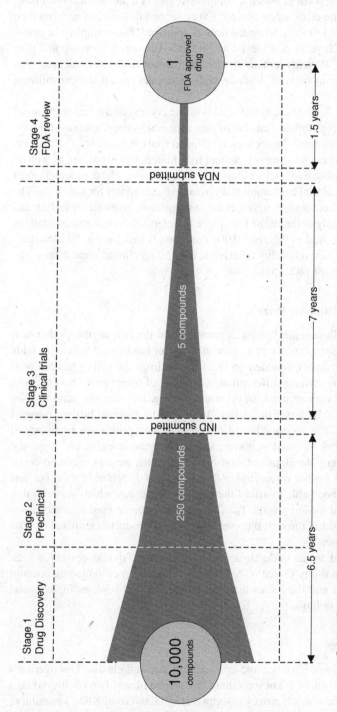

FIGURE 1.1 Drug discovery, development, and review process. (From Pharmaceutical Research and Manufacturers of America. Taken from: *Science, Business, Regulatory, and Intellectual Property Issues Cited as Hampering Drug Development Efforts*, GAO-07-49, U.S. Government Accountability Office, Washington, DC.)

Original Source: Pharmaceutical Research and Manufacturers of America. Taken from:
GAO-07-49 Science, Business, Regulatory, and Intellectual Property Issues Cited as Hampering Drug Development Efforts.
United States Government Accountability Office

Stage 1
Drug Discovery

Stage 2
Preclinical

Stage 3
Clinical trials

Stage 4
FDA review

10,000 compounds

250 compounds

5 compounds

1 FDA approved drug

IND submitted

NDA submitted

6.5 years

7 years

1.5 years

development. From the point at which a company registers a patent for a promising molecular structure, the clock starts ticking. Every second that is used up from then on represents potential lost sales when the drug is approved. For example, if a patent protection period of 20 years is achieved and it takes 10 years to develop and gain approval for the drug, 10 years remain in which to recover the costs associated plus an acceptable return on investment. Just one day's extra sales can often mean millions of dollars in the bank.

This pressure to make the best use of time is in the context of the fact that four of five compounds entering clinical trials fail to gain approval by regulators (as shown in Figure 1.1). As we shall see in later chapters, clinical trials are not cheap to run, and there is the associated manufacture of clinical trial materials to consider as well as many other indirect costs. Even before clinical trials can begin, 250 compounds must pass through preclinical trial evaluation to arrive at five candidates for the clinic. The cost of those 245 lost compounds, again, is not insignificant, given all the testing and data collection and analysis that must take place to determine safety and indications of purity and efficacy. Add to this the 10,000 compounds that need to be identified, selected, and screened for suitability to arrive at the 250 preclinical candidates—and yes, again, someone must pick up the tab.

1.5.2   Chasing the Ultimate Prize

No one is under any illusion that the development of new drugs is anything other than a game of chance. Despite this, the pharmaceutical sector has learned to beat the odds and has been a rich industry, founded on blockbuster drugs delivering jackpot winnings. Historically, the extreme differentiation born out of patent protection meeting patient needs created captive markets, premium pricing, and massive margins. Not just blockbusters but even lesser drugs have been able to generate healthy margins and massive returns. The industry has always argued that profits are necessary to compensate for the risk referred to above, and while gross margins are large, the profits, net of discovery, development, and marketing, plus general overhead costs, are necessary to fuel further research. Up to a point that is probably true, but this industry has always been able to afford the best of everything, which suggests that the balance is skewed toward profits. The industry has become used to a very comfortable financial position through the sale of marketed products facilitated by that vital regulatory approval.

Readers interested in an in-depth account of this area should consult a U.S. Government Accountability Office (GAO) report.[1] This is an enlightening account of drug development and the issues that will emerge in this book as fundamental contributors to SCM failings.

1.5.3   Times Change

In recent years, winnings have become ever more erratic and elusive. Discovering a totally new molecular entity is not something that can be planned and delivered on a schedule, no matter how much money is thrown at it. GlaxoSmithKline's mammoth research center at Stevenage in the UK was a major European construction project when it was built in the 1990s. How well has GSK's pipeline benefited from this endeavor? Suffice it to say that GSK is as active as any company in seeking compounds to license from the outside world. Where drugs have been discovered and entered development, the regulatory hurdles have escalated, making it increasingly difficult and time consuming to gain that vital approval. Official figures from regulators show disappointing decreases in approval numbers in recent years, and this is well documented in the GAO report.

Other factors have also been affecting revenue returns. Some governments and payers are pushing physicians to prescribe generic drugs rather than brands as soon as possible after patent protection expires. In fact, in the UK, where there is already a high percentage of generic prescribing by general practitioners (GPs), legislation was proposed to oblige the pharmacist to substitute a generic version if a GP has not already done so. It is not clear whether this will become law but does indicate that the pressure is on to move to less costly generic versions wherever possible. For innovators and patent owners, generics lead to shorter product life cycles and revenue erosion through lost sales. Innovators have retaliated through product life-cycle management aimed at producing extensions and re-presentations of the brand that can extend patent cover.

Branded products are also being attacked on price from stakeholders across the board. So far, that pressure is taking its toll, and strong stakeholder negotiation is likely to continue that trend. The pressure is on, therefore, for innovators to reduce costs and margins. The supply chain is one area where the spotlight is turning to seek out a cost advantage, and this is a key area for consideration in this book.

1.5.4 Costs Escalate

Although the potential rewards are still high, so is the development stake required to take part, and those costs continue to escalate. Estimates vary as to the cost of bringing a new drug to market, but $850 million to $1.9 billion seems to be generally accepted as a reasonable range. The major portion of this cost is the cost of failure: the failure to meet the demanding requirements for safety, efficacy, quality, and purity of a potential drug before it is allowed on the market. Understandably, then, the entire industry is concerned with avoiding costly failures, and business strategies and models have developed with this in mind.

1.5.5 The Driver for Changed Business Models

So in an environment of higher costs and lower returns, how has the industry evolved in response? Until the late 1970s/early 1980s, pharmaceutical companies tended to own much of the infrastructure required to bring a drug to market. From then onward, this concept of a traditional, vertically integrated business model was challenged severely as the big pharmaceutical companies began a wholesale exit from activities that were regarded as noncore to their business. The guiding principles were to reduce fixed costs and to release funds to channel into activities *perceived* to be more strategic, such as discovery research and marketing. The potential in this was to reduce the cost impact of compound failures while increasing spending on pipeline improvement and competitive positioning. Some more cynical commentators argue that the end game was to achieve higher, more predictable margins for shareholders in an already high-margin environment.

Manufacturing (including analytical testing) activities and distribution logistics were quickly identified as noncore, leading to a spin-out of people, facilities, and equipment into a rapidly growing contractor base. So began a massive and ever-spiraling move toward outsourcing in the industry. Plants and facilities that had previously been part of the larger pharmaceutical companies suddenly found themselves as third-party contractors having to survive alone beyond any transitionary arrangements that had been negotiated. They became service providers, charging fees for services to what were now their "sponsors." For these companies, the profitability of the contract rather than the success of the sponsoring pharmaceutical company had to become the first priority. So began the wave of outsourcing and third-party commercial relationships, which has followed an upward trend to this day.

The existence of this contractor base also made it possible to develop drugs without actually owning any of the facilities. From this, the business models now known as *biotech* and *virtual pharma* (because of their need to outsource to conserve cash) were spawned. In essence, these models are founded on compact teams of scientific and technical experts using contract manufacturing organizations (CMOs) and contract research organizations (CROs) to undertake the operational and transactional activities. The scientific and technical core team then sponsors and manages the transition of compounds through one or more stages of development. The value added is then offered for licensing in exchange for royalties and milestone payments, providing investors with an exit strategy.

There is a matter of definition to be clarified here before moving on. It is not unusual to witness conversations in which *biotech* has different meanings to the participants. For one person, it means a company operating in the arena of biological compounds. An other conversationalist will have in mind a small to medium-sized company developing drugs based on either chemical or biological compounds, the unifying factor being their dependence on investors for cash to operate the business. The definition used here refers to the latter, which is the way in which the trade associations are organized. For example, the majority of members of the UK Bio-Industry Association are companies working with small-molecule compounds.

Observations, Views, and Experiences of the Author

My first experience of biotech was when joining the company British Biotech in the mid-1990s. My principal responsibility as head of logistics was to establish a pan-European supply chain for two upcoming compounds in clinical development. Both compounds were small molecules and failed to reach the market. It was, however, an incredibly valuable experience for me personally because I learned a tremendous amount about drug discovery and development. The company had assembled an impressive team of scientific and technical experts, many from big pharma companies wishing to seek new and exciting challenges. This allowed me to learn about drug development, and how it affects SCM, from some of the best people in the field.

Readers can research the company history themselves. I mention it here because British Biotech was initially a European model for the biotech industry. Significant amounts of money were raised from investors (Including NASDAQ and NYSE investors). The share price rocketed as the investment was turned into clinical studies and data that showed apparent promising, even spectacular, results. That promise was dashed when the first compound failed to achieve regulatory approval and the second was found to have data that did not support further development in the direction intended. The critical mass of financial resources was not available to weather such a reversal of fortune, and the company was stopped in its tracks, becoming a shell of the company originally intended. Shareholders lost their investment, and the entire sector shuddered in response. This clearly exposed the risks as well as the opportunities associated with developing drugs with relatively limited resources. Nonetheless, although the appetite for investment in biotech companies has diminished, this is still a widespread business model to be explored here in a little more detail.

1.5.6 Biotech and Virtual Pharma

Table 1.1 is based on work that is contained in the UK government's commissioned report, "Bioscience 2015: Improving National Health, Increasing National Wealth"[2] [affectionately known as the "Big-T Report" after the team that compiled the report: the UK Bioscience Innovation and Growth Team (BIGT)]. The report foreword, written by the then UK Prime Minister, Tony Blair, demonstrated the importance attached to the bioscience sector as a driver of future economic growth. Although the description in the table taken from the report is aimed at bioscience (i.e., principally the biological and bio-processing sectors), it applies equally well to small-molecule companies.

This shows the progression that biotech companies make to fund a move through the phases of drug development. Companies have demonstrated that it is possible to develop a drug to market using the virtual model (Vanguard Medica was an early achiever, with Frovatriptan), but there are also potential issues that must be addressed. A major aspect is having sufficient funds to weather any of the delays that may occur due to unexpected safety issues. Under these circumstances, cash can run away quicker than the time required, and companies are at risk of "going to the wall." This encouraged a refinement of the biotech model aimed at reducing exposure to risk and so make it easier to attract investors. Enter the specialty pharma company. Such companies deal only in already licensed products or re-profile existing compounds with known safety profiles into new indications (e.g., disease areas) and thus reduce the risk of failure due to unexpected safety or efficacy issues.

The net impact of these changes is that the industry structure has transitioned. Large companies developing and manufacturing drugs to market for themselves have

TABLE 1.1 Biotech Company: Stages of Evolution

Stage of Company Evolution	Key Activities	Level of Funding	Example Sources of Funding
Idea development and validation Idea generation Seed funding	Secure assignment from university of IP, etc. Validate technology Develop commercial prototype products Carry out early preclinical trials	£50,000–£1 million	Seed funds: up to £250,000 Family/friend/angel funding: typically £100,000 VCs (seed specialists, biotech specialist funds) Small Business Research Initiative grants Investment funds aligned alongside research funding bodies
Early stage Startup/first-round VC	Start developing technology platform/product pipeline Broaden IP base Hire a management team and scientific group Start to engage in corporate partnering Secure premises and build company infrastructure	£1–£10 million	Startup-focused and broader VCs Very high net worth angels Other grants from £250,000 to £400,000 Collaboration between industry and research base >£100,000 Large international VC funds
Late stage Expansion stage Public companies	Build scale, roll out technology platform, continue with clinical development (even launch), and prepare for exit (probably IPO) Continue with expansion-stage activities, with ultimate aim of cash flow breakeven/profitability	Multiple rounds of VC funding £10–£50 million per round Large and variable	Large international VC funds Institutions willing to invest in private companies Pharma/biotech partners Debt Public markets: AIM, LSE, NASDAQ Pharma/biotech partners Debt

Source: UK government-sponsored report "Bioscience 2015: Improving National Health, Increasing National Wealth."
VC, venture capitalist.

been replaced by complex networks of independent companies operating through contractual arrangements that aim to limit risk and maximize reward. As biotech and big pharma companies seek to work more closely together to help fuel discovery research, this situation is only likely to be exacerbated. This has far-reaching implications for pharmaceutical supply chains. By way of exploration of this comment, I would like to introduce the first guest contributor, Dan Barreto. These views were captured from a conference call that I had with Dan one Sunday morning in between his frequent visits to Puerto Rico for his current company, C. R. Bard.

GUEST CONTRIBUTOR SLOT: DAN BARRETO

Responsibilities of Small and Medium-Sized Companies in Drug Development

I wish to speak about SMEs [small and medium-sized enterprises] researching and developing drugs but aiming to exit by handing over to big pharma (Johnson & Johnson, GlaxoSmithKline, Pfizer, etc.). The work done by an SME can set the future for the supply chain and affect the entire product life cycle. This work is the foundation that allows for a smooth transition from one stage to another. Going into a phase without completing all the tasks associated with the previous tasks creates additional work, forces parallel activities, and diminishes the strength of the process due to the multiplicity of priorities added to the process.

GMP [control of manufacturing; see Chapters 3 and 4] does not apply with full rigor in earlier stages [phases I and II], so reduced emphasis on meeting specific quality requirements is acceptable. However, the level of flexibility applied to a specific activity should be based on a good understanding of the need for control and management of current activities, and the potential need downstream of the data and intelligence gathered. When an SME hands over the baton to big pharma, if it is not in good shape, there can be major implications. Avoiding these potential consequences requires SMEs to take a longer-term view of GMP and also to consider characterization of the molecule, scalability, dosage-form selection, specification of materials, selection of suppliers, and so on.

When an IND [application to perform clinical trials in humans] is submitted and accepted, it is often difficult to change some potentially critical aspects. The reason for this is that the life cycle is perceived as a "one-way" approach in which any reassessment of work done previously is considered unnecessary, overwhelming, taxing, an indication of poor performance, and a potential showstopper for the project. This is a complete mistake, in my opinion. There should be an obligatory "Retrospective" review to assess any impacts on big pharma project time lines when issues are found. Time lines are often impossible to change, which can lead to taking risks to meet time lines and hope for the best.

This retrospective review should include documentation of notebooks (e.g., as scientists leave and data are lost). Good data and good documentation should be based on the relevance of the data that are being collected, whether they are for present use or for preservation as scientific reference in the future. Most companies do not appreciate that issues with products already in distribution may require a look back all the way to research and development as part of a comprehensive investigation or evaluation of the issues.

Dan's words are based on direct experience within both the FDA and senior industry leadership positions in quality control. They convey a word of caution for all SMEs developing compounds. They have a great responsibility on their shoulders to get things right before handing over to big pharma. In the same way that quality cannot be inspected into a product, due diligence cannot undo errors and omissions in the development process. Even if weaknesses are discovered, eradicating them is often too complicated to accomplish within time lines, resulting in suboptimal compromises made and undue risk incurred.

The underlying message is that supply chain issues are not just about counterfeit products entering the supply chain or concerns relating to distribution channel logistics—these are symptoms, not root causes. Throughout the book, the early formation of a supply chain will be a primary focus of attention. The point being made here is to place it on the agenda from the start and keep it there. To gain further clarification, it is necessary to examine an aspect of the history of pharmaceutical supply chains.

1.5.7   The Impact of History on Pharmaceutical Supply Chains

Prior to the more recent turbulent industry dynamic, when the world of pharmaceuticals was apparently simpler, the performance of supply chains received little attention. The logic was persuasive. The absolute necessity was to develop a supply chain capable of producing test materials to be used for clinical trials for regulatory scrutiny. The thinking behind this was: Why would anyone invest more money than necessary in a drug's supply chain before knowing that there was an approval to sell? A successful completion of clinical trials and subsequent regulatory approval would then open the door to gross margins that were orders of magnitude greater than the cost to manufacture the drug. For example, it would not be uncommon for a cost of goods to be only a few percentage points of the selling price. The justification for that has been mentioned above, but whether right or wrong, the ensuing mindset became: "Why bother about cost? Just do enough to gain an approval."

The results of such a mindset and the associated lack of attention led to the following being common for supply chains in the industry:

- Procurement policies and practices not focused on supplier performance
- Short-term tactical sourcing and outsourcing decision making
- Inflated inventories to protect against *any* lost sales
- Maximization of batch sizes to minimize cost per unit
- Extensive off-line testing and document checking
- Resistance to changing the status quo

Nor was this only an issue of cost and supply chain performance. The entire industry, through focusing on the regulator, did not connect sufficiently with their end customer in the way in which other sectors do routinely. This meant that there was a kind of "take it or leave it" approach to the customer. Some may challenge this assertion, but a justification is given in Chapter 2.

1.5.8   Specific Difficulties in Pharmaceuticals

There are, of course, difficulties that other sectors do not face, such as predicting the patient population applicable to a particular compound. For example, Viagra was originally trialed for angina, until reports of "unwanted" side effects began to appear—and the target market changed overnight! However, that should not be regarded as an excuse for ignoring potential patient needs in the drug development process. The exception proves the rule but does not make it; and the rule is that patient consumption of a medicine and the associated payment by the responsible party is the point at which value is realized. Vitally important though the approval and regulatory compliance aspects are, it is the supply chain that actually converts latent value into products in the hands of paying customers. We explore this in more detail in Chapter 2, where we look at value from the patient's viewpoint. For now, we should recognize that patients, payers, prescribers, regulators, health care practitioners, and other key stakeholders are demanding more of pharmaceutical supply chains. The bar needs to be raised for SCM in this vitally important sector—so next some background on SCM.

1.6   SUPPLY CHAIN MANAGEMENT IN CONTEXT

1.6.1   A Foundation for Moving Forward

Attention now turns to the second world, the world of SCM. To create a foundation for SCM it is important, first, to build understanding of the nature and characteristics of a supply chain, especially in relation to the *generation* of value (note that although we focus on the supply chain for products, much is equally applicable to the provision of services). It is all too easy to be taken up by the tools, techniques, and processes of SCM and actually lose sight of the main objective, which is to transfer value effectively into the hands of paying customers. This aspect needs to be addressed, as with many aspects of SCM, at the earliest possible stage.

In the same way that humans have evolved over the years but remain an interconnected network of bones, nerves, muscle, ligament, veins, arteries, and so on, supply chains are similar constructions, albeit millions of times less sophisticated. The issue is that supply chains have become increasingly networked and complex as business and technology have moved forward past the Industrial Revolution.

A Helpful Metaphor

When civilizations were making crude tools to kill, cook, and eat food, supply chains only extended to the fairly immediate surroundings or were within easy walking distance. These were still supply chains, however, requiring the finding and forming of raw materials into finished products. The principles of SCM would have been exactly the same as today. The hunter must know where the best sources of materials are, secure the necessary supply, transport it to the site of manufacture, form tools as required, store the materials ready for use, and maintain them in good order. The only difference is that all this would have been carried out by a single person in a confined area. It was indeed simple compared with today's challenges, but still a series of stages that needed to be undertaken to produce the end result of a valuable weapon or tool. If a source of supply, such as a particular kind of branch from a tree, was not available, production would stop. The interconnectedness was there then and still exists. Failing to recognize these relationships would be a recipe for starvation.

The message being conveyed here is that to be effective, supply chains do not need to be made up of multiple stages. In fact, imagine if our hunter decided to source his materials in the next village, or even in a different country; or he had his arrowhead forgings being molded in bulk in the next field, then being beaten into shape by a neighboring hunter who sold his services on the open market, then finally, received the beaten heads only to find that they didn't fit onto the spear shafts, which had been sourced offshore. Wouldn't you say that he had the best chance of producing a defect-free article if, to the extent possible, he kept it close around him? Rather than debate that now, time to move on. Food for thought, though?

1.6.2   The Impact of Complexity in Modern Supply Chains

Complexity has taken over by virtue of world markets consisting of customers who are demanding a multitude of product variants made from materials sourced in global networks. As far as the supply chain is concerned, though, the basic concept of interconnectedness still exists, as the metaphor aims to illustrate. Management of it is, however, considerably more involved. Perversely, it is only when this complexity is recognized that progress can be made in SCM. With this realization, quick fixes and flavors of the month are discounted immediately. Identification of root-cause issues and sustainable solutions becomes the only meaningful approach. A physician would not use a Band-Aid to treat an open wound requiring stitches. Similarly, corrective actions in supply chains require solutions commensurate with the scale of the injury. If there is nothing else to take from this book other than a clear understanding of the complexity of a supply chain and the need to follow a systemic path for solutions to problems, that will be a major achievement.

1.6.3   The Scope of SCM

By discussing the supply chain in terms of the above, hopefully it becomes clear that the supply chain has a broad scope. Each and every player—manufacturer, supplier, distributor, service provider—is part of the end-to-end supply chain. This may seem obvious, but it is surprising how many times *supply chain* is used to refer only to the flow of goods between facilities. In consequence, SCM is often associated with the logistics of moving objects from point A to point B. This is particularly the case with pharmaceuticals.

Observations, Views, and Experiences of the Author

I vividly remember a case in point that occurred during a client workshop several years ago. The assembled senior executives were a typical composition for a biotech senior team: a CEO, chief financial officer, VP of business development and licensing, and VP of pharmaceutical development. After the morning session, chatting over lunch, the VP of pharmaceutical development declared that her partner lectured in SCM at a university and could not understand why I had been called in to discuss matters so far ahead of launch (they were planning a phase II study, a critical stage for supply chain development). All through the morning session, I had emphasised the importance of using supply chain thinking in the development phase because the supply chain is "registered" and locked in after that.

This view appears to be the norm rather than the exception in pharmaceuticals. Mention the supply chain to many and the instant association is with trucks loaded with boxes of medicine moving between warehouses and hospitals, clinics, and pharmacies. As we explain later, this is true but it is only the tip of a massive iceberg. For the sake of clarity, therefore, the scope of SCM in this book is stated explicitly below.

SCM covers the design, management, and improvement of end-to-end supply chains. This includes all the stages and activities involved in moving raw materials through progressive stages to become products in customers' hands. All aspects of stewardship to achieve the above are included.

Stewardship is the operative word here, as it emphasizes that the entire organization has a role to play in the supply chain. Researchers, developers, manufacturers, and business support must all play their part. To do this, there must be some integrative presence in an organization, something that draws together the requisite strands to make the garment. These are the processes of SCM that should not be confused with the "function" of SCM. The function should be concerned that these processes are applied successfully and that interfacing roles have clearly defined expectations. It is for the business to decide on the supporting organizational structure to deliver those processes. This is where the SCM function can and should play a stewardship role.

Observations, Views, and Experiences of the Author

In my experience, there are often organizational tensions between personnel in certain key areas that affect the supply chain. Often, their roles are not clearly defined and agreed upon between them and they compete at the interface. These areas might be, by way of example:

- *Operations vs. production planning*
- *Engineering vs. procurement*
- *R&D vs. procurement*
- *Marketing vs. distribution logistics*

It would be good to think of these as creative tensions, but often they are not. Operations will make what they prefer rather than what customers demand; engineers will buy the most technologically interesting piece of equipment rather than the best buy to meet a purpose; R&D staff will use suppliers that cannot provide support on a commercial scale; and marketing personnel will want products in customers' hands next day without having provided forecasts. And it works both ways. Production planning overstates capacity; procurement "beats up" potentially great suppliers and fails to see the importance of scientific innovation; and distribution logistics insists on strict lead times that cannot bend to suit the customer.

I have rarely found people operating with malicious intent so as to purposely inflame these interfaces. The conclusion I have drawn from being intimately involved with these tensions over many years is that organizing to manage supply chains effectively is a tricky balancing act. Like a tightrope walker, an organization can only achieve success by keeping its eyes fixed firmly on the other side, which in supply chain terms is the end customer.

At this point I would like to introduce Nick Rich, an acknowledged international expert in supply chains and the associated management processes.

GUEST CONTRIBUTOR SLOT: NICK RICH

The Power of Integrated Supply Chains, by Design

If you look around you, you will probably find that the world's most successful businesses are part of integrated supply chains. These supply chains, value networks—call them what you will—are the result of design. The best product in the world can easily be eroded when it is matched by a poorly designed supply chain.

While product designers tend to determine what needs to be purchased, it is the supply chain specialist or multidisciplinary team that determines from whom, in what form, and what innovations suppliers and distributors can bring to new generations of products. A well-designed supply chain is therefore a source of innovation, organizational learning, and a continuous blend of improvement. Indeed, beyond the pharmaceutical and health care businesses lie organizations that have learned very well the benefits of a strategically aligned and designed supply chain—Toyota, Dell, Amazon, Tesco, and Wal-Mart being just a few. Equally, many businesses have suffered at the hands of a poorly designed chain that has damaged branding and eroded competitive advantage (just look at the use of exploited labor in the third world and its decimation of clothing and footwear businesses). It has been argued that if they want to maximize the returns on their relationship, no supply chain specialist can ever know enough about a supplier and no supplier can ever know enough about a customer's business.

With such a direct impact on the profitability, quality, delivery, flexibility, and corporate citizenship (to name just a few contributions to an organization's performance), it is important that supply chain designers understand the full range of methods and approaches to supply chain design, development, and coordination that are at their disposal and work out for themselves the optimal design. In my personal experience it is rare to find any one model that fits exactly or any individual tool that transforms a supply system. In addition, organizations have long memories, and rarely will supply chains be created from scratch. As such, the design process requires a mastery of adaptation and improvement processes so that any design matches the consumer market served by the product. Regulation also limits an industry in terms of compliance to procedures and governance, and this makes direct emulation of other sectors difficult. The paramount importance of safety in the pharmaceutical and health care sectors creates a three-dimensional puzzle for supply chain designers—a Rubik's cube if you like—where product needs, the right type of supplier, and the correct level of governance must be aligned with the needs of the market and time compression in serving consumers.

The modern world of the supply chain specialist (and the many other organizational departments that are involved with the design process) is a long way from the traditional images of the "company buyer," and with the pace of markets quickening, halving of product life cycles, and deregulation of markets, the role of the supply chain designer has never been more pivotal to the success of any business. If this makes the supply chain designers sound like strategic marketers—they are. They deal with a reverse marketing process and the integration of upstream supply chain operations to deliver what markets need profitably. The differentiator is not luck—in the modern competitive environment it is a new form of design that determines the effectiveness and efficiency of delivering global customer value.

It is likely that a specific optimization formula for any supply chain will require a mix of traditional scientific methods, a team-based approach with high levels of cross-functional management, high quality (total quality management/six sigma) and leaner, "waste-free" ways of working, whether it is to fulfill orders or to get a product to market more quickly. The strategy, structure, and relationships across the supply chain developed to deliver the highest levels of service are—I think you will agree—definitely the result of design.

This is a perfect scene setter for the SCM messages in this book. To draw particularly on Nick's final sentence, readers with a pharmaceutical background should contemplate the extent to which supply chains they are familiar with have been designed proactively. In my experience, those defining the supply chain through submission of a regulatory filing have scant experience of, and pay little attention to, the functioning of the final supply chain. It is not difficult or overly onerous; however, it does need people to do it at this stage. Anything later is too late.

1.7   THE HISTORY OF SUPPLY AND VALUE GENERATION

Tracking a detailed history of industrial supply and value generation is a daunting task and will not add value to the goals in this book. There is merit, however, in taking a brief, high-level view.

1.7.1   Division of Labor

At the dawn of the Industrial Revolution, Adam Smith, a well-known economist, wrote a book called *The Wealth of Nations*[3] in which he discussed his concept of the division of labor. Smith made a case for dividing work up into smaller packets so as to achieve the benefit of increased efficiency from specialization (as opposed to the example of the hunter in Section 1.6.1, who completed the entire task himself). It is a famous text and needs to be read to fully understand the reasoning. For the sake of this book, suffice it to say that this was the seed for increasingly complex supply chains to grow as parties to manufacture became disengaged from each other. This sparked a fundamental requirement to join the "divided out" activities in a coordinated and synchronized manner. This may have been the conception of today's complex supply chains.

1.7.2   Scientific Management

This idea of breaking tasks down to increase efficiency was developed further by F. W. Taylor in the early twentieth century. Taylor, who became known as the father of scientific management, worked his way up through the ranks as he advocated a more scientific approach to work to deliver the associated efficiency gains. There were numerous tales of how Taylor made dramatic improvements in human productivity through the use of systematic study and identification of new methods, such as the use of larger shovels in a steel mill!

The fundamental principles that Taylor developed can be summarized as follows:

- Use scientific methods, not rules of thumb.
- Select and train employees scientifically.
- Use detailed work instructions and supervision of employees.
- Plan and perform tasks based on scientific principles.

Taylor's principles were immensely influential in the world of industrialization, reinforcing and contributing to many of the assumptions underlying working practices, even today. The principles went on to become a foundation for the staff functions known as work measurement and method study, which subsequently became the discipline of industrial engineering (see Chapter 12). This approach to work, where human beings are regarded as factors of production that must be managed for productivity, remains an artifact in many organizations to this day and is discussed in more detail in subsequent chapters.

1.7.3 Mass Production

Henry Ford introduced mass production into the world with the Model T Ford and the assembly line, which depended on building high volumes of relatively inexpensive cars. The concept was to feed component parts made in high volumes to the production plant for assembly on a constantly-moving conveyor belt. Taylor's principles of scientific management fitted perfectly with this approach. These ways of working became the norm for businesses operating in the manufacturing sector. Pharmaceutical manufacture developed along similar lines in terms of organization and adoption of mass production methods to deal with the demand for blockbuster products.

1.7.4 The Japanese Revolution

It was not until the Japanese revolution that industry experienced any real threat to mass production operations. Companies such as Toyota, Honda, Nissan, and Matsushita adopted different ways of organizing and working in response to the economic devastation caused during World War II. Their new approach made them formidable competitors. This competition from the East, through higher quality and lower costs, forced certain sectors to respond radically in order to survive, and some still did not survive (e.g., the UK motorcycle industry). Pharmaceutical firms did not feel similar competitive pressure and to this day still operate, in the main, by the mass production model. There are moves afoot to change that, and history will determine if, when, and how that takes place. We hope to contribute to that.

It should be mentioned here that as I was writing the book, Toyota experienced some horrendous quality problems that severely questioned the company's reputation and status as the world's highest-quality producer. In my opinion, that should come as no surprise. There is an interesting metaphor that I sometimes use when in conversation with fervent advocates of a particular approach, such as lean, agile, or six sigma.

A Helpful Metaphor

Why don't we get away from these various pseudo-supply chain religions and focus on what is the best way to run production systems. Toyota has one that is world class, but ultimately it is not infallible. If we saw a budding athlete trying to become 100-meter world champion merely by emulating Usain Bolt, we'd say that he was mad! Our advice would certainly be that he should learn the fundamentals of athletics and practice them diligently. So why don't we get back to the fundamentals in improved ways of working?

Maybe it will help further to change the sport to one I am more familiar with—golf. I really admire Tiger Woods (who also recently fell from grace!) and love watching him play; what I look for is his relaxed address to the ball, slow, square takeaway, still head, straight left arm, good wrist position at the top, hands leading on the down swing, late hitting position through the ball, and a flowing follow-through. But I didn't learn those things from watching Tiger Woods. I was taught them by one of the millions of golf pros around the world who understand the fundamentals of a successful golf swing. So, in the spirit of the metaphor, it is with production systems: strong engagement with customer segments, clear understanding of means to value delivery, simple material flows, short lead times, minimal noise in communications, competent suppliers, and so on. I was never built to hit a golf ball like Tiger Woods can, but by learning the fundamental principles, I can play a passable round of golf.

The point here is that Toyota can get things wrong occasionally in the same way as any of the best in a field of activity can. The main thing is that by applying existing knowledge of the fundamental principles—return to the practice ground, some early nights, and an improved diet—recovery should be just around the corner. Anyone not taking the time to put in the hours on the fundamentals will never know what it is like to be in a position to recover. I cited the Toyota story here because we will draw substantially on the lessons learned from the Japanese revolution in production. No one should discount those genuine discoveries because of these unfortunate problems at Toyota.

1.8   THE DEVELOPMENT OF PROCESSES TO MANAGE THE SUPPLY CHAIN

As industrialization progressed, there began to evolve three separate camps with responsibilities within the overall endeavor of supplying customers. The first camp was concerned with acquiring goods and services from third parties on behalf of companies manufacturing products. The set of skills and activities involved in and responsible for third-party supply to a business (the extended supply chain) became known as *purchasing management*. The second camp was focused on physical conversion processes within the internal organization. The competencies involved here were linked to the manufacture, planning, scheduling, storage, and movement of goods in the converting facility and the management of all those engaged in the conversion process. This became known as *operations* or *production management*. The third camp was involved with moving products from business to business and eventually to customers. The relevant skill sets related to the international movement of goods and the associated commercial requirements. This became regarded as *distribution logistics*.

These three separate camps developed methods to manage those aspects of the supply chain that were of most relevance to them. Purchasing management focused on suppliers' supply chains. Operations management majored on internal manufacture, production control, materials handling, and inventory control of parts and materials. Distribution logistics targeted warehousing, inventory control of finished products, and transportation. The net result of three separate avenues to SCM has led to a fragmented history and little commonality of organizational structure, terminology, and methodology. This is open for debate, but the discipline of SCM must be one of the most poorly understood of all business functions.

Observations, Views, and Experiences of the Author

Over my career, I have been considered for many employment positions in SCM and have always been amazed by the differences in job titles, role descriptions, and relative reporting relationships. It has not been unusual to find companies looking for purchasing managers who are to report to logistics managers and them to find an exact reversal of the reporting relationship at another company; or virtually identical managerial roles being considered as part of purchasing, materials management, logistics, inventory management, manufacturing, or operations. These roles could be reporting to manufacturing, production, finance, or one of the three supply chain branches. This has been further exacerbated in recent times by the introduction of lean and six-sigma approaches, with an entirely new lexicon of terms and positions, such as "value stream manger."

The message here is that SCM has much progress to make before becoming a coherent set of business processes under a single umbrella. Readers should make allowances for this and expect to find disconnects, overlap, and duplication. As the discipline matures, this should be less and less the case. We aim to contribute to that higher level of appreciation.

1.9   LIFE IN SCM

It seems appropriate in this introduction to explain something about what life is like managing in supply chains. It is probably a bit like giving birth, in that unless you have done it, it is impossible to understand what it is like in practice—hence the value of a metaphor.

A Helpful Metaphor

To help understand life in SCM, consider the pilot of an oil supertanker. These ships have a momentum that demands respect. They have tremendous inertia born out of mass, structure and complex interconnections, presenting enormous difficulties for navigation and maneuverability. Any decision to alter course or speed, in even the slightest fashion, must be taken with due care and well in advance. There are physical constraints to what can be achieved. Timings missed are lost forever and can result in catastrophic outcomes. In a crash stop maneuver (full ahead to full reverse) it can take more than a mile to achieve standstill, and a turning circle requires similar dimensions. Spotting an obstacle at the last minute is not a prospect to relish!

Such is life in SCM. Activities are taking place "below deck" that are committed and difficult to change without causing problems. The difference between the ship and the supply chain is the fact that the ship is visible and it is relatively easy to understand the difficulties even in calm seas. The supply chain exists in the same way but is not visible to the naked eye because it has many layers and geographical locations.

The point of the metaphor is to help demonstrate the great difference between a customer demanding a product at will and the task of delivering that product. Dispatching to a pharmacy shelf or hospital dispensary is the result of coordinated activity begun months or even years earlier. Readers with a marketing background may have heard this message from their supply chain teams many times before! Can you imagine one of the ship's crew asking to disembark at an unscheduled port of destination because his mother-in-law was visiting one of the ports along the coast? We often are asked to do the equivalent of that in SCM and sometimes are forced to capitulate under pressure from senior management. The impact below deck will probably never hit the mother-in-law's radar screen or the senior managers.

1.10   MOVING FORWARD

The journey through the book follows a logical sequence that builds knowledge and understanding of the two worlds with a view to bringing it all together in a final chapter, Chapter 17, where we propose an entire range of prospective changes (some quite radical) that should eventually feed through into patient-centric supply chains. The book is arranged in three parts. Part I covers the current landscape in the pharmaceutical industry and SCM as practiced in the sector. In Chapter 1 we introduce aims and background and in Chapter 2 draw out the central focus that must be present for any chance of meaningful success—the patient. We discuss how well pharmaceuticals currently service patients through supply chains. We argue that it is essential to plot a course that is iterative in feeding patient experiences back into early-stage design for inclusion in improvement efforts.

Chapter 3 is an overview of the drug development process in sufficient detail to give the reader an appreciation of the risks, uncertainties, constraints, and obligations that companies have in developing pharmaceutical products. We aim to place current pharmaceutical supply chains into the context of the need for a zero-tolerance approach to patient safety. Change cannot take place unless the requirements of safe drug development are met. This is therefore a pivotal chapter for those wishing to participate in supply chain improvements. Whoever understands the way in which drugs are developed and is familiar with best-practice SCM has the potential to move mountains of underperformance. Those who cannot operate with the drug development fraternity in knowledgeable ways can make very little headway toward meaningful, sustainable change.

In Chapter 4 we look at both the chemical and biological specifics of the pharmaceutical supply chain, whose main object it is to deliver active substances to patients for therapeutic benefit. At one level, these supply chains are relatively straightforward compared with, say, the supply chain to build an aircraft. At another level, however, pharmaceutical supply chains have added complexities, in that materials and processes can be destabilized by unpredictable physical, chemical, and biological reactions and interactions. These uncertainties are highlighted and explored in this chapter.

In Chapter 5 we offer suggestions as to why pharmaceutical supply chains do not perform up to satisfactory levels. The analysis starts by tracing the stages of production, from initial supplies of material for safety testing through to full-scale commercial manufacture and supply to patients. It becomes clear that lost opportunities in the initial stages convert into major issues in later stages. Critically, we look at cause and effect, with a view to identifying root-cause issues rather than symptoms.

Part II begins with Chapter 6, where the supply chain is considered as a value proposition and consequent competitive weapon. It should become clear through the chapter that *supply* is actually the transfer to paying customers of value that has been created within an organization. This should set supply chain and associated management processes center stage to ensure that value is delivered and the cash is collected in return. This may be a difficult chapter for some drug developers to read at first, because it sets research and development as a support activity. Support does not mean second class, but it does mean that their engagement with the patient is vital to overall organizational performance.

In the remainder of Part II, Chapters 7 to 13, we turn our attention to the processes of SCM. In Chapter 7 we explain how the management processes should form a holistic set, each process operating in an integrated manner. It builds on the principles outlined by Michael Porter,[4] of focusing on the generation of competitive advantage though customer value and cost objectives. For this to happen, each player in the holistic must clearly understand the role and the key linkages within that role. In Chapters 8 to 12 we then explain each process set: production and inventory control; strategic procurement; transport, storage, and distribution; information systems and improvement, respectively. In Chapter 13, practical ways of using the processes in previous chapters are described. A suggested framework for action and remediation is proposed and a case study is explored.

Part III is about preparing to change and executing on that. The initiatives to adopt exemplar working practices within the pharmaceutical industry are examined in Chapter 14, and progress to date is critiqued objectively. This includes FDA's Critical Path Initiative and the International Conference on Harmonization (ICH) guidelines Q8 to Q10 (see Chapter 3 for further details).

In Chapter 15 we define the concept of exemplar thinking and move through the various approaches that have emerged over the years; we also consider whether there is a thread of common "systemic" truisms running through many of the initiatives, such as total quality management, world-class manufacturing, and lean thinking.

The most important chapter is probably Chapter 16. We explore individual behavior, organizational leadership, and culture as the underpinning movers of all meaningful improvement. These aspects result in organizational behavior: that is, people doing the right things or, indeed, the wrong things. Doing the right things consistently can result in improvements that make a difference to the lives of patients. We all know what doing the wrong things means.

As noted earlier, in Chapter 17 we return focus to the patient to relate the text to possible new and improved ways of working on the supply chain and in the industry for enhanced patient outcomes. For many, the supply chain may have no relevance to their current perception of patient outcomes, which is heavily biased toward unmet medical needs. The overall message in the chapter is that this industry should redefine patient outcomes as the complete experience a patient encounters when receiving pharmaceutical treatments and medicines. To achieve this, there must be an organizational change in engagement with patients from an early stage. This means redefining research and development as the single process entity *design*. Too long has the sector had steel walls between the "R" and the "D." Some may argue that this is not the case, but evidence suggests otherwise. Reading the chapter will reveal much more about the thinking here, but as an initial thought, what if the combined entity *design* were responsible for taking a drug to the prototype stage: that is, proving that the drug has manufacturability and is delivering acceptable and differentiated benefits to patients? That is what other sectors insist on with their products. It may be difficult or even impossible—but it may be far easier and effective than many believe. Throughout the text we will study the additional complexities and nuances of pharmaceuticals and ask: Are they *that* impossible to address? All this, and more, will be explored throughout the book.

2 Plotting a Course to Patient Value

2.1 WHY FOCUS ON PATIENT VALUE?

Like any other business sector, the pharmaceutical sector must generate profits in order to survive and grow. This is the reality of the business world. No organization, no matter how altruistic in nature, can incur costs without generating revenues to cover those costs and also to provide for investment in the future and the associated return to investors. There may be a question of "reasonableness" in relation to profits, as mentioned in Chapter 1, but pharmaceutical firms have generally been very successful in generating profit. The revenues necessary to generate those profits can only come from paying customers: that is, patients or those responsible for payment on behalf of patients.

Release of value therefore does not take place until the body or person responsible for payment hands over the cash. Up until that point, all value is latent. This is an extremely important point to bear in mind. *Value* is a hard measure in the same way that cost is. Valuations of compounds at the various stages of research and development are predicated upon an eventual commercialization by way of a working supply chain invoicing customers and receiving cash. Without the supply chain, revenues (release of value) cannot be earned, no matter how incredible a scientific breakthrough or market strategy may appear. Is the natural corollary, therefore, that patients are ultimately in charge? Some would say no, insisting that patients do not know enough about medicine to influence the activities of pharmaceutical companies in their scientific endeavors. Others take the opposite view, asserting that medical knowledge is not necessary—that patients should still be able to articulate their specific needs such that pharmaceutical companies can frame their activities around patients. I frequently encounter these opposing positions, which has brought me to the conclusion that the answer lies somewhere in between. Traditionally, however, the balance appears to have been heavily skewed away from patient involvement. To explore this further, we should look at where the patient fits at present.

2.2 WHERE DOES THE PATIENT CURRENTLY FIT?

In Chapter 1 we touched on the "alleged" lowly status of the patient perspective in drug development and continued the theme in Section 2.1. Interestingly, as likely

Supply Chain Management in the Drug Industry: Delivering Patient Value for Pharmaceuticals and Biologics, By Hedley Rees
Copyright © 2011 John Wiley & Sons, Inc.

users of medicines during our lifetime, most of us should have an opinion, and should therefore be able to identify closely with patient needs. Clearly, when in pain or under threat from disease, access to a curative medicine can provide intense relief, and in this respect the value of medicine is well understood. Aspirin and penicillin are notable examples of the transformative potential of medicines. These were not developed in detailed consultation with prospective patients, and no one would argue that they should have been. There was an obvious market and the products sold themselves. So why shouldn't drug developers go on looking for cures without reference to patient needs? The answer is that drugs are never perfect, especially when first launched, for all sorts of reasons: for example, inappropriate dosage forms, side effects, interactions, and suboptimal efficacy. This is not a bad thing in itself, because some issues emerge only after a product is launched, as is common to all sectors of industry. However, if a comparison is made with these other sectors in terms of how customer experiences are reacted to, an interesting perspective emerges.

Observations, Views, and Experiences of the Author

I discussed this aspect with Robin Jaques, a partner in the consultancy S. A. Partners.[1] *Robin had previously been head of procurement at Dyson Appliances Ltd., a highly innovative UK domestic appliance company (Sir James Dyson, the owner, advises the UK Conservative Party on innovation in business) and procurement manager for landing gear at Airbus UK (formerly part of BAe Systems). I asked Robin what he would suggest was different between pharmaceuticals and other sectors. He thought for awhile and then came out with this insight. "When, say, an aerospace company launches a new plane to its airline customers, that is the beginning of a second phase of product development. The plane must obviously be commercially attractive to airlines, safe, and fit for its purpose at entry into service, following several years of certification testing with air-worthiness authorities, but based on in-flight experience and feedback from airline customers and consumers experiencing the product, there is a second rapid introduction of improvements: sometimes to fine-tune the original concept, often to push its performance envelope further to enhance the value for the airline and the consumer. After this period, further evolutions of the product are planned in line with technological advances, legislative changes, and competitive threats—meaning that on a product that may be manufactured for 20 years or more, the job for product developers is never complete."*

This raises an open question of how effective the drug development *process* is at understanding the needs of their customers (patients) for increasingly safe and effective drugs and identifying what changes need to be made to improve the products. I suggest that the process is not very effective, to say the least. That is all well and good and probably close to the mark, I hear readers remarks, but what has this to do with SCM? The answer is that modern supply chain philosophies, almost without exception, place understanding of the customer value position as the fundamental starting point. A supply chain built to deliver that proposition is thus designed proactively through inclusive product design and development methodologies. These "customer-inclusive" methodologies do not exist, to any meaningful degree, in the world of pharmaceutical research and development.

Observations, Views, and Experiences of the Author (continued)

I have received feedback from industry colleagues disagreeing strongly with the view expressed above, and this has sensitized me to the need for a full explanation of what is meant here. It is not to suggest that the patient knows better than the medical professionals, nor that the patient should be able to demand magic medicine for the price of a bag of sweets. The meaning is that the foundation of successful business is the long-term satisfaction of customer needs at an affordable price. Therefore, if one observes an industry sector that has a history with little evidence of customer engagement, that would appear to fly in the face of conventional wisdom and be worthy of some examination.

This leads to a key factor. Historically, pharmaceutical markets have enjoyed extended periods of patent protection where competition is severely restricted. The reason for this is well known. The unfortunate side effect is that the industry focuses on attaining approval, at the expense of measures to assure long-term competitive positioning and customer satisfaction. The regulator is the gateway to success and, as such, the primary customer of drug development companies. The patient is, at best, a prospective beneficiary—a possibly "desperate" person who will eventually benefit from groundbreaking discovery and development of a drug for an unmet medical need. But because the regulators' views are binding and omnipotents they are the true customers of medicines, in my opinion.

This is not to say that regulators have engineered this situation, because they clearly have not, and in many respects I'm sure they would prefer that it were different (see Dr. Woodcock's comments in Section 14.1). However, since the approval of the regulatory filing is the ultimate objective and the regulatory authorities call the tune on that, so the "customer" is defined. The product is the regulatory filing: the common technical document *as it is termed (see Chapter 3). Industry regards the regulator as a parent in a relationship that could almost be termed a "reward-based dependency."*

If true, how could this have happened? One reason is the peculiar situation in this industry, where it is not uncommon to discover a compound that began development for one patient population and later is found to work in a totally different patient population (as with Pfizer's Viagra). Development could be well along the way before the customer is even identified. How, then, could the product be developed with the customer in mind?

There is clearly a mindset dimension to this situation. The current mindset is that serendipity is so prevalent in drug discovery that any attempt to build acceptable margins around patient satisfaction would be destined to failure. The counter to that

*may be that lower but more predicable margins founded on broad-based customer
satisfaction could be a sustainable alternative over the long term. This is an aspect
that is developed further throughout the book.*

To begin the examination we examine the views of a few guest contributors. The
first contributor, Jo-anna Allen, extends the argument that the sector does not engage
properly with its patients, suggesting that it does not engage effectively with the key
patient interface: marketing.

GUEST CONTRIBUTOR SLOT: JO-ANNA ALLEN

Marketing Perspective in Pharmaceuticals

In my experience, marketing is involved too late in the research and development
of drugs. The search for medicines to meet unmet clinical needs means that the end
user is secondary to the clinical data which prove that a drug is working. This is
compounded by the fact that sometimes drug discoveries are stumbled across as they
are developed with one disease area in mind but are licensed for something totally
different (e.g., Viagra, Provigil). This leads to a "take it or leave it" approach, where
marketers and sales people are allocated responsibility to market and sell a new
product over which they had very little influence. To me, this situation is unique to
pharmaceuticals; in other sectors marketing would represent end-user needs and play
a key role in research and development.

The situation described above often sees the marketer's role subordinated to designing product packaging to make products more appealing or to differentiate from
the generic version when products come off patent. A company with a popular treatment for dysmenorrhea launched a day pack designed to be discrete for women. The
only problem was that the cost of 30 generic tablets was the same as that of a day pack
containing 9 tablets. Again, marketing's ability to question such a cost differential
in-company is extremely limited; also, such initiatives are often used to extend the
life cycle of a product and are viewed cynically by health care practitioners.

The issue of design is potentially compounded by who we think the customer
actual is, and whether we develop products with the person who buys them in mind
or the end user of a product. Although the salesperson on the ground may think of the
patient when selling the product, the customer is the person who buys or prescribes
the drugs. Certainly, in the new UK National Health Service (NHS), the customer
is moving farther away from the patient. In the good old days, the salesperson was
one person away from the end user. In the new NHS, the person who buys the drugs
may be three or four times removed from the end user. Perhaps the challenge to the
industry is to define who the customer actual is, the buyer or the patient! There are,
of course, examples of better practices being adopted. The treatment of diabetes is
one such area where development is very much centered on the patient. Examples of
this are the move to insulin pens, allowing diabetic patients to inject more discretely

in public. Companies continue to work in this area for the benefit of patients, inhaled insulin being one such initiative, although success in this area still awaits, with some launched products already having been withdrawn from the market.

Vaccines and injectables both attract some consideration to both the end user and customers, but a benefit to one group may be a disadvantage to the other. Needle-stick injuries and the associated problems have led some companies to design retractable needles. While this offers a benefit to the injector, the injected commonly complain of an increase in pain as the needle retracts. One company had to withdraw a vaccine with a retractable needle because of the high level of patient complaints and went back to the regular prefilled syringe. Involvement of both user and receiver at the design stage could help prevent some of these costly mistakes.

This came as something of a surprise to me, even though I had been working with marketing teams in pharma for some time. I had always assumed that there was much greater engagement than this evidence suggested. On reflection, however, this assumption was based on knowledge of the workings of *other* sectors. In general business operations, companies tend to have varying levels of success with direct engagement of end customers in the design process, but typically, marketing can facilitate a degree of meaningful input on behalf of customers. To hear that even marketing staff found it difficult to make a worthwhile contribution was a sobering thought. Some people working in the sector may well disagree with these comments, and let us all hope that there is a working model to be shared for the benefit of all.

2.3   WHY IS IT NECESSARY TO PLOT A COURSE?

Reading the above it should become obvious why a course is necessary. Other sectors, such as those noted in Section 2.2, have proved that the required and essential business focus does not happen by chance. It is the result of well-planned, well-coordinated, and well-executed activities across organizations, focused on customer satisfaction. The Japanese led the way during their postwar efforts at regeneration. This created a competitive environment in those sectors, so that for many it was "respond or go to the wall." Meaningful change to quality, cost, and delivery performance resulted in those sectors meeting the competitive challenge, and these changes have for the most part been sustained.

Pharmaceuticals has not been subject to similar competitive pressures to date due to the extreme differentiation and other historical factors noted earlier; also highlighted earlier is the fact that change is on the horizon as stakeholders demand more from their medicines, blockbusters become increasingly difficult to find, and generics steal postpatent profits. This would suggest that prudent innovative pharmaceutical companies need to become proactive and behave as if competitive pressures exist. This is the only way to ensure long-term sustainable success in a changing world, and must start with patient value.

This does not mean cutting corners or acting with undue haste. In fact, experience from the exemplar sectors proves that the opposite is the case. More time and effort needs to be spent in the early stages of design and development, where the roots of any product and the associated supply chains are sown and cultivated. Racing for the clinic without proper consideration of the end result required is a formula for failure; and as explained in Chapter 1, this is a sector where failure is never far away.

Before investigating this further, it may be enlightening to gather some additional perspectives by way of second opinions. To start, let's listen to Brian Williams.

GUEST CONTRIBUTOR SLOT: BRIAN WILLIAMS

A Practicing Retail Pharmacist's View and Patient Packs

For many years, pharmacists in the UK have wielded their scissors, cutting and snipping at perfectly sensible patient packs and giving their patients an assortment of off-cut blisters. What is this man talking about, you may ask? Well I am referring to original package dispensing or, more precisely, the lack of it. Twice in the recent past, both the pharmaceutical industry and the pharmacy and medical professions have agreed to move over to patient packet prescribing and dispensing. On the last occasion, in the late 1990s, an initiative was stopped in its tracks by the department of health on grounds of excessive cost, although many argued that this was exaggerated.

Let me give you a couple of examples. The synthetic penicillin amoxicillin is probably the most widely prescribed generic antibiotic. The original blister packs of both the 250- and 500-mg capsules come in packages containing 21 capsules. This is fine for a dose of one capsule three times a day for seven days. But many physicians prescribe a course of treatment for five days, so 15 capsules are required. This necessitates that the pharmacist cut and remove six capsules from the original carton. The options are either that the 15 capsules be placed in a new plain carton, supplied by the pharmacy with an attached dispensing label, or that the 15 capsules be dispensed in the original package and a home found for the remaining six capsules. The first option requires the provision of an additional patient information leaflet, such as photocopying the original, as only one is supplied in the original package. For the second option, the six remaining capsules can be placed inside a second unopened pack of amoxicillin capsules, which will now contain 27 capsules (21 plus 6). If a further prescription is received for 15 capsules, then after removal, only 12 capsules will remain in this carton, so the original packaging concept starts to collapse. Furthermore, batch identity is now effectively lost and there will be packs of the same product on the shelves containing different quantities, with an inherent potential for dispensing errors. Surely, there is an overwhelming need for the pharmaceutical industry to address this problem and supply amoxicillin in original packs of both 15 and 21 capsules.

Another area of concern is that the industry has not agreed on how many tablets or capsules should be packaged for a month's supply. This is normally either 28 or 30. However, apart from calendar packs, the pharmacist must dispense the quantity written on the prescription, so that if 28 tablets are required and the original pack is in 30's, two tablets are cut and removed from the blister and placed in another unopened pack on the shelf. Of course, the reverse also happens: 30 tablets are prescribed and only an original pack of 28 is available. In this instance, two tablets are cut from a second original pack on the shelf to provide the right quantity. The situation is self-perpetuating and covers the entire range of products; for example, 120 tablets may be prescribed against package sizes of 112, 56 capsules are prescribed against package sizes of 60, and so on. The big danger, of course, is that the two capsules cut from, say, a 10-mg blister may be moved to a pack containing 25-mg capsules, or that one product is returned into a package of a completely different product that has a similar name.

Most pharmacists believe that breaking up original packets of medicines to dispense the exact amount prescribed is a significant problem, contributing to waste as well as being time consuming. The potential for mixed batches, the provision of patient information leaflets, and the feeling that snipping tablet strips is unprofessional all contribute to the frustration that pharmacists feel with the lack of resolution of this problem.

So what needs to be done? The principles underlying original package dispensing—compliance, assurance, safety, and effectiveness—have not changed. The UK government needs to be persuaded to implement original package dispensing: first, allow pharmacists to supply the most suitable original package for a given prescription and be reimbursed accordingly; second, to agree on a uniform package size for a month's supply; and third, to make it easier for physicians to prescribe in original package sizes, such as by agreeing to changes in their computer software.

Unfortunately, we are still waiting. As long ago as 1958, Arthur Chamings pointed out at a British pharmaceutical conference that 80% of prescription medicines were being dispensed in original packets in Europe and North America. The Royal Pharmaceutical Society has now pledged to campaign for pharmacists to be able to dispense medicines in original packets, and we hope that they will be successful this time.

Observations, Views, and Experiences of the Author

Hopefully, Brian's comments speak for themselves. He did, in fact, tell me about the lunacy of this when I set up my own independent business in 2005. We both had held senior positions in pharmaceutical production for many years and could not understand it. No one from marketing had ever beaten our doors down to seek solutions to their patient and dispensing problem, because clearly, they did not know that it existed. It is difficult to think of any other sector with so little knowledge of how their products were used in the channel through to the end users. There was also a unique selling point waiting to be grabbed if any one generics producer had offered a packet of 15 tablets as part of its portfolio.

This is not even just a "lost opportunity" story—it is a huge compliance risk. That was the original driver for patient packs—to stop pharmacists from having to break them down into smaller units that could become mixed up with other products. That gap has still not been plugged.

The logical question from Brian's observations in the field, therefore, is who *is* actually collecting intelligence in relation to pharmacists and patients use of pharmaceutical products? Certainly, in the UK, it is not the pharmaceutical companies; otherwise, they would surely have reacted. What happens outside the UK is not something the author has explored in any depth, but given the global nature of pharmaceutical companies, if it doesn't happen in the UK, it is probably not happening in other markets.

Next we hear from Katie Wood, who provides a clinical operations perspective.

GUEST CONTRIBUTOR SLOT: KATIE WOOD

Formulating Products with the End in Mind

"Would you tell me, please, which way I ought to go from here" said Alice to the Cheshire Cat. "Well," replied the Cat, "that depends a good deal on where you want to get to!"[2]

Drug discoverers would do well to heed these words. The best compound with the greatest potential as a drug is worthless if it cannot be translated into a clinical formulation. So much time and effort is put into early drug discovery and into making molecules "druggable" that often the appropriateness of the final drug delivery is overlooked until late in the process, by which time clinical trials are under way and a change in formulation will have a major impact on both time lines and budgets and hence on the overall development program and eventual time to market for the drug.

The regulatory chemistry, manufacturing, and controls (CMC; see Chapter 3) must not be ignored. This is information that is detailed within any regulatory submission during the clinical trials in drug development as well as ultimately in the marketing information and labeling. To make a change at any late stage is a big deal, as it can be even early in the process! Consider the example of an IND (investigational new drug) application submitted where a capsule had been developed in four dose strengths but all the capsules were of the same size and color, with no distinctive markings on them. It was back to the drawing board for the drugmakers, with both a delay in time and an increase in budget before the IND was finally approved!

The considerations are many, and guidance should be sought from those in regulatory affairs, clinical, marketing, and competitive intelligence in order to gather the information required to develop a product which in the 10 years it may take to get it to market will still be in an acceptable form for the prescribers and patients for whom it is being developed. All the considerations are beyond the scope of this commentary; however, at the outset we must always ask some fundamental questions: What type of disease is being targeted, and how is it manifested? For example, would a patient with arthritis cope with having to self-administer an injection or count several small tablets out of a bottle? Would a patient with esophageal cancer manage to swallow several large capsules or tablets, or a patient with diabetes be able to swallow a powder formulation which can only be dissolved in lemonade or a sweet diluent? Is the drug best given as a capsule or tablet, using a needle-free device for self-administration at home, or intravenously under the supervision of a physician in a hospital setting? Is the drug going to having pediatric labeling, in which case even greater thought needs to go into the formulation, for children are not little adults, neither in their physical development nor in their understanding of the importance of taking a medication that may taste "yukky" or be difficult to chew or swallow.

The second most important concern when considering the most acceptable formulation for a drug is the potential marketplace. As the world becomes smaller and the global markets more open, it is a necessity to consider the buyer! Would an enema or suppository formulation be accepted well anywhere? Would it be possible to market pharmaceuticals using bovine materials in India? Stability and shelf life also need to be considered if, for example, the market for a drug is likely to be large in countries where there are extremes of temperature and the drug may have to travel over long distances and potentially sit at airports for extended periods! If all of the foregoing considerations are not made early in development, there is a risk that the drug may be very effective but unmarketable!

These were words from a key stakeholder in the supply chain! Those operating in clinical trials, as Katie does, appreciate the costs and difficulties associated with starting on the wrong course or of changing in midcourse. They see a patients' reactions to an inappropriate dosage form and witness their incredulity that a company could develop a product so divorced from their own particular circumstances. What, in fact, happens with any comments or complaints from patients as a drug trial progresses? Are these fed back into the target profile for the product? Is corrective action then taken at the point where things can be changed relatively easily? As we now see below, there is nothing in the drug development process that requires consideration of these factors; and we now also know that the marketing team is not going to intervene on the patient's behalf.

Next we hear from an expert in the world of U.S. pharmaceutical channel distribution, Ron Krawczyk. Ron's input refers to the application of his deep experience of channel networks to influence some of the issues of engagement that he sees in his everyday work.

GUEST CONTRIBUTOR SLOT: RON KRAWCZYK

Connecting Patient to Product Through the Distribution Channel

Connecting the product to the patient should be of the utmost priority for the pharmaceutical or biotech manufacturer. That includes accessing the role and value of any and all service providers and intermediaries involved. This became very clear to all of those involved as we initiated a project to define the optimal solution for the design of a distribution strategy. We were focused on developing a distribution strategy for a product that was to be used for the treatment of children with a behavioral disorder.

It was an oral tablet, quick dissolving, and for all intents and purposes seemed as though it would fit right into the current distribution channels, with the main point of access being the retail pharmacist. This sounded logical and was a correct assumption. Everyone was eager to get started and more eager to complete the distribution model.

It was enlightening to all when we began to define the objectives for the design of the distribution strategy. That exercise involved all of the senior leadership team as well as key stakeholders within the organization. The purpose of defining the objectives was to be clear that in the design of an optimal solution, all strategies and tactics aligned with the objectives or else we needed to reconsider what we were designing. Key product and market assumptions were understood—or were they? I consulted my trusty diagram showing U.S. pharmaceutical distribution channels (Figure 2.1). This chart is very easy to understand, with the manufacturer at the top, the list of influencers along the left-hand side, and the intermediaries clustered together in rows between the manufacturer and the patient. I really like this arrangement, because it is manufacturer centric. It is a broad statement, I know, although most manufacturers that I work with always put themselves at the top and the patient or prescriber at the bottom. I like to turn that around and start with the patient, the site of care, and the prescriber!.

When we began to discuss the patient for whom the product was being prescribed, the conversation soon became very interesting. Let's assume that they were children, aged 5 to 16 years. Remember, I mentioned a behavioral disorder, so let's begin with some key assumptions. The patients did not drive nor did they visit the prescribing physician on their own. Market research showed that the typical child suffering from

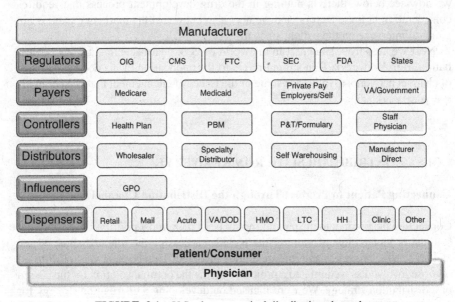

FIGURE 2.1   U.S. pharmaceutical distribution channels.

this disorder was not an only child and was often being cared for by a single (divorced or unmarried) parent, usually the mother.

This is where it really became interesting. Rather than speaking about the product and the retail outlet, it is important to identify the "patient journey" and in this case to include the mother or primary caregiver. The point at which the product meets the patient is what we needed to solve for. Also, market research showed that parents would be very interested in having the prescription mailed to their homes rather than driving to a pharmacy with the children in the car to pick up the medication. The next step was to further define the prescription and package size. Understanding that the medication was to be titrated on a two-week interval, we struggled to find the correct package size for the retail outlet to dispense that was going to meet the needs of the prescriber and be consistent with the product label. This was not as easy as we had imagined. If you begin to compare the patient journey to the diagram of the channels, it becomes obvious that additional work needed to be completed. No longer were we designing a distribution strategy; we were now working on creating a solution for the distribution of the product that considered not only the physical, financial, and transactional flows, but focused on the patient and the patient journey. So we abandoned the distribution strategy for a better-thought-out plan and created a channel strategy focused on our four P's—patient, provider, payer, and pharmacist—that indeed matched up to the company's objectives.

This solution was not created by any one person; it involved many people from across the company to define the optimal solution to meet the needs of the patient and in this case the caregiver. The solution required a holistic approach and an in-depth look into the patient's journey as well as a lot of common sense. This was a very good example of the need for the manufacturer to begin with the patient and design a channel strategy inclusive of how and where the product would be sold so that all patients have the necessary access to the product.

2.4   UNDERSTANDING HOW THE COURSE IS PRESENTLY SET

To gain a proper understanding of how this disconnect occurs, it is necessary to go to the start of the development process. The regulatory authorities define a route to application and approval for conducting clinical trials and marketing of drugs (refer to Chapter 3 for details and references). In the United States, it is a new drug application (NDA) for chemicals and a biologics license application (BLA) for biologicals. In the European Union it is a marketing authorization application (MAA). The result of a successful NDA/BLA/MAA is a label claim approved by the regulators. This claim is incredibly important to the market potential for a drug. It is the differentiator and can make or break a compound. Particularly if a drug is the second or later to reach the market, the claim should be superior to that of the drug innovator; otherwise, there should be little rationale for use of the alternative product (unless it costs less, and using cost as a differentiator would be regarded by the innovator industry as the kiss of death for the profitability of that class of compound).

The label claim that a drug developer is aiming to achieve is (or should be) set out in a target product profile at the beginning of development activities. FDA's labeling regulations (21 CFR 201.56 and 201.57; see Chapter 3 for more on 21 CFRs) require the following information:

- Description of the drug
- Clinical pharmacology
- Indications (disease state) and usage
- Contraindications
- Warnings
- Precautions
- Adverse reactions
- Drug abuse and dependence
- Overdosage
- Dosage and administration
- How supplied
- Animal pharmacology and/or animal toxicology (if necessary)
- Clinical studies/references (if necessary)

It is not until well down the list that mention is made of anything other than a medical parameter, and then it is the only one: how supplied. In practice, this means how many tablets or dosage units will be in a box or container and what the container will be. The multitude of other things about the product's makeup and supply requirements are contained within what is known as the CMC section (CTD Module 3 or quality section; see Chapter 3), which is compiled by technical specialists focused on supporting strictly medical parameters. There is no process of which I am aware to factor patient and other related stakeholder needs into the final approved product for sale. Since the label attained is the differentiator for the marketed product, all attention is focused there.

Observations, Views, and Experiences of the Author

Whenever I am asked to help a company prepare for launch of a product, I have to get to know where the project team is with things. This means collecting a vast array of information required to define the end-to-end supply chain at the current state of development, such as suppliers used and locations, projected approval dates, material specifications, validation status of batches made, product structures, and special requirements. Almost without fail, this is the first time that this will have been done. I've stopped being surprised by this, although it would be nice to experience such a surprise. The information always exists, but no responsibility has been allocated for translating it into supply chain information. This disconnect between the various stages of manufacture is amplified further by the almost total absence of connection with the commercial demand for and use of the product. Not that there haven't been attempts to make this happen, but marketing has never been involved until this stage, so no vehicle exists to make it happen. The result is a severely debilitating disconnect for the end-to-end supply chain.

The next speaker we hear from is Jack Shapiro, a person in constant contact with real patients who has a very deep understanding of their needs and views.

GUEST CONTRIBUTOR SLOT: JACK SHAPIRO

The Pharmaceutical Industry and Patient Relationships

At least four trends have helped to sour the relationship between the physician and his or her patient, and I'm afraid that we, the pharmaceutical industry, have had a big hand in this.

1. Never forget that we live in a post-Vioxx world, a world that saw physicians get mud on their faces and hurt their rapport with patients (not to mention their rapport with us, the industry). Every subsequent product recall or bad news flash about a prescription drug has added to the problem. Better researched drugs, phase IV studies that actually take place and are completed, and timely reporting of ADRs (adverse drug or device reaction) might help—but don't count on it.

2. Let's face it: Physicians hate our TV ads and hate it when their patients refer to them. The only good news is that some physicians have a bit more trust in those Web sites for patients that are more complete and seem to be more objective, but not always. Unfortunately, that's not a feeling shared universally, and many physicians wish we'd stop that, too.

3. Too many of our drugs are basically expensive me-too drugs that offer minimal, if any, advantages over earlier compounds. Physicians know this and patients eventually figure it out and can't understand why their doctor is making them pay so much for so little. High-tier co-pays don't help this problem.

4. We make a classic mistake as an industry in thinking that consumers have a clue what we're talking about. In focus group after focus group, I hear questions regarding incredibly basic things that we in the industry take for granted, such as: "What is an OTC drug?" "What does 'OTC' mean, and how does that differ from a prescription drug?" "What's a generic drug, really? What does 'generic' mean, and how does that differ from a drug that's not generic?" And perhaps my favorite: "What's an NSAID? What does *that* mean?" Do you really think that in the precious 6 minutes that a primary care physician has to spend with a patient, he or she can deal with all this? I don't, and I'm worried about our industry's future.

Some dramatic food for thought here! If Jack is right, and who would argue to the contrary, patients are a confused group resigned to *not* understanding how this industry works. If the patient does not know what a generic drug is and that in most cases it is identical to the innovator product, he or she will not make an informed choice. The patient will probably not push for the cheaper product in the way that normal markets work to drive efficiencies up and costs down. Notice also, from Jack's comment, the role that marketing is playing in all this—the promotion of existing products. It begs the question how much marketing is involved with the development of those existing products. Readers can make up their own minds on that.

2.5 CAPTURING VALUE FOR PATIENTS

To finish the chapter, let's comment on value for patients, since the end market is made up of patients. Even though they are often supported financially by a third party such as government or an insurance company, patients ultimately decide what they like and what they don't like. So, hypothetically, if a pharmaceutical company were interested in taking the *long-term* needs of patients into account when formulating a business strategy, how should they go about it? Joshua Bashford is just one example of an industry professional with some ideas.

GUEST CONTRIBUTOR SLOT: JOSHUA BASHFORD

Some Innovative Ideas for Pharmaceutical Companies

Engaging patients with their treatment process can spur interest in learning about their disease and encourage a more active role in their treatment. Technically savvy patients can realize support via a Web-based platform for disease management sponsored by pharma company A which provides a patient with a wealth of available features, such as a diary to log symptoms, information related to their illness, side effects to monitor, reminders for taking medicine, and links to social media for forums or groups of people with similar illnesses. Such a platform could also include behavioral tracking, such as food, drink, and exercise for people with metabolic disorders. Patient involvement would also provide company A with a feedback mechanism for continued safety and efficacy, drug adherence and cessation, population data, and more. In addition, a similar platform could provide a portal for the primary care physician to assess outcomes without seeing the patient. If this opened up to many (thousands) of patients, primary care physicians could see how one patient tracks with others who have similar illnesses and/or comorbidities. In the end, this would improve outcomes, establish repeat traffic to company A's Web site by both physicians and patients, and provide the company with a continuous stream of data for safety monitoring.

What a perfect platform from which to develop differentiated products, both innovator and generic. When their BID (twice daily) treatment regimen is causing some degree of drowsiness, how many patients would love their drug, to become a "once at night" treatment. The drug would turn instantly from a negative to a positive. Not only would it help the patient's medical condition, it would also encourage a good night's sleep. As a patient, I'm going to go with that product every time, no matter how cheap the competition. The same goes for branded drugs with suboptimal issues in certain key patient use areas.

These suggestions made by Josh therefore appear to be potential win–win–win–win outcomes. The pharma company benefits by having a better relationship and connection with patients to feed into their processes. Patients have access to far more information on their conditions and treatment options. Physicians get increased support with patients and personal education on pharmaceutical products. Even payers should benefit: from better connected thinking among the other three stakeholder groups.

The specifics of this piece from Josh are not, of course, meant to be prescriptive in any way. They are included here to demonstrate the kind of thinking that needs to be encouraged and shared among all players in the sector.

This concludes the case for the defense of paying and paid-for patients.

3 Pharmaceutical Drug Development

3.1 DRUG DEVELOPMENT'S ROLE IN THE SUPPLY CHAIN

The title of this first section may be surprising to some. It continues the theme of drug development having no purpose without a commercial supply chain. The converse is also true, of course, but one of the things that this book attempts to tease out is some of the deep-rooted, unspoken assumptions in the sector that inhibit attempts to make meaningful improvements in quality, cost, and value. The one targeted here is that thinking about the supply chain comes after a drug is developed. Hence we focus here on what drug development should do for the supply chain. We begin with some personal content.

Observations, Views, and Experiences of the Author

In 2005, I became an independent consultant in pharmaceutical SCM, having spent over a decade in permanent roles with biotech companies (SMEs) helping to launch drugs in global markets. When my employer, OSI Pharmaceuticals, decided to shift their manufacture and supply chain efforts from the UK to the Long Island, New York, headquarters, I took the opportunity to go it alone. Armed with a severance package, I set about developing client business. The article that follows is something I wrote as part of my attempt to build awareness of SCM in the sector and also to promote my own newly packaged service proposition. Some of the earlier sections in the book have drawn on the sentiments, but it is included here in full.

Registering a Drug or Building a Value Stream?

Historically in pharmaceuticals, performance of the supply chain has been a low priority. Blockbuster drugs with secure markets and "silly" margins meant that the focus was always on the scientific and technical aspects of registration and supply. As long as the drug was approved and patients received the drug manufactured to the regulators' satisfaction, then job done. However, vitally important though the science is, it is the supply chain that delivers the value—and there are signs that key stakeholders are demanding more.

Supply Chain Management in the Drug Industry: Delivering Patient Value for Pharmaceuticals and Biologics, By Hedley Rees
Copyright © 2011 John Wiley & Sons, Inc.

The global pressure to contain health care budgets is focusing on prescription medicine, which in turn spotlights the cost, efficiency, and effectiveness of drug manufacture. The current FDA initiative to introduce process analytical technology (PAT) is evidence of regulators responding. This is a positive start to facilitating improved ways of working in the supply chain to favorably affect quality, cost, and lead time. At a recent conference in the Netherlands, Jon E. Clark, associate director of policy development for the Center for Drug Evaluation and Research at the FDA, is quoted as saying: "There should be a way to protect the public without slowing CMC innovation and continuous improvement."

The question now is: How will the industry approach the opportunity, and any further opportunities, to modernize the supply chain? The plain fact is that welcome as PAT is, the concept that quality cannot be inspected into a product has been applied in other industries for many years. Industry sectors such as aerospace, electronics, and automotives have been attacking process variability and raising process understanding and capability for several decades. Quality has increased and costs have been reduced dramatically. This has taken place as an industry-driven imperative: working within the bounds of safety standards and regulation, but pushing the boundaries of modernization. This has not always been the case in pharmaceuticals.

"Batch and queue" manufacture (see Chapter 7); campaign scheduling; multisourcing procurement policies; large, capital-intensive, inflexible machinery; and maximization of batch sizes are just some examples of "cultural" practices within pharmaceuticals that impede the adoption of world-class methods. It will take more than just the regulators to bring about modernization; the entire industry must attack the inertia built up over many, many years.

As demonstrated by the exemplar sectors above, however, the starting point is not in currently established supply chains. It must be at the design, development, and registration stage of a medicinal product. It is estimated by researchers at Cardiff Business School (John Bichino)[1] that over 80 percent of cost is locked into a product at the design and development stage. In pharmaceuticals, because of the historical inertia to change, it is probably significantly higher.

The message is clear, then: For meaningful improvement, scientific and technical staff must work closely with supply chain practitioners and other relevant parties to help secure responsive, cost-effective, and risk-mitigated supply chains to compete on the world stage. This should not wait until a drug has been registered but should start as early as possible in the CMC development process by developing and implementing SCM best practices to expedite such development and definitely before registration-oriented or pivotal clinical trials. This will be the case particularly as the more virtual business models of drug development become increasingly prominent. Such developments present huge opportunities to harness the increasingly high-caliber third-party contract supply base and reduce overall risk in progression, provided that complexity and cost are managed carefully. Resources for these companies are preciously scarce, guaranteeing that that will always be the case.

So, moving to our topic: Registering a drug or building a value stream? I suggest that CMC development must reset the line of sight—from supply of drug to the clinic and gaining registration, to building a patient value stream: capable processes and suppliers, streamlined logistics, flexible plant and equipment, shorter cycle times, effective flow of information, and reduced waste. All these factors can and should be addressed at the CMC development stage, as they are equally germane to development progression and success as a commercial product.

*To use the words of Jon E. Clark once again, from the same conference: "The phar-
maceutical industry has one of the most technically advanced discovery organizations,
but remains more conservative when it comes to using 'cutting edge' technology in
manufacturing." Hopefully, the wind of change is upon us!*

*I have not changed my views since 2005. In fact, my view has grown stronger
since writing that. The gauntlet has been thrown down, but evidence of fundamental
change in the traditional ways of developing and making drugs is difficult to find.*

With this insight in mind, the remainder of this chapter is about establishing a
baseline of understanding of drug development. To do a more comprehensive job of
this, and cognizant of my nonspecialization in this area, I am pleased that Patrick
Crowley agreed to help.

Pat and I act as consultants for Alacrita,[2] and this is how we began our work on
this chapter.

What follows is our joint account (but all scientific and technical questions should
be addressed to Patrick!).

3.2 INTRODUCTION TO DRUG DEVELOPMENT

Before a drug is administered to humans it must be assessed in what are generically
termed *preclinical studies* in animals, ex vivo (e.g., tissue studies) and in vitro tests.
Such activities usually follow the handover from discovery research of a chemical or
biological entity that shows the potential to cure or alleviate an ailment or disease.
Early preclinical studies are focused on providing information to enable a decision to
be made to begin clinical studies in humans as the first step toward transforming a compound to a possible medicinal product. Nonclinical development groups have broader
assignments, however, and remain involved in development programs throughout all
clinical assessment phases and beyond. Other functions participate increasingly as
development proceeds, so that a commercial product can be made available (if the
program is successful) and documented evidence is assembled and presented to regulatory agencies, demonstrating that a drug is safe, effective, and suitable for marketing.

Following handover to development personnel, discovery teams return to focus
on finding a follow-up compound or possibly a material for another indication.
Discovery research can be creative and relatively unstructured, since the aim is
to explore new and uncharted regions. In contrast, development must be defined,
rigorous, and controlled. In no other (legal!) sector are novel substances administered
to human beings with as yet unknown effects on vital organs and various other bodily
nooks and crannies. Thus, development programs are highly regulated. They must be
underpinned by good science, concern for patient well-being, and strict compliance
with ethical, quality, and various procedural standards. Regulatory bodies that are part
of sovereign governments must approve study protocols, can demand specific quality
standards and safeguards, and need to be informed of any significant events. No
matter how potentially effective a drug is, if it is not safe or does not meet acceptable

standards of performance and purity, there will be no license to market. Regulations designed to ensure such safety, quality, and efficacy are discussed later in the chapter.

Attrition rates at the discovery–development interface can be very high. It has been estimated that 245 of every 250 candidates for development fail to surmount preclinical evaluation hurdles. Furthermore, a novel molecular or biological entity emanating from a drug discovery program has to survive a long and complex journey to become a medication to cure or alleviate a particular disease. Programs:

- Are long lasting (where the drug survives the various hurdles)
- Are expensive
- Need to be carefully coordinated so that activities are aligned, feedback from such activities is rapid, with responses to any findings communicated to stakeholders in a timely and well-considered manner.

Regulatory requirements can also be considered as hurdles in the development program. Agencies are involved in virtually every facet of programs. Nonfamiliarity with requirements and of their diversity can slow evaluation and progression. Timeliness and diligence are predicated by the fact that the novel material has to be dosed to humans in clinical studies to determine whether it is efficacious and safe. Plans and processes have to be in place so that any unexpected findings are communicated to regulatory agencies and other stakeholders in a timely and considered way. Trials running concurrently may need to be redesigned or suspended until investigations are complete. In a more general sense there is a need for coordination, communication, and prompt decision making across all facets of pharmaceutical product development. Hence, disciplines such as project management, supply chain management, and data collection and analysis (among others) play key roles.

Program alignments are best understood by first considering the activities and roles of the various development functions. This is best done by starting with the end product in the form of medication taken by or administered to a patient and considering the various activities necessary to make such a product available.

3.3   THE MEDICINAL PRODUCT

A medicine contains an accurate dose of a drug in an easy-to-use and easy-to-administer form (e.g., tablet, injection). For the drug to attain the status of "medicine," the following objectives must be attained:

- The drug must be shown to be safe.
- The drug must be shown to be effective.
- A process for manufacturing the drug substance has to be developed, along with controls to assure its quality.
- The drug product has to be developed for clinical studies in the first instance and ultimately as the commercial product.
- Controls for the quality of drug substance and drug product need to be developed concurrently with other aspects of the development program.

The roles played by the various product development disciplines to attain these objectives will be discussed next. Activities and interactions are best understood by considering clinical trials as the pivotal activity. Contributions by nonclinical development functions are then considered. Finally, their roles in making commercial product available are considered.

3.4   CLINICAL TRIALS

Clinical trials to establish safety and efficacy can vary in size, duration, and patient types, depending on many factors, not least the clinical condition and patient groups. However, they tend to progress in the following sequence:

- Phase I trials: studies in healthy human volunteers
- Phase II trials: proof-of-concept studies in patients
- Phase III trials: studies to definitively show efficacy and safety at doses and dosage regimen intended for commercial products.

Such studies require input from and coordination across many clinical and nonclinical and regulatory departments.

3.4.1   Phase I Trials

Phase I (sometimes termed *human pharmacology*) studies are (with rare exceptions, such as anticancer agents) performed in healthy volunteers in the controlled setting of a clinical unit. They are designed to provide information on:

- Whether the drug is absorbed (if dosed orally)
- The drug's metabolism and distribution throughout body tissues
- How readily the drug is removed, transformed, or excreted from the body

It is usual to begin phase I studies by administering very low doses. If there are no untoward effects, dosing may be increased to a level of something like 10% of the "no effect level" derived from the animal safety studies (Section 3.5.1). Volunteers are screened comprehensively before, during, and after dosing. Measurements of components in blood and tissues are made, as well as various physiological tests (e.g., heart rate and blood pressure). Biomarkers are being used increasingly to provide early indications of efficacy, intolerance, or other drug-related effects. It is also now common to genotype subjects so that genome-associated effects can be ascertained, affording better patient selection for the later efficacy studies. Figure 3.1 summarizes how activities are aligned, sequentially and in parallel, in programs leading to phase I clinical trials. Similar interactions occur in subsequent trials.

Volunteer studies do not usually provide evidence of therapeutic effect: Healthy volunteers are not burdened with the specific clinical condition. However, they provide an estimate of dose frequency (depending on rate of removal from the body) and

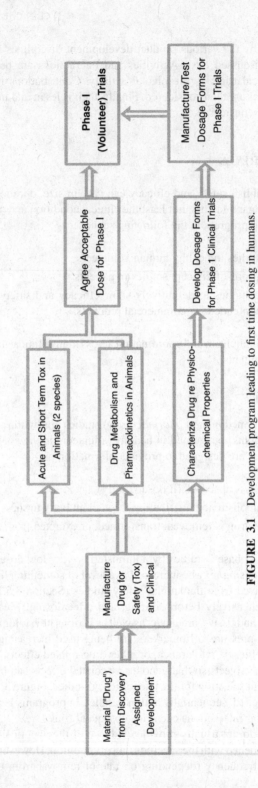

FIGURE 3.1 Development program leading to first time dosing in humans.

on maximum tolerated dose. Additional phase I studies may be performed at any time during the overall development program to explore a particular facet of human pharmacology, to determine whether a change in the drug formulation affects how the drug is absorbed (bioavailability) and handled (pharmacokinetics) or to explore performance in a specific category of patients (e.g., elderly or specific genotypic patients).

3.4.2   Phase II Clinical Trials

Phase II clinical trials are usually designed to determine whether a drug has the therapeutic benefit predicated by research and preclinical studies. Trials may be subdivided into sequential IIA and IIB programs, the former possibly designed to establish "proof of concept." Phase IIB studies focus on a narrower dose range or frequency to prove efficacy conclusively and to provide guidance on dose and dosage regimens for the subsequent phase III clinical trials. Phase II trials on cancer medications may be designed to provide sufficient information for registration and approval as a product, if warranted by the clinical results. Phase II studies usually employ more plasma and tissue sampling for clinical and safety-relevant relevant markers than do later, larger trials. Compound attrition rates are high, usually because efficacy is not demonstrated. It is not unusual for trials to be repeated, using differing patient subsets, or dose- and time-related variables that were not explored in the first trial.

3.4.3   Phase III Clinical Trials

Phase III trials usually involve large patient numbers, encompassing many centers, countries, and continents. They are designed to provide conclusively that a drug is effective and safe. Because of the greater numbers, there is a greater likelihood of an adverse event being manifest in a tiny cohort of patients. Alternatively, clinical measurements while a trial is in progress may be so impressive that it would be unethical to continue dosing with placebo (the control in most such trials). Organizations need to have systems in place to capture, report, and analyze information readily so that steps can be taken to safeguard patient well-being.

3.4.4   Other Clinical Programs

Phase 0 Trials   These recently designated trials are intended to expedite the clinical evaluation of new molecular entities in oncology drug evaluation. They involve the administration of a single microdose of drug, the dose being too low to elicit a therapeutic or untoward effect. Studies require less preclinical information than normal (e.g., reduced manufacturing and toxicology testing) and are used to help select a single entity for progression from a number of candidates. Such selection may be based on pharmacokinetic performance being akin to that in the discovery animal model, which indicated efficacy potential. Phase 0 studies may be considered as "pre-development" (being used by discovery groups to select a candidate for progression to development).

Commercial Product Clinical studies do not stop when a compound progresses to a medicinal product. Phase IV studies, trials to evaluate suitability for patient and disease subsets and comparative studies with other medications, are all likely. Observational studies and pharmacovigilance data mining can also identify noteworthy patient responses. Nuances of drug behavior may be uncovered that were not evident in the precommercial clinical trials. Advances in molecular biology, receptor pharmacology, and better understanding of the clinical conditions may also identify new opportunities for modifying delivery by reformulation so that the medication is more effective, safer, or more convenient. Many great medications comprise such second-generation products as Toprol XL and Wellbutrin XL, where more convenient dosing and full daily cover are provided by modifying release from the dosage form. Most clinical trials are blinded and placebo controlled, to minimize the risk of biased outcomes. General considerations applicable to the design, purpose, and performance of clinical trials are contained in ICH Guide E8.[3] Activities associated with the setup, management, and reporting of clinical studies are addressed later in the chapter.

3.5 RELATED DEVELOPMENT PROGRAMS

Clinical programs provide the ultimate test of a drug's safety and efficacy. They are also usually rate limiting to overall progression. Therefore, the activities of nonclinical groups should, where possible, be designed and executed to stay off this critical path. However, nonclinical groups are pivotal, and can be rate limiting, to making commercial products available in the event of successful clinical trials. Next we discuss the functions of the following groups and their interactions: safety evaluation (toxicology), drug metabolism and pharmacokinetics, chemical and biopharmaceutical development, analytical sciences and quality functions, and pharmaceutical development.

3.5.1 Safety Evaluation (Toxicology)

Before a novel material can be administered to humans it must exhibit a clean bill of health in both animal studies and in vitro assessments such as genotoxicity screens. Toxicity can take many forms but may be broadly categorized as acute and chronic toxicity. Early studies focus on acute (single dose) and repeat dosing effects: testing protocols designed to determine a safe starting dose in humans. Requirements are country specific, but in the general sense the administration of a single dose to humans (in phase I trials) requires that no untoward effects are demonstrated following repeat dosing for up to four weeks in two animal species, rodent and nonrodent. Repeat dosing in humans requires animal studies of longer duration (details vary with country). A dose to humans will be very low at the outset and guided by *no toxic effect levels* (NELs) established in the animal studies. Animal testing requirements for clearance for human dosage are provided in ICH Guide M3(R2).[4]

If the compound continues to show promise, longer and more detailed animal toxicology studies are warranted. These include studies to identify and explore the effects on particular target organs that then merit detailed consideration and assessment in follow-up animal studies and careful monitoring in clinical studies in humans. Studies mandated by regulatory agencies include:

- Acute toxicology
- Subacute or chronic toxicology
- Genetic toxicology
- Reproductive toxicity
- Carcinogenicity studies
- Immunotoxicity
- Phototoxicity

Additional information on drug safety is available from FDA[5] and ICH[6] databases.

Long-term animal safety studies and those focusing on specific facets of toxicology usually proceed in parallel with clinical trials (where there is sufficient cover from the earlier animal safety studies to support the ongoing trials). If a finding from these ongoing studies in animals raises concerns, the impact on the clinical program (redesign or termination) needs to be considered. Good science also ordains that, when warranted, investigative studies be performed to explore a noteworthy finding, validate a change in the drug substance mode of manufacture, or ensure that a previously unseen impurity is not hazardous. A finding in animal studies or in patients may also elicit a request from regulatory agencies for more detailed investigations (e.g., effect on a specific organ or tissue). Generally, in such cases there is dialogue between the agency and the organization to agree on the study design, duration, animal species, and the observations and measurements that will be appropriate. Issues can also arise with commercial products requiring comment or exploratory studies by the safety evaluation group. Hence, like other nonclinical development groups, safety evaluation personnel remain involved throughout a development program and product lifetime.

3.5.2 Drug Metabolism and Pharmacokinetics

In addition to biological and clinical effects, it is necessary to generate information on other facets of a drug's behavior in animals and humans. Such knowledge concerns:

- How the drug is absorbed (unless administered parenterally)
- Where it is distributed in the body
- How the body transforms (metabolizes) the drug
- How quickly and by what route drug and metabolites are eliminated from the body

Studies to elucidate these behaviors (collectively termed ADME) are performed in volunteers, in patients, and in animals, so that species with metabolic pathways and clearance routes comparable to those in humans are selected for the longer-term toxicology studies. Such work requires analytical expertise to identify and quantify the metabolites (and intact drug) in biological fluids and tissues to determine levels, rates of disposition, and clearance. Other activities that come within the purview of drug metabolism and pharmacokinetics include but are not limited to the following concerns:

- Dosing to humans (and sometimes to animals) requires that a drug be formulated in a suitable dosage unit. The effect of formulation on absorption (bioavailability) and time course (pharmacokinetics) in the body needs to be assessed.
- During clinical programs, samples may be taken from patients for evaluation (e.g., blood sugar in diabetics, inflammatory mediators in rheumatoid arthritis and other inflammatory diseases). Methods need to be developed and used to determine the presence and level of such biomarkers for efficacy or toxicity.

Like other drug development functions, drug metabolism and pharmacokinetic involvement continues throughout the development time span and beyond.

3.5.3 Chemical and Biopharmaceutical Development

A drug substance [also termed an active pharmaceutical ingredient (API) or active substance] needs to be available to fund such development activities as:

- Safety evaluation
- ADME work (developing animal models and analytical methods for drug determinations in biological fluids)
- Developing and providing dosage forms for clinical trials and ultimately for commercialization
- Analytical method development

Hence, a process for making a novel material must be developed and stocks prepared. An initial route of synthesis may be developed from the information provided by discovery scientists. At the same time, process chemists ("route scouts") consider whether this original mode of manufacture can be scaled up to higher volumes without altering the nature and performance of the compound. If scale-up is not possible, a more efficient, scalable, and safer mode of manufacture must be developed. However, the route provided in discovery may be retained throughout early and mid-development so that the program maintains momentum. Regulatory agencies expect that understanding of compound manufacture will increase as the development program progresses. It is accepted that in the early stages, prior to human use, there will be unknowns to be identified through iterative processing, probably at a small scale (this is a critical point of influence). However, compounds for administration to humans must be prepared, characterized, and tested such that quality is assured and there are no characteristics that could threaten the safety and well-being of trial participants.

Samples of drug-related impurities, metabolites, or other drug-related structures may be required for analytical development, testing in animals, or use as markers (reference materials) for determining their presence in biological fluids or in drug and drug products (e.g., in stability programs). Chemical development is responsible for the development of a route of preparation and for supplying such materials. Work may be performed in-house or at contract organizations. If the drug continues to progress, the process for drug manufacture at a commercial scale must be transferred to a commercial facility. Factors additional to synthesis and purity then become increasingly important. If the drug is a synthetic compound, it may be assembled from other structures by routes that are hazardous (e.g., hydrogenation, Grignard synthesis), employ volatile and/or flammable organic solvents, and use toxic reagents.

The mode of manufacture needs to be designed so that safety during processing and purity in terms of freedom from hazardous residues in final material is assured. The drug must also be suitable for continued processing leading to a drug product. Hence, properties such as polymorphism, particle size, or aggregation need to be explored and controlled if necessary. The drug must retain its quality (be stable) and be made by a process that is cost-effective. If the drug is a biopharmaceutical, or even a small molecule derived from fermentation, the same requirements (except processing) apply, as a drug substance or drug product may pose unique demands. Most biopharmaceuticals are administered parenterally, so need to be sterile. Being structurally fragile, they cannot be sterilized by the harsher technologies (autoclaving, heat, or irradiation). Hence, they must be manufactured as sterile bulk material which is then processed aseptically to drug product. This is particularly challenging, as "live" cells are usually the source of the active ingredient. Culturing these provides friendly environments for the growth of bacteria, fungi, and so on, and as a consequence, endotoxins, mycotoxins, and viruses can be carried through the process. Standards for cleanliness are high, and processes to remove or inactivate biological and nonbiological contaminants need to be developed and validated. Clean-room technologies, chromatographic purification, and concentration processes such as reverse osmosis feature prominently with such materials. Manufacturing cycles for biological and biopharmaceutical products can be as long as six months, and quality assessment testing is usually more comprehensive (i.e., more tests) than it is for small molecules.

3.5.4 Analytical Sciences and Quality Functions

Assuring the quality of a material or product involves much more than testing the finished article (important though that is). Quality also concerns controlling starting and other input materials, the environment for product manufacture, and the operating limits (process parameters) for each stage. It also encompasses the overall management of the process and facility. These include:

- Operating procedures
- Change control systems

- Training programs
- Systems for recording and checking
- Processes for quality alerts and root-cause investigations where an incident occurs
- Corrective and preventive action systems to remedy an unsatisfactory situation or operation

Many of these are procedural, but some require determinations or measurements that inform as to the state of a facility or equipment, completion of a process stage, or the quality of an intermediate, or provide evidence to explain an incident. For such operations and eventualities, methods need to be developed and shown to be fit for the purpose. Quality systems and test methods need to be in place to monitor and assure the suitability of material destined for use in animal safety or clinical programs. Methods must also be developed and suitably characterized for use with commercial product. Performance characteristics such as robustness, reproducibility, and sensitivity need to be defined so that departments charged with routinely monitoring component materials and commercial product are aware of the method capabilities (and limitations).

3.5.5 Pharmaceutical Development

The patient does not take (or is not administered) drug per se, but a unit containing an accurate dose of the drug. The dosage form must also meet other quality standards (e.g., be sterile if intended for injection). Dosage units are usually required for phase I studies in volunteers (i.e., early in the program) and from there through to commercial products. Drug properties and dosages determine the selection of other materials in the formulation, their levels, and possibly the process for manufacture. In early clinical trials the effective (and safe) dose is not known (it is not even known whether the drug is efficacious). Hence, it is usual to develop dosage forms containing a range of drug contents for trial use. Clinical trials are usually blinded so that neither the patient nor the clinical assessor is aware of the treatment regimen. Units containing different doses must therefore be identical in appearance, as must any placebo formulation. A commercial product, in contrast, requires visual differentiation (e.g., size, color, shape) if different strengths are available. Hence, units for clinical studies may not be suitable as commercial product. Separate formulations for commercial use need to be developed (when the dose is known). These must evoke the same in vivo effect as the clinical units, so must be evaluated for impact on bioavailability (if dosed orally) and stability on storage. Analytical methods must also be modified to take account of changes.

Pharmaceutical development personnel, along with manufacturing groups, are responsible for designing the process for the commercial product. The process must be aligned with commercial manufacturing capabilities and technologies. At a suitable time (usually during or before phase III trials) the process is transferred to a commercial site, necessitating scale-up studies. It is also necessary to define operating limits for each stage, quality standards for input materials and intermediates, and specifications and limits for finished products to ensure adequate and consistent quality. Hence, in common with the other nonclinical disciplines, pharmaceutical development functions need to be aligned with activities in clinical and other nonclinical functions.

The foregoing summary of the roles of nonclinical functions does not encompass the full range of interunit interactions. Many associated and subtasks underpin each activity. Furthermore, no program runs exactly to a preordained master plan. False starts, restarts, and roadblocks can and do occur. There is a need for strong project management to ensure that activities are aligned, choke points and conflicts are addressed and resolved, and contributing units support the overall program in a coordinated manner.

3.6   MANAGING CLINICAL PROGRAMS

Clinical trials may be confined to a specific region or country (e.g., trials on parasitic infections), to a limited number of clinical centers of excellence (e.g., oncology treatment centers), or to developed countries. In many other (probably most) cases, studies can virtually span the world. Regardless of reach, it is imperative that the principles and best practices of supply chain management be brought to bear on how studies are initiated, managed, and reported. Furthermore, supply chains for clinical programs can be considered as "two-way." Trial protocols (including changes made while a trial is in progress) need to go from the center to the trial site. Dosage forms need to go the same way. In return, samples of biological fluids may need to be sent from the trial center to the R&D center for analysis. Data and information generated at the trial center (including alerts) must also be relayed back to the trial coordinating center. Such a supply chain can be more complex than many other commercial activities in which flow is one-way.

Operational complexities associated with setup, running, and reporting clinical studies are best understood by considering the clinical program as the core activity, as it provides definitive evidence for drug safety and efficacy. Programs require several "inputs" to generate such information, which we describe next.

3.6.1   Patient Recruitment

Patients are recruited for trials through clinical institutes such as university or teaching hospitals, regional centers of clinical excellence, clinical opinion leaders, who can persuade clinicians working in the therapeutic area to participate, and through general medical practitioners. State organizations (e.g., the U.S. Army) or nongovernmental agencies (e.g., the World Health Organization) may also sponsor and participate in trials. Participants identify and recruit suitable patients and ensure that the appropriate dosing, clinical monitoring for effect, and reporting are carried out as defined in the trial protocol. Trial centers may be scattered across continents and countries. Recruitment can vary widely from original estimates. Dropouts, noncompliance with regimens, and possibly a need to shift dosage (if the protocol allows) are common. The possibility of an adverse event is omnipresent, and procedures for prompt reporting to a clinical advisory committee (or similar body), regulatory agencies, and so on, need to be in place. Study suspension or termination may need to be considered, but this is not straightforward in conditions or treatments where patients are stabilized on the trial drug and withdrawal might be hazardous.

3.6.2   Clinical Trial Setup and Management

It is clinicians' responsibility to safeguard the well-being of patients and do nothing that might cause harm. Hence, every clinician who provides or monitors patients needs to be made aware of the purpose of the medication and study, previous experience with the drug (e.g., in earlier trials, in animals), potential side effects, and actions to be initiated in the event of unexpected findings. Clinicians and associated staff need to be aware of and be comfortable with the dosing and evaluation methodologies specified in the test protocol, with the case reports that need to be populated (by the patient or monitor, depending on the trial), and with reporting schedules and time lines that need to be complied with to ensure overall alignment with other facets of the trial.

During a trial, the recruitment rate may not proceed as planned or promised. Other centers may need to be brought on line to keep the program on schedule. Changes to trial protocols during the study may be warranted by unexpected benefits as well as by side effects. The active drug might be significantly more beneficial than the placebo. Denying such a benefit to patients receiving placebo or a comparator drug would be unethical, so the trial protocol may need to be altered. Such possibilities need to be covered by preagreed protocols, with agencies advised of developments (and amendments) in a timely manner. Clinical trials require good and timely communication, coordination, and interaction with country-specific regulatory agencies. Trials in multiple countries (possibly with different regulatory emphasis) can be especially demanding. Consequently, it is important to understand the makeup of regulatory agencies, their charters, and their involvement in drug development, approval, and the commercial environment. Such roles are discussed in the following section.

3.7   REGULATORY AFFAIRS AND AUTHORITIES

Most pharmaceutical companies have units with specific responsibility for regulatory affairs [although the activity can also be outsourced to contract regulatory organizations (CROs)]. Regulatory affairs personnel, coordinate all aspects of R&D and commercial operations pertaining to regulatory requirements. This group is responsible for gathering and assembling information that forms the basis of new drug applications, clinical trials applications, and updates for existing commercial products, and acts as the prime interface with regulatory authorities.

Virtually all countries have agencies charged with national stewardship of the development, marketing, and general use of pharmaceutical products. Responsibilities encompass but are not restricted to:

- *Approval and stewardship of clinical trials.* Agencies have to be satisfied, from the information provided by the trialist, that the drug is unlikely to do any harm, that the trial is warranted because of some unmet clinical need, and that there are systems in place to ensure that patient selection, monitoring, and reporting (including reporting of serious adverse events) is performed to the requisite standards.
- *Assessment of applications for authorization to market a medicinal product.* Such assessment follows clinical studies to show safety and efficacy.
- *Pharmacovigilance programs.* These programs are necessary to detect untoward effects or emerging trends for commercially available medications.

Awareness of global requirements and more nuanced regional and national variations is vital when managing development programs and commercial operations. The roles of the major agencies are discussed below. Readers are encouraged to become familiar with the guidelines associated with various facets of development that are readily available on agency Web sites, such as:

- The U.S. Food and Drug Administration (FDA) and associated *Code of Federal Regulations* Title 21 (CFR 21) regulates the largest pharmaceutical market in the world, the United States. Guides, updates, and alerts can be accessed on the FDA Web site,[7] as can CFR 21.
- The European Medicines Agency (EMA[8]), the regulator for the European Union.

The FDA, the EMA, and the Japanese regulatory agency (the Ministry of Health and Welfare) cooperate to harmonize requirements [through the International Conference on Harmonization (ICH)[9]]. The ICH has developed a series of guidelines for various facets of the drug development process and a common structure for documents requesting approval to market: the *common technical document* (CTD) (see Figure 3.2 for the CTD pyramid). This harmonization process remains ongoing, so readers should refer to the respective Web sites for the most up-to-date guidance documents, as these are amended regularly (see also Section 3.7.3).

3.7.1   Regulator in the United States: The U.S. Food and Drug Administration

The FDA (in the Department of Health and Human Services) is responsible for protecting public health by assuring the safety, efficacy, and security of human and veterinary drugs, biological products, medical devices, food, cosmetics, and products

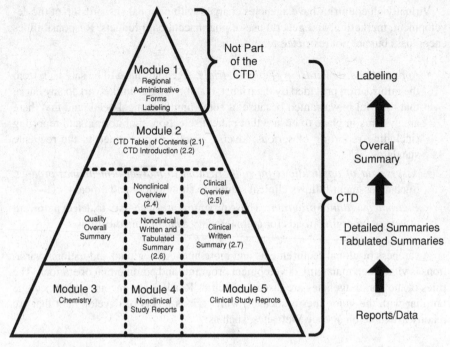

FIGURE 3.2   The CTD's pyramid structure. (From the FDA Web site.)

that emit radiation (among others). Organizations and individuals are legally bound to comply with FDA and CFR requirements; noncompliance can have sweeping consequences. The FDA has a reputation for being uncompromising in upholding regulations in pursuit of public safety.

Various centers within the agency relate to different areas of responsibility. The centers applicable to pharmaceuticals are the *Center for Drug Evaluation and Research* (CDER) and the *Center for Biological Evaluation and Research* (CBER). CDER regulates nonprescription [over-the-counter (OTC)] and prescription drugs, including biological therapeutics and generic drugs. When federal regulation of drugs was begun in 1848, only imported drugs were addressed. In 1905 the American Medical Association launched a private, voluntary means of controlling a substantial part of the drug business, and this remained in place for over a half-century. Drug regulation has evolved considerably since President Theodore Roosevelt signed the 1906 Pure Food and Drugs Act.

CBER regulates biological products for human use under applicable federal laws, including the Public Health Service Act and the Federal Food, Drug, and Cosmetic Act. CBER protects and advances public health by ensuring that biological products are safe, effective, and available to those in need. CBER also informs the public on the safe and appropriate use of biological products.

Title 21, **Code of Federal Regulations** The regulations in force in the United States, 21 CFR, are maintained and updated by the FDA and are accessible at the FDA Web site. Two areas are especially important to the subject matter of this book:

1. Regulations covering the licensing (approval) process for drugs. These are contained in 21 CFR 310, 311, and 312 and are discussed in Section 3.7.3.
2. Good practices in clinical (C), laboratory (L), manufacturing (M), and distribution (D) activities, commonly termed *GxP*. The prefix *current* (c) is applied to the terms to designate that the latest version of regulations must be applied. The specific regulations with the greatest impact on supply chains relate to manufacture and distribution (cGMP and cGDP), although cGCP and cGLP must always be considered where relevant. The sections of 21 CFR that cover cGMP and cGDP are:

   - 21 CFR 210: Current Good Manufacturing Practice in Manufacturing, Processing, Packing or Holding of Drugs; General
   - 21 CFR 211: Current Good Manufacturing Practice for Finished Pharmaceuticals
   - 21 CFR Part 11: Electronic Signatures

The importance of an understanding of these regulations as they apply to supply chain management cannot be overemphasised. There are two main reasons for this: first, to avoid any contravention that would result in supply chain failure; and second, and often less well recognized, to facilitate successful implementation of beneficial improvements. All too often, sponsor companies steer clear of change to avoid falling foul of the regulations.

3.7.2 Regulator in the European Union: The European Medicines Agency

To cover this section, Jill Bunyan, an experienced regulatory professional who also works under the Alacrita[10] banner, has agreed to contribute the EU regulatory overview.

GUEST CONTRIBUTOR SLOT: JILL BUNYAN

Overview of EU Regulations

The European Medicines Agency, headquartered in London, is responsible for the protection and promotion of public and animal health through the evaluation and supervision of medicines for human and veterinary use.

- The EMA reviews applications for European marketing authorization for medicinal products under the auspices of the *centralized procedure.* This mode of registration enables companies to submit a single authorization application to the agency. If granted, the centralized (or "community") authorization is valid in all European Union (EU) and EEA–EFTA states (Iceland, Liechtenstein, and Norway).

- All medicinal products for human and animal use derived from biotechnology and other high technology processes must be approved via the centralized procedure. So must medicines intended for the treatment of HIV/AIDS, cancer, diabetes, neurodegenerative diseases, autoimmune and other immune dysfunctions, and viral diseases. Designated "orphan " medicines (i.e., those intended for the treatment of rare diseases) are also evaluated under the centralized process.
- Similarly, all veterinary medicines intended for use as performance enhancers, to promote the growth of treated animals, or to increase yields from treated animals are assessed via the centralized procedure.

For medicinal products that do not fall under any of the foregoing categories, companies can submit an application for a centralized marketing authorization to the agency, provided that the medicinal product constitutes a significant therapeutic, scientific, or technical innovation, or the product is in some other respect in the interest of patient or animal health. The safety of medicines is monitored constantly by the agency through a pharmacovigilance network. Applications for other medicinal products for human use can be submitted nationally, that is, to the regulatory authority of an individual member state, or by the decentralized or mutual recognition procedures if authorization is required in more than one member state.

EU Regulations, Directives, and Guidelines   The body of European Union legislation in the pharmaceutical sector is contained in Volumes 1 and 5 of *The Rules Governing Medicinal Products in the European Union*[11]:

- *Volume 1:* EU pharmaceutical legislation for medicinal products for human use
- *Volume 5:* EU pharmaceutical legislation for medicinal products for veterinary use

The basic legislation is supported by a series of guidelines published in the remaining volumes:

- *Volume 2:* Notice to applicants and regulatory guidelines for medicinal products for human use
- *Volume 3:* Scientific guidelines for medicinal products for human use
- *Volume 4:* Guidelines for good manufacturing practices for medicinal products for human and veterinary use
- *Volume 6:* Notice to applicants and regulatory guidelines for medicinal products for veterinary use
- *Volume 7:* Scientific guidelines for medicinal products for veterinary use

- *Volume 8:* Maximum residue limits
- *Volume 9:* Guidelines for pharmacovigilance for medicinal products for human and veterinary use
- *Volume 10:* Guidelines for clinical trial

Medicinal products for pediatric use, orphan and herbal medicinal products, and advanced therapies are governed by specific rules.[12]

Since introduction of the first European Community Directive (Directive 65/65/EEC) in 1965, a plethora of directives, regulations, and guidelines have been published. Knowledge of these terms helps to understand the requirements.

- A *Directive* is a legislative act requiring member states to achieve a particular result *without dictating the means of achieving that result in the member state.* It must be implemented into national legislation before being enforced.
- *Regulations* are self-executing, binding in their entirety, and applicable to all member states.

Other terminology with respect to EU governance (e.g., decisions, recommendations, opinions) is less relevant to pharmaceutical operations and is not discussed here.

To facilitate the interpretation of the legislation and its uniform implementation, numerous guidelines of a regulatory and scientific nature have additionally been adopted. Although these are purportedly simply "guidance" or "advice," deviations need to be explained and adequately justified in license applications.

Directive 2003/94/EC of October 8, 2003[13] laid down the principles and guidelines of good manufacturing practice for medicinal products for human use and investigational medicinal products for human use. This directive has been transposed to separate national legislation in each country, and some countries have published useful (local) guidance on GMPs [e.g., the MHRA's (UK) "Orange Guide"].

3.7.3 International Conference on Harmonization

The International Conference on Harmonization of Technical Requirements for Registration of Pharmaceuticals for Human Use brings together the regulatory authorities of Europe, Japan, and the United States and experts from academia and the pharmaceutical industry to discuss scientific and technical aspects of product registration and to propose common guidance and processes for the evaluation of requests for product approvals. The object of harmonization is to reduce or obviate duplicate or unnecessary testing during the development of new medicines. This should lead to more economical use of human, animal, and material resources, and to reduce delays in the global development and availability of new medicines while maintaining safeguards on quality, safety, and efficacy to protect public health. To fulfill its mission, the ICH produces guidelines for use by member states. Europe and Japan fully mandate the use of a common technical document for presenting information when requesting approval to market (see below), and the FDA "highly recommends" use of the CTD but leaves the decision to the submitting sponsor company's discretion.

Despite such harmonization efforts, variations in interpretation and application of guidelines persist among regulatory assessors. Thus, it may be advisable to confirm understanding of requirements directly with regulatory agency staff where ambiguity exists. Such consultations are common with and encouraged by the FDA in particular. Meetings prior to clinical trials, prior to registration, or where a noteworthy event merits dialogue afford opportunities for information exchange and establishing common ground. Maximum use should be made of such a facility.

Common Technical Document   The *common technical document* (CTD or eCTD) is the vehicle by which participating regulatory agencies obtain information from a company seeking approval to market a product. The concept of a CTD has been developed by the ICH in an effort to make review more efficient and to save sponsors cost and time when working with different application formats for the various countries. The pyramid structure in Figure 3.2 (taken from the FDA Web site)[14] shows a diagrammatic representation of the makeup. There are three assessment areas: quality (CMC), safety (nonclinical), and efficacy (clinical). Similar but less detailed assessments apply to an application to start clinical trials in humans: investigational new drug application (IND) in the United States and clinical trial application (CTA) in the European Union.

A CTD should provide a regulatory assessor with a comprehensive picture of a drug's profile, performance, and development history. With respect to the intended process for commercial manufacture (drug substance and drug product), detail must be provided for each operation and input that can influence quality or processing characteristics. This includes but is not limited to specifications, suppliers, contract manufacturers, analytical testing methods, process descriptions, critical process parameters, manufacturing batch details, excipients, and packaging components and closures.

Requests for information on any omissions or for clarifications may be made by the regulatory assessor during review of the application. These must be answered satisfactorily by the sponsor company prior to approval. Drugs that receive approval must then be manufactured and tested for quality according to the information submitted. Changes must be carefully controlled and, where appropriate, regulatory approval obtained before implementation. Compilation of a CTD is a major undertaking and the final submission can run to many, many thousands of pages. It can be regarded as a product in itself, with the regulator as the customer. Development must be organized and resourced so as to populate the CTD with the required information. Otherwise, compilation becomes rate limiting to filing and approval.

Sections 3.8 to 3.10 were written by Patrick Crowley as a nonsupply chain specialist with no input from me. The really pleasing aspect of this is that Patrick's comments demonstrate a deep appreciation and understanding of the significance of SCM that I believe is required of drug developers around the world.

GUEST CONTRIBUTOR SLOT: PATRICK CROWLEY

3.8 SUPPLY CHAIN MANAGEMENT IN DEVELOPMENT PROGRAMS

Supply chain management principles and practices can be used advantageously during new product development. These are not limited to physical commodities but are equally relevant to many processes for information flow, such as communications concerning clinical programs, assembly of information for regulatory submissions, technology transfers between R&D and manufacturing operations, and interfaces with contract organizations. Accounts are provided here on such activities, with potential for SCM-related enhancements.

3.8.1 Dosage Forms for Clinical Trials

Each clinical center needs trial materials for issuing to patients. These may comprise: the test medication, possibly in a number of strengths (doses); a placebo if the trial is blinded (usually the case), and comparator medications (for comparative trials), usually blinded. Comparator drugs need to be modified to make then visually indistinguishable from the novel (test) drug and placebo. For example, the comparator (e.g., a tablet) might be inserted in a capsule or broken down (milled) to granules which are then encapsulated. The test drug would also be provided in capsule form. It may be possible to obtain an intermediate (e.g., granules) from the organization marketing the comparator and to compress it into a tablet that is visually indistinguishable from the test drug. Such modifications could affect drug stability or bioavailability. Tests are required to reassure that there has been no untoward effect.

3.8.2 Packaging and Labeling

Clinical studies on a novel drug may be designed to evaluate the effect of dose frequency: for example, to compare a twice (BID) or three times daily (TID) dosage with a once-daily (OD) regimen. Blinding requirements necessitate that neither patient, clinician, nor trial center professionals be aware of what medication is being taken by an individual patient. This requires that a patient on a TID regimen take three doses of active drug daily. A patient on OD dosage takes one dose of active drug and two units of placebo, to maintain the blinded nature of the study. Patients in the BD arm take two actives doses and one placebo. Special packaging configurations may be required to ensure patient compliance. Such a pack might comprise rows of blister pockets, each row representing daily dosage as follows:

- *TID:* a row of three units (daily dose) comprising active doses in the three pockets
- *BD:* a three-pocket row containing two actives and one placebo
- *OD:* as for BID/TID but containing one active and two placebos

Such individualized configurations may also be employed where different doses of active drug are used, or where comparators may have different dose regimens for the test drug in the study. Dosage forms and packaging meeting such requirements need to be conceptualized, developed, and assembled in house or on contract. Pharmaceutical development personnel must carry out the requisite investigative studies and prepare, package, label (in country-specific languages), and ship to clinical centers (or oversee these if done on contract). The visually identical nature of such supplies means that packaging and labeling be carefully controlled so that mix-ups do not occur.

Managing such a supply chain requires not only the timely preparation of blinded presentations as outlined above but also close communication between clinical operations teams and pharmaceutical development personnel in case stocks run out at a particular center because of better-than-planned patient recruitment or because shelf life is exceeded. Replacements need to be provided rapidly. Good trial-wide inventory monitoring and control systems could enable procurement of replacement stock from centers where recruitment is slow, as this could be done far more rapidly than sourcing direct from the pharmaceutical development staff. Such "swapping" is not without complexity, as materials may be labeled in different languages or center identifier codes, but, if the possibility is considered at the outset, there may be ways to surmount such obstacles.

Findings during clinical trials sometimes mandate that a new strength of product, not envisaged when planning the study, needs to be assessed. Trial momentum could be put in jeopardy by such unexpected developments. Supply chain risk mitigation might involve preparing additional dosage strengths or stocks of an intermediate to hold in reserve for rapid conversion to the new strength. It may be impossible to cover every possible scenario, and the development, manufacture, and supply of such new trial material units cannot often be done quickly because of the aforementioned complexities or because of the manufacturing time frames required for some materials (manufacture of a biopharmaceutical usually takes about six months). Close coordination and communication among stakeholders, together with imaginative supply chain management, can obviate or minimize delays.

3.8.3 Drug Substance Procurement

Novel active ingredients for the manufacture of dosage forms for clinical trials cannot be purchased off the shelf. They must be made in house or on contract. The mode of manufacture may still be under development, so a less than efficient synthesis may need to be used. This can be expensive, leading to pressures to minimize stocks. However, reserve material is needed in case of unexpected changes in demand (as outlined above). Stocking policy for drug and dosage forms needs to be agreed upon by all stakeholders so that supply and programs are not compromised by shortages. Starting materials or intermediates for assembly of the drug substance may be novel (i.e., not available commercially). So may the materials used to prepare biopharmaceutical materials. Policies for procurement and stocking such materials need to be considered, developed, and implemented.

3.8.4   Quality Considerations

Dosage forms (actives, placebos, comparators) used in clinical studies must meet the same quality requirements as those for commercial medications. Such materials need to be tested for quality after manufacture and in stability programs to determine storage conditions and "use-by" periods. This, in turn, requires appropriate testing methodologies. Hence, analytical methods need to be developed, stability studies run, and storage, handling, and transport precautions identified and implemented so that the quality of trial materials is not compromised. Such quality standards need to be proposed to, and prior agreement obtained from, regulatory agencies in countries where trials are being run.

Medications being evaluated in the trials need to be prepared under the aegis of good manufacturing Practice (GMP), and quality testing must be carried out according to the requirements of good laboratory practice (GLP). Regulatory agencies such as the FDA will inspect organizations as part of the license review process for compliance with these requirements. To obviate problems in these areas, quality assurance groups from the R&D organization regularly audit centers, and facilities during development to determine compliance with guideline requirements and to agree on corrective plans to remedy any deficiency identified.

Clinical trials need to be set up, monitored, and reported according to the principles of good clinical practice (GCP). These requirements are wide ranging, encompassing clinical centers, suitability of Clinical and other support staff, recording, validating and transmitting trial-related findings, and the conversion of such data to knowledge. The relevant GCP guidelines as defined by the ICH are identified as GCP E6(R1).[15]

3.8.5   Data Collection and Transmission

The diligent recording and collection of clinical measurements on a new drug's safety and efficacy, and its timely submission to central data processing and evaluation functions, is not usually considered to be part of supply chain management. Yet if clinical trials are rate limiting in the path to commercialization, the collection and transmission of such information is no less important than where supply concerns physical commodities. The same concepts apply with respect to reliable and timely delivery to the customer. Historically, data collection and conversion to knowledge and decision making was haphazard and slow. However, pharmaceutical R&D organizations are now adopting innovative approaches to improving trial design and knowledge collection at all stages of clinical programs. Information technology (IT) networks are now widespread and can greatly improve remote data collection, transmission, and analysis. There has been a concomitant improvement in response capability to important incidents or findings. Adaptive clinical protocols are designed at the outset to facilitate rapid responses (such as protocol amendments) to findings. Such developments in clinical research and the enhanced response capability that IT affords facilitates a "virtual" supply chain that can enhance the quality of clinical programs and the timeliness of completion. This in turn enhances efficiency and compresses time lines in a rate-limiting development activity.

3.8.6   New Product Filings

From the foregoing comments it will be evident that nonclinical areas are intimately involved in supporting clinical trials. Concurrently, these same (nonclinical) functions must consider the overall objective, including the provision of commercial product after approval by regulatory agencies. Such approval follows an application (NDA or MAA) to the relevant agency, with information and data to demonstrate that the drug and the medication containing it:

- Have been shown to be safe and effective.
- Can be made in a facility and by a process that assures quality.
- Are subject to tests and limits to assure that each batch is of the requisite quality.
- Retain quality during transport, storage, and use. Shelf life requirements can span several years, due largely to centralization of manufacturing capability and the worldwide nature of markets.

The assembly and presentation of information supporting a request for approval to market is, as already stated, a complex exercise, with inputs from many groups throughout an organization (i.e., R&D, manufacturing, commercial, etc). Input is also required from external organizations. Contract organizations may have been utilized in the development program. Even if this is not the case, it is necessary to procure and submit information concerning:

- *Drug substance manufacture:* from providers of reagents, solvents, intermediates, process aids, and containers for storage and shipping.
- *Drug product manufacture:* from providers of excipients, containers and closures (primary packaging), secondary packaging, and labeling materials.

While the assembly of information in filings is usually coordinated by regulatory affairs staff, there is a need for overview and review by data-generating departments as well as the provision of information to sustain claims for efficacy, safety, quality, GMP, and so on. There is also a need to provide overview "expert reports" or quality overall summaries for key areas (usually safety, efficacy, and quality). The exercise is considerable.

3.9   MANUFACTURE AND SUPPLY OF COMMERCIAL PRODUCTS

Making a new product available requires the following coordinated activities between development and other groups, either in house or external:

- Designing a process for drug substance manufacture.
- Designing a process for product manufacture (in house or by a contract manufacturer).

- Procuring (or preparing) product components (including packaging and labeling).
- Defining quality standards and limits for input materials, facilities, operating variables for each stage of manufacture, packaging materials and operations, and so on.

Materials (drug substance and drug product) for clinical studies are usually prepared on a pilot scale, as requirements are relatively modest compared to those of commercial product. Commercial manufacture usually employs larger-scale plant and processing equipment. Equipment may have differing principles of operation (although designed to achieve the same effect). Different solvents may be preferred to mitigate safety risks. Process parameters need to be redefined to reflect scale and operational differences: for example, (1) cooling or crystallization rates in drug substance manufacture, or (2) process times for the various suboperations (e.g., mixing times for solids during dosage-form manufacture, or spraying rates when coating particles or dosage units such as tablets). Such variables can conceivably affect drug or product quality, so need to be validated with processing "windows" (limits) established and defined. Possibilities are usually evaluated and variables defined first on a pilot scale. Technology transfer campaigns then determine performance on a commercial scale in manufacturing plants. Testing (e.g., analytical and other) methodology is also transferred to commercial quality control laboratories. Products made at scale in this way are then tested for compliance with specifications and stability studies are initiated to assure that quality is retained for the duration of the shelf life claimed.

Regulatory agencies carry our preapproval inspections as part of the evaluation process. Inspectors visit sites of manufacture to examine the data generated on scale-up as well as the quality systems proposed and other controls mandated by GMP requirements that need to be in place for routine manufacture. Development (chemical and pharmaceutical) units work jointly with manufacturing and quality groups before and during technology transfer and subsequently if issues are encountered that need to be remedied (troubleshooting). Such support work can continue, when warranted, throughout the lifetime of the product. Planning, organizing, and coordination are vital to ensure that programs run according to plan, that materials are available throughout the program where required by the various activities, and that urgent events are responded to in a timely and considered manner.

3.10 SUPPLY CHAIN MANAGEMENT FOR COMMERCIAL PRODUCTS

Supply chain management practices illustrate how complexity can be managed during development and when preparing for commercial product launch.

3.10.1 Manufacturing Site Selection

R&D and commercial groups may perform development and manufacturing activities in house, with contract manufacturers, or by using a mixture of in-house functions and outsourcing. Policy may change during development or at any time in the life of a commercial product due to business events (e.g., mergers), changes in strategy, loss or acquisition of in-house capability, and so on. Such changes may be associated with starting materials for a drug substance, intermediate, or finished material (drug or drug product). In some instances it may be necessary to construct a new manufacturing facility specifically for the new product. The timing of such a major investment is crucial, as for materials such as biopharmaceuticals it may be necessary to use material from such a new commercial site in the pivotal clinical program (or in a proportion of the trials).

3.10.2   Outsourced Facilities, Materials, or Test Methodologies

A supply chain policy relying on external providers needs to be backed up by information that such a facility has the capability to meet demand, is fit for the purpose, and has the requisite quality systems in place. Contracts need to be agreed upon and in place concerning opt-out scenarios, prioritization of work, incident notification, and stockholdings, among many other items. Backup providers may also need to be considered and would also need to be validated and certificated.

3.10.3   Shipping and Storage

Shipping may not be confined to sending finished products to market. It is not unusual for intermediates and drug substances to be shipped between sites, countries, and continents, to take advantage of capability, capacity, and economics or even proximity to key starting materials (drugs such as quinidine or topotecan are sourced from plants indigenous to remote regions). The manufacture of dosage units in one country, to be packaged closer to market, is a widespread practice. Transnational and transcontinental interflow of starting materials and product components is also commonplace. Management of such supply chains requires not only that the right quantities be in the right place at the right time; novel materials may pose additional challenges:

1. *Safety.* The pharmaceutical agent itself (drug) may pose hazards. Oxidation (aerobic and nonaerobic) potential can render a material explosive. A poorly sealed or ruptured container can leak hazardous material to the environment. Studies should explore the potential for such behavior. Their impact then needs to be considered, and packaging, storage, and transport conditions need to be defined, communicated, and implemented.

2. *Drug product quality.* Some diseases are indigenous to remote and poorer regions. Sophisticated transport and storage facilities may not be in place at the tail end of supply chains for clinical or commercial medications. Special containers or transport may be needed for temperature-sensitive products such as vaccines to protect them from hostile climatic conditions.

3. *Special transportation.* Biopharmaceuticals are inherently fragile, and intermediates usually comprise aqueous solutions and thus need to be shipped in a deep-frozen state. Packaging, cooling, and temperature-monitoring devices and recording systems

will probably be required. Prior information also needs to be generated to assure that shipped materials withstand stresses accompanying air freight, road transport, or security-monitoring technologies. Customs barriers also need to be managed.

4. *Regulatory liability.* A CTD constrains the sponsor company to the supply chain details submitted during the application to market the product. Sourcing strategies and supply chain structure (architecture) must be identified and committed to in the CTD. Postapproval changes must be managed by change control processes concordant with cGMP. Regulatory approval may be necessary before implementation. A business case to effect such changes can be difficult to build, and hence change inertia occurs. The critical corollary is that robust and cost-effective supply chains be defined during development (i.e., prior to registration). The application of supply chain thinking during development is something that does not happen in the industry as a matter of routine, but the benefits of such a strategy are obvious. The company sponsoring the license application is responsible for making sure that changes and notification are managed properly. Contractors have much to offer by way of advice and guidance, but the ultimate responsibility lies with the sponsor. With this comes the requirement for skills and experience to manage such change processes successfully. Companies using the more virtual business model can sometimes miss this aspect when resourcing a business.

3.10.4   Conclusions

Managing drug evaluation and development programs requires an enormous breath of expertise, ranging from the purely technical to activities more usually associated with commercial operations. Each program poses different challenges, so cannot be run to a rigid predesigned template. A wide range of skills, experience, and innovation are required to ensure that activities are coordinated, risks are mitigated, and incidents are managed appropriately. The flow and packaging of materials and information is complex but amenable to regulation by applying the precepts of supply chain management. This can have a significant effect on efficiency and duration of programs, leading to "faster to market" time lines. Hence, SCM experts should be intimately involved in development programs from the outset and continuously propound approaches to reduce waste and shorten lead times at every stage.

4 End-to-End Pharmaceutical Supply Chains

4.1 INTRODUCTION

This chapter begins with some words of Dan Jones, chairman of the Lean Enterprise Academy in the UK and author, along with Jim Womack and Daniel Roos, of a now world-famous book, *The Machine That Changed the World*.[1] Some years ago I signed up to receive Dan's regular email updates. One of the earlier ones referred to Dan's excursion into the world of pharmaceutical manufacture. He estimated that the end-to-end supply chain was probably twice as long as the 319 days it took to get a well-known fizzy drink from mining of the bauxite for the aluminum can, to filling the shelves at Wal-Mart. I recently asked Dan for more background on the makeup of his number, and below is his response.

> The point is this. As part of one of my walks and talks I virtually walked the end-to-end supply chain for a typical pill. It turns out that processing the ingredients for the pill takes about six different processing steps in different facilities and often in different locations, each separately scheduled and subject to the same scheduling delays you get from batch production systems making to forecast. So in all this takes about a year to work its way through the system to the pill plant. There the ingredients are mixed and made into pills and packed and palletized—taking about 30 days from door to door. Then it goes through between three and five different warehousing steps, including the warehouse belonging to the retailer or hospital. Then it gets dispensed and used. It sits about 11 months in these warehouses! Very similar to auto parts in a pre-lean parts distribution system! So a total supply chain throughput time of two years. This is not actually unusual for many manufactured products as it turns out. A great opportunity if the pharma guys were ever short of cash!

These are sobering words coming from a leading world expert in the field, don't you think? So now we have it on good authority that there is potential for pharma to have a tremendous impact on cash consumed by the supply chain. If money were not enough incentive, there is a far more powerful one: The compliance risks in these ever more complex supply chains driven by mass outsourcing have increased enormously. There are now thousands of companies developing and marketing drugs, controlling their supply chains with varying degrees of competence. Some of these companies

Supply Chain Management in the Drug Industry: Delivering Patient Value for Pharmaceuticals and Biologics, By Hedley Rees
Copyright © 2011 John Wiley & Sons, Inc.

are small, very small. They may not have any professional supply chain management presence at all at their disposal. This does not, however, change the obligation they have for the supply chain.

4.2   WHERE DOES RESPONSIBILITY FOR THE SUPPLY CHAIN LAY?

As the various stages and players emerge through the supply chain, it is all too easy to forget where the buck stops in respect to keeping the whole thing on track. Below are some extracts from an article I wrote for *Pharmaceutical Formulation and Quality*.[2] Although the article is primarily about virtual pharma, the sentiments apply across the board. Some extracts from the article are included here.

> The company sponsoring the investigational new drug/new drug application (IND/NDA) filing is responsible for compliance along this entire supply chain. Contractors must, of course, pass the due diligence GMP/quality audit, but, in addition, the working supply chain must be compliant at each and every stage, with nothing falling through the cracks. This means investigation of out-of-specification results and appropriate (root cause) corrective and preventive actions; complaints handling; technical documentation review and approval by suitably knowledgeable and qualified personnel; and closely controlled documentation. Supply and quality agreements must bind players in the chain together so there is maximum alignment between standard operating procedures (SOPs) across organizational boundaries.

> Supply and quality agreements will, in the main, be between the sponsor company and each company entity in the chain, making coordinated action along the supply chain a logistical nightmare. Who holds the responsibility for making this arrangement deliver compliant drug to site or markets?

The article then draws on the experience of Dan Barreto (who appeared in Chapter 1):

> "Sponsor companies have important obligations to meet all regulatory filing expectations," said Dan Barreto, staff vice president of quality at C.R. Bard, Inc., former international vice president of cGMP Compliance at Janssen Pharmaceutica, and a former FDA supervisory investigator. "Supply chain contractors play a vital role in meeting those obligations on a continuous basis, but they must be proactively managed to deliver since the ultimate responsibility inherently resides with the sponsor company."

> The sentiment is echoed by Marla Phillips, Ph.D., director of the Pharmaceutical Technology Institute at Xavier University (Cincinnati). Dr. Phillips asserts: "In the Preamble to the 1978 GMP [Good Manufacturing Practice] Regulations, the commissioner made it clear that the contracting firm owns the goods and the contractor merely performs a service. The responsibility for release against the registered information and GxP [good working practices] compliance rests with the contracting firm."

> As vice president of quality assurance and regulatory compliance at Endo Pharmaceuticals (Newark, Delaware), Dr. Ranjana Pathak is highly experienced in the world of

pharmaceuticals and has practical experience with the FDA's expectations: Endo had a (successful) four-day FDA inspection in 2006.

"A quality system for a [virtual] company is a subject close to my heart," Dr. Pathak says. "A [virtual] company needs to have the systems in place which can enable them to ensure that the product distributed will be safe and effective." In filing with the FDA, companies must ensure that the data supporting the application is authentic and that there are systems in place at the sponsoring site that will continue to monitor data generation. In order to comply with FDA regulations, companies must also implement a rigorous record review program and a meaningful audit program. A complaints program—in which the care management organization informs the sponsor of all complaints and adverse events are handled in a timely manner—should also be in place. The sponsor must ensure that the validation program, including cleaning, process, and equipment, is carried out in a timely manner. Once the drug is approved, the company must set up an annual product review program."

The answer to the question of responsibility is therefore clear. Throughout drug development and beyond, it is the company sponsoring the applications for licenses that is held accountable. Once approved, it is the company holding the license to market, awarded by the competent authority, which is culpable. This is a crucial point to bear in mind as the chapter progresses.

4.3   SPONSORING COMPANIES, LICENSE HOLDERS, AND THEIR SUPPLY CHAINS

In the earlier chapters we emphasized the importance of taking a holistic view of supply chains. Figure 4.1 depicts the stages involved in the end-to-end supply chain required to produce a traditional small-molecule drug. Initially, we focus there because most of the commonly marketed drugs were developed and are produced as small molecules by means of chemical synthesis. Earlier we noted the rapid growth in drugs made from biological compounds of far more complex structure, known as *large-molecule drugs, biologicals*, or *biologics*. The power of these drugs is their potential to use the biological systems of nature to develop remedies that fit in with the natural workings of the body. The manufacture of biologicals is significantly less predictable and prone to variability than that of small-molecule products. They are also, typically, significantly more expensive to make, with supply chains that complicate the already complex modern-day supply chain of small molecules. So we treat biologicals as a separate section following from small-molecule supply chains. Many of the regulations of GxP and product licenses apply to both and are covered in the initial section. The biologicals section (Section 4.11) will then focus on the very special issues in the manufacture and supply of these products.

Since I am not a scientist or experienced in the manufacture of biologically derived products, Stephen Ward has kindly agreed to coauthor this chapter and provide firsthand scientific and commercial insight into this challenging, exciting, and key class of products. Readers wishing to focus initially on this area should move

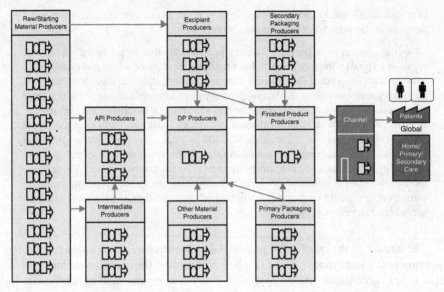

FIGURE 4.1   End-to-end pharmaceutical supply chain.

to Section 4.11. It should be borne in mind that Sections 4.7 to 4.9 are common to both.

4.4   SUPPLY CHAINS FOR SMALL-MOLECULE PRODUCTS

Hopefully, the reader is now converted to the interconnectedness of every level or entity in the supply chain. Any one of these stages has the potential to bring a supply chain to its knees, and the farther upstream problems occur, if not identified and rectified immediately, the more difficult and time consuming it is to recover. It is also important to bear in mind that these stages often involve companies that are totally independent of one another. They are businesses focused on delivering value for their shareholders, and if that is at the expense of others in the supply chain, then so be it (at least according to the cynics among us). True, it is in the long-term interest of all the players to support the end game, but short-term goals (and profits!) are notorious for overriding the long term, and this must always be borne in mind.

So what does this mean for a pharmaceutical company sponsoring an application to license a drug for manufacture and sale to patients? It means that they have a tough job on their hands. As sponsors, they are held totally responsible for that end-to-end supply chain; there is no hiding place. It is not a defense to argue incompetence or ignorance on behalf of a contractor—it is the sponsor's responsibility to ensure that contractors are competent and provided with all the relevant information relating to the product's manufacture. Every out-of-specification result and temperature excursion must be investigated, documented, and corrective action initiated and closed out. Processes and systems must be validated (prove they do what they are intended to do; see Section 4.9.4) and documentary evidence collected. Good practices (GxPs) must be adhered to, and agreements must be in place. There is quite an extensive list, which we expand on later. The main point being made here is that while all the organizations involved will have the relevant competencies and act with goodwill, the sponsoring company or license holder is held accountable. By way of example, consider the actual case study below.

4.4.1   Case Study

This case study relates to a small company sponsoring a phase III study being run at U.S. investigator sites. The compound was a re-profile of a generic compound with a good safety profile. The supply chain comprised active ingredient sourced in a EU country, shipped to UK for tableting into blisters, shipped to another UK site for clinical trial packaging and blinding, and then transferred to a U.S. distribution center awaiting release to clinical trial sites.

There were many potential issues related to this arrangement. Picking on one by way of example, the clinical trial supplies shipped from the UK to the United States were sent with the necessary calibrated data loggers (monitors of temperature throughout the entire journey). When the temperature recording charts were downloaded at the receiving destination, they showed there had been three 1-hour temperature excursions up to 45°C. The freight forwarder was unable (or unwilling?) to explain what had happened. The research data on the impact of this type of elevated temperature on the integrity of this product (stability data) were still being collected. The analytical chemists could not put their hands on their hearts and say that the product was still within specifications.

What we did in practice was to have samples drawn from representative portions of the shipment and have them shipped back to the tablet manufacturer under "cool" conditions. On receipt, the manufacturer performed assays (tests) on the samples and confirmed that there had been no adverse effect on the product, and this was fully documented as an investigation and closed out by our qualified person.

The point of this case study is to emphasize that even with a supply chain made up of fully compliant companies operating to the best of their ability, there must be oversight of the working supply chain as events occur between the interfaces. Companies operating the virtual model may not have picked up the issue at all since there was no routine chain of communication between the sponsoring company and the company discovering the defect (a well-known CRO is the United States).

These obligations must be honored in a climate where supply chains are becoming ever more networked and globe spanning. In cases where sponsoring companies own all or most of the supply chain producers, with a single shared quality control system, the task is challenging but achievable. Even when sponsoring companies do not own most of the facilities, but are resourced internally to manage the outsourcing, the task is possible. There is a point, however, where the critical mass of a sponsoring company cannot realistically support their obligations for compliance due to lack of cash or resources or both. This is an important consideration that I believe should be addressed.

Returning to the topic, in this chapter we consider the scope of the supply chain and lay responsibility squarely on the sponsoring or license-holding company. This is especially applicable to the obligation to apply due diligence from start to finish, across all stages, as shown in Figure 4.1. In addition to that, we highlight the distinguishing characteristics and issues at each stage and the potential impact on SCM. The two must go hand in hand before improvements can be applied in the sector.

So, where do we start? Perversely to some perhaps, we start at the end.

4.5   STARTING AT THE FINAL DESTINATION

A critical aspect to remember in the proper design and management of supply chains is the "end" at which to start. For reasons that will become clear later, the pharmaceutical sector likes to start at the beginning and work forward. This is a logic that works well in many scientific situations, but not in supply chains. The logic should always start with the patient (or end customer in other sectors) and work backward. This allows the route to customer satisfaction to be plotted with the necessary milestones along the way. The converse creates a potential for the important milestones to be driven by events rather than customer need. This means that the starting point is a patient in the primary care, secondary care, or home setting, presenting indications of potential ill health or disease. In the event that a pharmacological solution is appropriate, a medicine is prescribed to target the problem. For this to be effective, the drug must enter the patient's body.

4.6   HOW DRUGS ENTER THE BODY

For pharmaceutical products to perform their function, they must enter the body in some way. Coincidental with supply chain terminology, the industry calls this a (drug) delivery system. The prime component of a drug delivery system is the dosage form. For many presentations, the delivery system is also the dosage form. In the case of, say, an injection, the delivery system will be a needle or syringe, and the dosage form will be the solution in the vial or ampoule containing the active ingredient. Possible drug delivery systems and dosage forms include the following four types.

1. Oral
   - Pill, tablet, or capsule
   - Specialty tablet, such as buccal, sublingual, or orally disintegrating
   - Thin film (e.g., Listerine PocketPaks)
   - Liquid solution or suspension (e.g., drink or syrup)
   - Powder or liquid or solid crystals
   - Chewing gum
   - Natural or herbal plant, seed, or food of sorts (e.g., marijuana such as that found in "special brownies")

2. Inhalational
   - Aerosol
   - Inhaler
   - Nebulizer
   - Smoking (often in natural herb or freebase powder form; e.g., tobacco or marijuana and cocaine or methamphetamine, respectively)
   - Vaporizer (usually to vaporize natural herbs such as marijuana)
3. Parenteral injection
   - Intradermal
   - Intramuscular
   - Intraosseous
   - Intraperitoneal
   - Intravenous
   - Subcutaneous
4. Topical
   - Cream, gel, liniment or balm, lotion, or ointment, etc.
   - Ear drops (optic)
   - Eyedrops (ophthalmic)
   - Skin patch (transdermal)
   - Suppository
   - Rectal (e.g., enema)
   - Vaginal (e.g., douche, pessary)

From this it should be clear that there are many, many ways that a drug can be delivered into the body. Each method has its own particular advantages, and disadvantages and careful selection of a dosage form and the manner in which it is delivered to the patient can be critical to the success of a medicine.

4.7   DESIGN OF DRUG DELIVERY SYSTEMS

It may be helpful at this point to explore this topic with the help of an expert who has plied his trade in a world familiar to most, if not all, of us—the world of chewing gum! His name is Niels C. Kaarsholm and here he explains the science of developing drugs in the chewing gum sector.

GUEST CONTRIBUTOR SLOT: NIELS C. KAARSHOLM

Chewing Gum as a Drug Delivery Vehicle

Nicotine Chewing Gum   Chewing gum as a vehicle for delivering active pharmaceutical ingredients (APIs) is well established for nicotine replacement therapy

(NRT), used to facilitate smoking cessation.[3] First developed in the late 1960s, nicotine chewing gum became available commercially in 1978. Initially it was sold by prescription only, however, in most countries it is now available over the counter (OTC) in pharmacies and drugstores. Together with lozenges, patches, inhalers and mouth sprays, nicotine gum forms the NRT OTC category, which generated more than $1300 million in total worldwide sales in 2008. Of these, nicotine gum is the largest single entity, representing about one-half the total NRT OTC segment, and growing.

Nicotine delivery by chewing gum remains an active, evolving field with new generations of products being developed continuously based on improvements in texture, taste, and flavorings as well as a time action profile of the nicotine anticraving effect. Indeed, the success of nicotine gum would suggest that the gum format represents an attractive opportunity when exploring new delivery modalities as part of the life-cycle management for existing oral drugs in an effort to provide the patient with new advantages in terms of convenience, efficacy, and/or safety.

Other Active Pharmaceutical Ingredients in Extruded Gum   The feasibility of co-formulating APIs in general with chewing gum is met with some technical challenges originating from the process by which chewing gum is traditionally produced. The characteristic component of all chewing gums is the gum base, which is a complex mixture of elastomers, natural and synthetic resins, fats, emulsifiers, waxes, antioxidants, and fillers.[4] The initial step in the manufacturing process involves softening of the gum base at a temperature of 50 to 60°C in a mixer using slowly turning blades. Sweeteners and flavors are added together with the API during this process. From the mixer the warm mass passes onto cooling belts and then moves on to the rolling site, where it is extruded into a carpet of gum. This carpet is rolled out to the correct thickness by a series of rollers before it is scored into single pieces. After appropriate conditioning the gum is finally ready for coating. As a chemically inert molecule, nicotine "survives" the warm mixing process and releases intact and reproducibly upon chewing of the final gum. In contrast, many other potential APIs undergo chemical change when exposed to the complex gum base mixture at elevated temperature. As a result, the necessary reproducible release of intact API from the gum is often difficult to obtain.

Compressed Chewing Gum   The use of compression technology has provided a solution to the technical problem of mixing API with gum base at elevated temperature. In this procedure pelleted gum base (with particle size in the range 0.2 to 2 mm) is simply mixed with bulk sweeteners, flavors, APIs, and other excipients, and the dry mixture is compressed directly into tablets.[5] The tablets may comprise one or two layers with the gum base pellets and the API either premixed or separated, and a tablet coating may be added as needed. The resulting compressed tablets have excellent mouth-feel; after a brief crunchiness the tablet behaves like regular gum within seconds. The compression procedure obviously reduces unwanted chemical reactions of the API expected with the warm-mixing extruded gums. However, in comparison with regular tablet compression, the presence of the gum base pellets requires focus on the content of uniformity. Also, the bulk sweeteners are typically hygroscopic; hence, humidity must be controlled carefully during production and packaging of the tablets.

Appropriate APIs for the Compressed Gum Format   The CMC (see Chapter 3) challenges of formulating APIs in gum format typically comprise stabilization, taste masking, and release. The release of API from the gum may be controlled within a range by varying the size and amount of gum base pellets included in the tablet. Stabilization of the API may be affected by granulation and by various complex formations. Often, it is a question of controlling the migration of humidity within the tablet and across the air–solid interface. Taste masking is an art on its own. Many APIs have an unpleasant taste (e.g., bitter, astringent or metallic); hence, complexation and encapsulation techniques are important as well as a setup for systematic sensory testing, preferentially using a professional taste panel. The challenge of masking taste also depends on dose, of course. The therapeutic dose of many APIs is too high to allow efficient taste masking in the gum format.

When competing against a simple tablet, the success of the gum format ultimately rests on the ability to provide an advantage to the patient in terms of convenience, efficacy, and/or safety. Chewing gums containing fluoride for prophylaxis of dental carries, chlorhexidine as local disinfectant, and vitamins and/or food supplements have been available for some time.[6] Clearly, the ease of administration without the need for water adds convenience to the entire segment emphasizing frequent or "on-the-go" administration. Obvious "convenience" candidates for gum formulation would include antiobesity agents (e.g., Orlistat) and antireflux agents (including proton pump inhibitors). Additional advantages in terms of efficacy could be derived from improved local effects. Agents to treat sore throat (e.g., benzydamin, flurbiprofen, ambroxol) and cough and cold (phenylephrin) belong in this category and would seem to fit nicely with the gum concept. Finally, the gum format would seem to facilitate buccal delivery, which may provide advantages in terms of faster onset of action and/or reduced dosing. In addition to nicotine, agents to treat migraine (e.g., triptans) or erectile dysfunction (e.g., sildenafil, vardenafil, tadalafil) are candidates in this category.

Conclusions   Nicotine in smoking cessation has firmly established chewing gum as a drug delivery system. With the introduction of compressed gum technology, it is now possible stably to incorporate and release most APIs in the gum format. A number of proof-of-principle trials have been carried out demonstrating bioequivalence between API as delivered by gum and by traditional tablet.[7] Several drugs and therapeutic areas exist where the potential of the gum delivery system may be exploited to provide a unique life-cycle management opportunity to the benefit of the patient as well as for the brand.

The object of including this piece from Niels is twofold. First, it highlights the thought processes and particular challenges involved in developing a production process for a drug delivery system. Once the process is defined, it must be adhered to strictly; otherwise, the drug may not perform as required when it enters the body. Any change would require repetition of the thinking processes and confirmation that there is no adverse impact on product performance and impact on patient safety.

The second objective is to highlight that this as an innovation in drug delivery that has been around for some years and has barely been considered by the industry. There must surely be patient populations that would be better served by this system: for example, people with swallowing difficulties or aversion to more invasive delivery systems. Niels refers to this opportunity. To take this forward, however, would mean pharma companies spending on development work that may take their eye off the search for products to cure "unmet medical need" (i.e., blockbusters). Is this more evidence of patient needs taking a back seat?

4.8   WHAT THIS MEANS FOR THE SUPPLY CHAIN

The work in Chapter 3 describes how the pharmacology of a drug must be completely understood and the drug designed to meet exacting criteria. There is little or no room to maneuvre when the drug is manufactured. The careful measurements and parameters must be reproduced religiously every time a batch is produced. Any change or unexplained difference at any stage can have a significant impact on a drug's safety, efficacy, or quality or any combination of the three.

This is a fundamental principle on which pharmaceutical supply chains are based and is the driver behind the good working practices referred to in Chapter 3. The requirements associated with these good working practices in the supply chain, which principally are contained within good manufacturing practice and good distribution practice, are covered here in overview. The object of the overview is to sensitize those unfamiliar with the regulations to the basic requirements that affect the application of SCM in pharmaceuticals. These relate predominantly to the constraints that exist that are nonnegotiable and also to those that appear to exist but are not a strict requirement. It is important to emphasize that this is a two-way street and is a real opportunity for improvement to take place (especially with respect to quality by design and process analytical technology). As with any competent authority's regulations concerning specific circumstances at any point in time, readers should always seek the relevant professional advice.

4.9   KEY ASPECTS OF GMP AND GDP IN RELATION TO SCM

4.9.1   Organization

The regulations require that a quality control unit be established whose responsibility it is to approve or reject materials and check and approve relevant documentation. There must be a clear organizational reporting relationship that allows the quality unit to be independent of the production function so that no undue influence can be brought to bear when difficult decisions about product disposition have to be made. For example, rejection of a batch of product can have dramatic cost implications, in terms of both the material lost and the potential opportunity cost of sales revenue forgone. Commercial pressures can therefore be intense, and in the opinion of the regulators, organizational separation is the only sure way to ensure that patient safety comes first.

Other aspects of organization cover the need for personnel to be properly qualified, trained, equipped, and informed of their job requirements. Staff must have relevant knowledge and experience of the areas in which they work and their résumés must demonstrate that and be available for inspection. Standard operating procedures (SOPs) should be written and approved only by suitably qualified staff. Those working to SOPs should be kept abreast of the latest versions and training given, where relevant, in any changes to working practices. Training files must be kept up to date to provide evidence of training and competence to perform duties to the required standards. There must also be sufficient numbers of personnel available to carry out tasks. This may seem irrelevant to regulatory compliance matters, but in practice, it is absolutely vital.

4.9.2 Quality Management System

The regulations require that SOPs be established for all aspects of GxP. These SOPs, together with policy and guidance documents, should make up a fit-for-purpose management system to assure product quality. These must be carefully documented and controlled, made available to all relevant staff, who must be trained and confirm that they are competent to work under the SOPs. In recent years, there has been a move from the regulators to broaden quality systems and utilize the principles of ISO 9001/2 and similar systems. ICH Q10 is intended guidance for companies that wish to develop their quality management systems along best practice lines.

4.9.3 Quality and/or Technical Agreement

EU regulations require that a written contract is in place between companies where services are provided by a third party undertaking activities that may affect GxP. In the regulations, this agreement is referred to explicitly. ICH Q7A, 16.13, states: "There should be a written and approved contract or formal agreement between a company and its contractors that defines in detail, the GMP responsibilities, including the quality measure of each party."

For example, if a company is sponsoring a clinical trial and wishes to have the API made by a third-party contractor (a CMO), they will be the contract giver and the contract manufacturer will be the contract acceptor. Similarly, if the contract manufacturer outsources the delivery of its service provision, there must again be a contract in place. In the United States, this contract, commonly termed a *quality agreement*, ensures that obligations for quality assurance activities such as reporting and acting on out-of-specification results are clearly defined. The supply agreement will then normally contain the specifications, process, and working methods.

In EU countries, the contract document, more commonly called a *technical agreement*, includes both the quality procedures and the technical information relating to specifications. This has led to a degree of confusion between the two areas. In practice, both work when the supply agreement and quality/technical agreement are taken together. Personally, I prefer to see the technical information and quality procedures in a single document, to enable easier documentation of changes. This is because the supply agreement rarely changes once executed, whereas technical details and quality arrangements tend to change more frequently. This makes it better to have a *quality and technical agreement*, which becomes a working document that is properly updated under change control.

4.9.4 Validation

Validation aims to confirm and document that the output from a process or operation is as specified. In the case of a press producing tablets, for example, the producer must prove that under defined and documented production conditions, the tablets manufactured will consistently meet specifications. There are a number of stages to validation that follow the development life cycle:

- *Design qualification:* confirms that the design meets requirements
- *Installation qualification:* confirms that the installation meets requirements
- *Operational qualification:* confirms that the operation meets requirements
- *Process qualification:* confirms that the entire process meets requirements

Validation should be carried out to a protocol, sometimes called a *master validation plan.* 21 CFR Glossary defines a validation protocol as: "a written plan stating how validation will be conducted and defining acceptance criteria. For example, the protocol for a manufacturing process identifies processing equipment, critical process parameters and/or operating ranges, product characteristics, sampling, test data to be collected, number of validation runs and acceptable test results."

Although validation is vitally important in ensuring that product is produced as intended, it can also be extremely prohibitive to change, since it is a resource-hungry activity. One possible solution is that instead of defining processes as a single set of parameters, the development stage actually explores a range of the most relevant parameters (critical quality attributes) to define a "design space." Then validation would be required only if operations extended beyond the space. This is the one of the key principles of quality by design, explored in Chapter 15.

4.9.5 Change Control

Changes to any aspect of the supply chain must be carefully controlled. This involves assessment of the impact of any proposed change on safety, efficacy, and quality of the product. Companies are required to have a standard operating procedure that defines all the responsibilities and activities involved. Many companies form a change control board, so that assessment can be made more easily with all the key personnel present. The main stages are as follows:

- Define the change clearly.
- Perform an impact or risk assessment.
- Make a cross-functional review.
- Identify needs for validation, verification, and other risk mitigations.
- Sign-off on the implementation plan.
- Implement change according to the plan and document accordingly.

Historically, pharma companies have been averse to changing anything that would require authorization by the regulators. The reasons and counters for this is something to be considered in the light of the opportunity for improvement.

4.9.6   Stability

Products tend to degrade over time under the ravages of temperature and humidly effects, for example. Stability is a measure of how quickly or slowly that happens. Some compounds are as "stable as old boots," as the term goes. Others may last only days or weeks. In general terms, biological compounds are far more sensitive than small molecules to temperature and humidity. This means that cold chain storage and transportation is a major consideration in biologics. This does not mean that it is never a concern in small molecules. In the early stages of development, where relatively less is known about the stability profile, the evidence may not exist to assume that a compound is not temperature or humidity sensitive. This means that material may need to be stored and transported under controlled temperature conditions. This is an important point for those responsible for the supply chain to bear in mind; it is a compliance risk that has grown in recent years. Clearly, it is important to know the profile of degradation for any product so that it is not consumed in an inferior state. The ICH has established guidelines for stability testing that govern this area. Stephen Ward expands further in relation to biologics specifically in Section 4.11.5.

4.9.7   Investigations and CAPAs

Any out-of-specification result or unplanned deviation must be investigated to find the root cause, which must then be corrected through corrective and preventive actions (CAPAs). Pharmaceutical companies are required to document the investigation carefully and not close the file until a satisfactory solution to the quality issue has been identified, approved, and implemented. It is the responsibility of the trial sponsor or license holder to ensure that this happens. If the manufacturer is the sponsor or license holder, this will be covered under the quality system SOPs of that company. If the manufacturer is under contract, this must be covered within the quality and/or technical agreement (see Section 4.9.3)

4.9.8   Customer Complaints

Companies must monitor records and respond to customer complaints relating to products. They should then have a process of correcting any deficiencies identified and reporting any matters relating to safety to the appropriate competent authority (see also Adrian Hampshire's contribution in Section 11.3.4).

4.9.9   Traceability and Recall

Traceability and recall are classic supply chain concerns. As a product is made and distributed, it is possible that quality defects could be identified in one of two ways:

1. A finished product in the marketplace could be found to cause adverse patient events or to exhibit some other unacceptable problem.
2. A constituent material in the product could be identified (by a supplier or manufacturer) as being of suspect quality.

In either case, the supply chain must be halted while investigations take place. This requires identification of all the batches of product that could be involved and taking them out of the system by quarantining them. To do this, there needs to be forward (in case 1 above, where did the product go to) and reverse (in case 2 above, where did it come from) traceability. This now provides a basis to look at the various physical stages of production, storage, and delivery along the entire supply chain shown in Figure 4.1.

4.10   OVERVIEW OF THE STAGES ON ROUTE TO PATIENT DELIVERY

The descriptions that follow may be a great disappointment to engineers, chemists, biochemists, biochemical engineers, wholesalers, pharmacists, and all the other disciplines engaged in making and distributing pharmaceuticals. By necessity, it can only be an overview, and as with all overviews, it will not satisfy the demands for intimate detail. This section therefore comes with a "government" health warning that this is not a do-it-yourself guide to making and supplying medicines. There are huge scientific, technical, and regulatory challenges involved in the practical world of drug production and delivery to patients. All we can do here is to identify the stages and discuss some of the considerations that affect SCM.

Figure 4.1 is a schematic of the stages involved in the manufacture of small-molecule compounds. In accord with the concept of starting at the patient end, we begin with the distribution channel.

4.10.1   The Distribution Channel

As a patient, it is comforting to know that access to medicines is as immediate and convenient as possible. Since the manufacturers historically made the product in large batches and patients typically needed only one or two packs, there was a gap to fill in getting the product to millions of patients in diverse locations; also, manufacturers did not want to have the hassle of collecting money from these millions of patients and dealing with all the other aspects of managing payments. So the wholesaler emerged as a willing intermediary in the supply chain. Wholesalers purchased the product from manufacturers and made their living out of the messy business of getting product to patients (or secondary care sites) and dealing with the payment transactions. In return, the wholesalers charged a percentage markup on the product selling price.

This makes the wholesaler the party charged with getting the product from the manufacturer into patients' hands. By this stage, all the science and technology in the product performance is completed. The requirement from then on is careful storage, handling, tracking, and commercial accounting of the products so that no unintended harm or damage is done to any and all parties concerned. Typically, to get the product to patients, wholesalers must deliver to locations that are available to the patient. These are likely to be, for example, community pharmacies, supermarkets, drug-stores, hospital pharmacies, clinics, physicians' offices, and primary care facilities. Increasingly, direct delivery to patient homes is becoming a preferred option.

It is beyond our scope here to delve into the detailed workings of channel flows: physical, information, and money. They are extremely complex and require the specialist help of those who spend their lives working in the area. One such expert is Ron Krawczyk[8] of Blue Fin Group, who served as a guest contributor in Section 2.3. Strategies must be devised and implemented based on a detailed understanding of requirements, and critically, patient value must be at the forefront.

Figure 4.2 shows a schematic of the flow of goods and financial transactions involved in a typical U.S. distribution channel. In principle it seems relatively straightforward; in practice it is extremely complex. For further details on this subject, readers should refer to the Kaiser Family Foundation publication *Follow the Pill*.[9] What follows is a summary from the report on the four key players.

1. *Pharmaceutical manufacturers*. Manufacturers have the most influence on prices. They establish a wholesale acquisition cost (WAC), which is the baseline at which wholesalers purchase the drug products. Discounts and rebates may be applied.
2. *Wholesale distributors*. Consolidation has left the top three wholesale distributors with almost 90% of the wholesale market! They typically sell to pharmacies at WAC plus some negotiated percentage. They may also facilitate negotiation of discounts between manufacturers and customers.
3. *Pharmacies*. Pharmacies negotiate discounts and rebates with manufacturers and wholesalers based on sales volume and market share. They also negotiate with pharmacy benefit managers for inclusion in their networks.
4. *Pharmacy benefit managers* (PBMs). PBMs account for approximately two-thirds of U.S. prescriptions written. PBMs aim to deliver savings for their customers (payers) through cost containment programs.

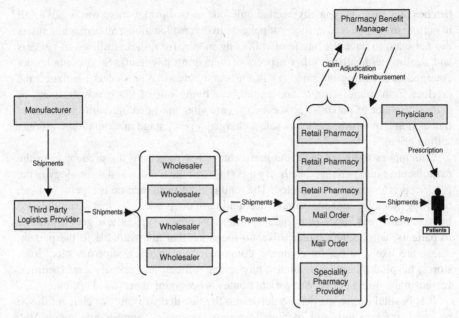

FIGURE 4.2   Typical flow of goods and payment in the U.S. distribution channel. (Compiled with assistance from Blue Fin Group.)

The report goes on the stress the complexity and poorly understood nature of the channel for pharmaceuticals, which leads to dramatically varying prices.

The stage prior to this is production of drug product.

4.10.2   Drug Product Production

Secondary Packaging   The final stage of product production is secondary packaging. This involves labeling and packing into presentations suitable for patient use and filling into shipping outers ready for transfer to the distribution channel. None of the packaging is in contact with the product or able to affect product integrity. All printed matter must be closely controlled to ensure that the labeling on the product is as approved in the license. This includes purchased materials and materials printed in-house. Materials are typically based on paper, board, corrugated packaging, and overwrapping films of different types.

At the secondary packaging stage, the drug product is enclosed in primary packaging (see below), so the threat to product integrity is much less. This reduced risk is, however, countered by the need for the labeling and all associated text to conform strictly to the information that has been registered with the regulators; also, mislabeling can have a dire effect on patient safety if it leads to a product being identified incorrectly. The majority of product recalls are related to mislabeling or packaging issues, so there remains a substantial element of noncompliance risk.

In supply chain terms the challenges of secondary packaging lay in the complexity of end-item variants [stock keeping units (SKUs)] and the lead time of origination of packaging artwork and the associated approvals. Particularly in EU countries, where virtually every country has its own language pack for each product presentation, the range of different SKUs passing through the secondary packaging lines can be extraordinary. In addition, with such a variety of packaging component items, each in different languages, the mix of components delivered to the site of production can be vast. This is one area where the makers and suppliers of production equipment would be well advised to develop smaller, more flexible equipment solutions.

Primary Packaging   Next to consider is primary packaging, the precursor stage to secondary packaging. The primary packaging operation concerns the encasement of the drug product in suitable materials to protect the integrity of the drug product. This means that the packaging must be capable of protecting against the impact of moisture, humidity, and light, for example, to the extent required by the nature of the product as determined through development. These materials would typically be a bottle and closure, sealed aluminum foil blisters, sachet, vial and stopper, and so on. Once contained in the primary package, the product must remain stable over the registered shelf life of the product (see the discussion of stability testing in Section 4.11.5).

The supply chain challenge relates to these items that are more difficult to source, higher in cost, and have a longer lead time. The specifications may be required to meet demanding performance criteria that only a limited number of suppliers can achieve. This means that the purchasing portfolio positions tend to be either strategic or critical, calling for a different approach to secondary packaging.

Another characteristic of this stage is the need to schedule production runs in cognizance of production constraints. The issues of batch changeover and potential cross-contamination are normally greater here.

Drug Product Production   The stage prior to primary packaging is conversion of the active ingredient (API) into the drug product through processes such as blending, mixing, and forming. The product output is quantities of tablets, soft-gel capsules, or a bulk solution, for example. To be able to produce a suitable product, the API must be mixed with other ingredients that facilitate the requirements for drug delivery. For solid-dose products these are known as excipients, which means they are not part of the mode of action for the drug but are there to help the processing and delivery of the drug.

These three stages can be carried out independently or in a connected series. If they are independent, there must be adequate and validated containment to cover the period they are held awaiting the next stage. For example, tablets held in bulk prior to being packaged into blisters must be kept in containers that prevent any adverse effect on stability. It is always preferable from a supply chain best practice viewpoint to join the processes so that the temptation to make larger quantities and hold them in store is avoided. This leads to the batch and queue issues discussed later. Amazingly, some companies do not just separate these operations inside the production walls;

they actually separate them between facilities. So we see tablets produced in bulk, filled into shipment containers, and sent thousands of miles to another facility, where they are received, inspected, stored, and eventually loaded on the lines for primary packaging. Sometimes they even go a second round as the primary packaged product is filled to bulk and sent again on its way.

Some of the larger CMOs have even consciously decided to make the separation in the name of specialization up to a particular stage of dosage forms. Hence, clients are forced to send their products on journeys to secondary packaging—whether they want to or not.

4.10.3   Primary Product Production

Active Pharmaceutical Ingredient and Key Intermediates   The primary product section of the supply chain has its roots firmly in the world of fine chemicals manufacture. Those that have entered into the arena of pharmaceutical manufacture and supply have needed to invest time and resources in meeting the standards of regulators for compliance with good manufacturing practice (GMP) and good laboratory practices (GLP), and to a lesser extent, good distribution practice (GDP). The sector has seen an increasing requirement for GxP upstream from API to pivotal, key, and earlier stage intermediates to the extent that it has become problematic to supply pharmaceutical materials without GxP embedded in operating methods. Over time, of course, this has had a negative impact on costs. (See also Chris Oldenhof's contribution in Section 5.5.1 for some unfortunate competitive side effects.)

From a supply chain viewpoint, suppliers to branded pharma are have historically been in a strong position by virtue of the degree of exclusivity afforded by their presence in the regulatory filing. In generics, of course, the situation is totally different. Since these companies' heritage is based in the competitive world of chemicals, they tend to be skilled negotiators and commercially aware. These are often testing supply markets for those engaged in procurement; also to be borne in mind is that this sector is capital intensive and utilization is a key driver. This can be an advantage in times of overcapacity, but of course, a cause of concern where capacity is limited. When this is the case, costs and lead times tend to go up and out, respectively.

Raw and Starting Material Producers   Refer to Sections 4.11.2 and 4.11.3.

4.11   MANUFACTURE AND SUPPLY OF BIOLOGICAL ENTITIES

As noted earlier, the section on biological production is authored by Stephen Ward. Stephen and I met as fellow members of the UK Bio-Industry Association's Manufacturing Advisory Committee. It was only after a couple of meetings that, by chance, I realized that Stephen was a fellow Welshman. He had developed the perfect Oxford English accent through his earlier exit from the Principality, whereas I had retained

Welsh residency long enough for the accent to stick for life. From the first meeting we were strong allies in advocating the use of twenty-first-century modernization approaches (notably, quality by design) in the development of drugs—singing from the same hymn sheet, as some would say.

As a committee, chaired and inspired by Brendan Fish (now at GSK, previously Medimunne), we went on to run a one-day workshop, in London, for SMEs in biotherapeutics wishing to learn about the quality by design approach. We both spoke and had a really enjoyable and successful day.[10]

Before handing over to Stephen, it should be mentioned that the level of detail is comparatively deeper here than in most other sections of the book. There are two reasons for this: first, this is an extremely complex area; and second, because it demonstrates how much science is linked inextricably with successful supply chain management approaches. Stephen has faced those challenges and found workable solutions without any formal training in the discipline.

GUEST CONTRIBUTOR SLOT: STEPHEN WARD

4.11.1   Manufacture and Supply of Biological Products

Over the last few years, there has been a significant increase in the importance of biological-based products (often termed *biopharmaceuticals*, *biologicals*, or *biologics*). Once the domain of innovative biotech companies, they are now playing a more important role in large pharma pipelines. Although the reasons for this switch are many, including patent expiry, pressure from generics, and underdelivering R&D pipelines, the upshot is that very complex molecules are now becoming more commonplace within both SMEs and large organizations. It is expected that the current market for biopharmaceuticals will increase from $125 billion in 2008 to $203 billion by 2015.[11] Senior pharma executives often speak about wanting pipelines to be 25 to 30% biopharmaceutical. Clearly, the development, manufacture, and delivery of these new medicines to patients brings a range of challenges to the supply chain professional, some of which are unique while others can be resolved using prior supply chain knowledge. In this section we provide an overview of the biological supply chain and to highlight troublesome areas.

4.11.2   Types of Biological Products

A new type of product began to to be developed in the 1970s and 1980s based on the ability of scientists to introduce a piece of desired DNA into a cell (gene cloning) and for the cell to use its in-built machinery to express that gene to produce the protein of choice; this is known as *recombinant technology*. This platform has allowed the biotechnology industry to grow to over 4700 companies in 2008.[12] Not all biotechnology products, however, are based on recombinant technology. Biological products are often protein based, but can also be composed of nucleic acid, sugars,

TABLE 4.1   Overview of Biological Products

Type of Biological	Description
Monoclonal antibodies (mAbs)	Recombinant proteins of exquisite specificity for a preselected target which can induce a range of effects (e.g., block a cell receptor, activate a cell receptor, activate the immune system).
Hormones	Classic examples such as human growth hormone and insulin.
Cytokines	Small proteins that help orchestrate the cells of the immune system. For example, G-CSF is used to stimulate the immune system to make more white blood cells.
Vaccines	This reenergized product class includes vaccines to protect against a range of infectious agents as well as for use in a therapeutic context to treat existing disease (e.g., chronic viral infection or therapeutic cancer vaccines).
Gene therapy	Virus constructs are often used to deliver, and ultimately overcome, a patient's faulty gene.
Cell-based medicine	A fantastically hot sector, often termed *regenerative medicine*. Cells or tissues are the product, and are introduced to reverse a disease state or replace cells that may have been lost due to injury or medical intervention.

or, indeed, all three! Biologicals cover an array of medicine types as detailed in Table 4.1; I have included the new cell-based medicines, which are expected to become a huge class of innovative medicines in the future.

Unsurprisingly, biological products, especially advanced medicines such as cells, are challenging (but rewarding) to develop. An extensive array of biological and operational factors affect the ability of the process to generate products of the desired activity and quality. To find a logical path through these process factors, risk-assessment tools can be very useful not only to improve operational success, but also to identify process variables which may have an impact on the effectiveness and safety of the resulting product. These inputs can then be investigated in the lab to determine which are indeed important, and perhaps most critically, use multiparameter experimental approaches such as design of experiment (DoE) statistics to understand the complex interaction between process parameters and their effect on the product. This results in a much better understood process and product, allowing the manufacturer more operational flexibility within a data-derived set of operational limits known as a design space (see Chapter 14).

A broad review of how to generate every type of biological is not within the scope of this section; instead, I shall focus on the generation of a "common" biological such as a monocloncal antibody. The overview of the biological development process shown in Figure 4.3 illustrates the many steps common for recombinant biologicals and cell therapies. I have used a very rough rule to divide the process into bite-sized segments.

Stage 1.   The production cells used can be either microbial, such as bacteria or yeast, or eukatyotic, such as from insects or mammals. A whole raft of scientific,

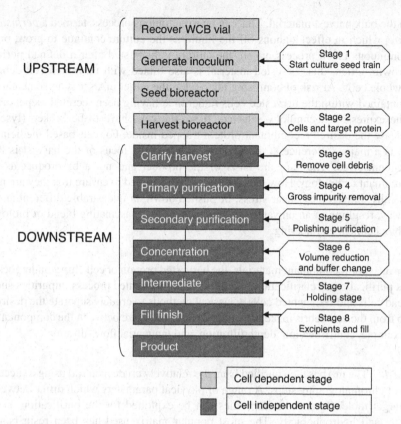

FIGURE 4.3 Manufacturing process for a recombinant monoclonal antibody.

regulatory, clinical, and commercial issues need to be evaluated when choosing between the available technologies. However, the engine that is harnessed to produce the active material is cellular. With recombinant technology, the cell is clearly a by-product of the process and needs to be "controlled" for only a defined portion of the process prior to it being purified out. In contrast, cells that are manufactured for cell or tissue therapy are the product themselves, and the process requires that these cells be retained in a "healthy" state for much longer, often encompassing environments outside a GMP wrapper and therefore extra challenging. Issues common to both approaches do exist; I shall highlight where they diverge and cell therapy–specific challenges appear. Cells from a defined cell bank are taken and expanded under aseptic (sterile) conditions using defined growth media and supplements through a "seed train." This series of culture steps will produce enough cells to seed a large culture vessel or bioreactor.

Stage 2. The mAb product secreted from the cells during their growth phase into the surrounding nutrient media are recovered from a large culture vessel or bioreactor to form the bulk harvest material. This can be a continuous process, termed a *perfusion culture*, which in effect siphons off the liquid as the culture continue to grow, or a discontinuous batch process, where the culture is harvested after a defined period of growth. Often, this harvested material is also mixed with unwanted cell debris and whole cells. At risk of confusing the reader, the target mAb may in some cases be contained within the harvested cells rather than having been secreted, depending on the expression technology selected. If so, the cells have to be broken (lysed) to release the desired recombinant protein trapped inside. For cell-based medicines there is a major difference at this process point, as the focus of the harvest is the cells themselves: They are the basis of the product and not a by-product as in recombinant technology. How these cells are then handled to ensure that they are not physically damaged by shear stress, or pushed down an undesirable differentiation pathway, resulting in an unwanted cell phenotype, is a fascinating blend of biology and biochemical engineering.

Stage 3.   For recombinant materials, the harvested protein or cell slurry undergoes a gross purification or clarification to remove bulky unwanted process impurities such as dead cells and fragmented cells. Classical methods to crudely separate the desired mAb from the cell debris make use of the difference in size between the components: for example, centrifugation, depth filtration, and tangential flow filtration.

Stage 4.   The mAb is then purified from the relatively crude material using a succession of chromatography steps. A range of physical parameters which differ between the target molecule and the impurities can be exploited for the purification: size, charge, and hydrophobicity. The most popular matrix used has been resin beads packed into columns, but several suppliers are now challenging this, with various membranes that have adsorbtive surface properties such as chromatography resins, but with an enhanced flow rate. The first step (primary purification) often utilizes the specific nature of the target protein to isolate it from the complex slurry; it is often called *affinity purification*. Subsequent detachment of the target from the matrix often involves a low pH. This is useful, as holding the partially purified material in this buffer can also neutralize any inapparent viruses that were endemic within the producer cell line, or indeed, introduced in any agents or buffers.

Stage 5.   The harvested material (eluate) may then have to be concentrated and the buffer adjusted before the second series of chromatography steps is performed to remove any residual process impurities, such as host cell proteins or nucleic acid that may still be present; this is often called *polishing chromatography*.

Stage 6.   Again, the eluted material will need to be concentrated and put into the buffer that will constitute the final formulation filled into the final container system. Prior to the final fill-finish step, a second viral-removal operation, usually passing through a membrane filter, is undertaken by way of a belt and braces.

Stage 7.   Due to the complexity of the process operation, a holding stage may need to be introduced to allow the purified material to be transferred to the relevant site (or department) which has the specialist expertise to perform the fill-finish operation in a sterile manner.

Stage 8.   The final container–closure system may be of various designs: for example, a stoppered vial of various forms, or a syringe. The container closure system, dose form (lyophilized, liquid or frozen), and storage/onward-shipping conditions will depend on the stability of the material to heating, freezing, and light. The type of clinical setting and target patient population may also dictate the fill-finish and temperature-controlled shipment system employed; this should be identified at the start of the project when the target product profile is determined.

4.11.3   Starting Materials

Where Does the Supply Chain Start?   It is often easy to think instinctively of a supply chain as the GMP and GDP machinery to manufacture and deliver intermediate or finished product. For biologicals, the supply chain can start much earlier in the product life cycle. For example, the cells used to generate the recombinant product or the virus backbone of a gene therapy product may be sufficient for early research to generate proof-of-concept data, but totally inappropriate for generating clinically safe material. As is often the case, the gene sequence has to be reintroduced (recloned) into a regulatory-compliant and validated host cell. On the face of it, this seems a relatively easy undertaking. Caution must be exercised, however, as the host change can have a range of consequences on the safety and efficacy of the product, both intended and unintended. For example, alterations in glycosylation patterns, changes in immunogenicity (ability to induce an immune response in humans), plus changes in biological activity can occur for a purified recombinant protein following host change. This is even more evident where cells are the active component. Unless comparable cells can be derived after proof of principle has been shown (which is not easy to show since cells express over 30,000 genes!), early researchers have to ensure that the cells they isolate can be developed into a regulatory-compliant therapy. Impressively, the broader regenerative medicine community realized this fairly early in the sector's development, and great efforts are made to ensure the suitability of starting materials used in the procurement of tissues and cells from donors such as growth media, transport buffers, and supplements. Such advanced cell therapies are now covered by an extensive set of EU regulations[13] and the U.S. *Code of Federal Regulations*,[14] which cover the development activity before GMP manufacture to ensure not only that patient ethics are maintained, but also that cells free of communicable disease are harvested, identified, and stored. The supply chain can clearly be very elongated indeed for cell therapy, with academics intertwined with GMP (illustrated in Figure 4.4). The innovator company bringing the product to market is responsible for ensuring that all raw and starting materials, process intermediates, and final product are of the appropriate quality to ensure not

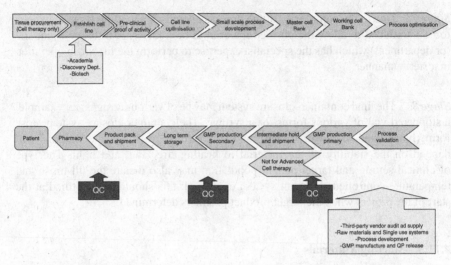

FIGURE 4.4   Development life cycle for a biological product from early research.

only patient safety, but also a commercially viable product. Expanded supply chains inevitably result in more complex supplier audits and due-diligence inspections.

Cell Banks   The overview of the biological development process shown in Figure 4.4 illustrates the many steps common for recombinant biologicals and cell therapies. The bedrock of biologicals are the cell banks: the *parental cell bank*, which can often be a very small number of vials frozen at the start of the project (which may not leave the research department if the project goes awry!); the *master cell bank*, really the crown jewel of the project, composed of several hundred vials characterized and tested extensively for infective agents within both in vitro and in vivo systems; the *working cell bank*, used as the starting point for manufacture, which is also tested for infectious agents, but not as extensively; and the *end-of-process cell bank*, harvested at the end of the process, which is tested to ensure the genetic stability of the producer cells over the life of the process and to check for the lack of any adventitious contaminants introduced during manufacture.

4.11.4   Raw Materials

There are several key raw material types common across most biological processes, the timely availability of which has a key impact on the ability not only to deliver various intermediates to the next unit operation, but also to ensure that material is of sufficient quality, potency, and most important, safety.

Growth Media and Supplements   To allow the producer cell to grow to the cell mass required within a suitable reactor type requires a complex mixture of sugars, amino acids, and growth factors in a sterile liquid buffer. These components can be

TABLE 4.2   Pros and Cons of Pre-prepared Liquid Medium

Advantages	Disadvantages
Ready to use	Increased storage capacity needed
Company quality control requirement reduced	Frozen and/or cold storage over a longer period
Inventory management simpler	Shorter shelf life
WIFI system requirements reduced or removed	Increased cost
Buffer filling and filtration requirements reduced	Container-leachable data over longer periods required

supplied directly in liquid form for combination on site, in powder for reconstitution as needed, or indeed in both forms. Clearly, the choice of format depends on many factors, such as process scale, local storage capacity, site liquid-handling capacity, company philosophy, and commercial considerations of price and supply strategy (see Table 4.2 for some advantages and disadvantages of preprepared liquid medium). For processes developed by SMEs, the infrastructure, skills, and analytical methods are often not present within the organization to handle sterile media preparation. Also, it is likely that liquid media formulations would have been used during process development and/or pilot-scale manufacture, resulting in early "buy-in" into a liquid formulation for the process. Indeed, the increasing use of single-use or disposable units within a process coupled to modular clean-room design fosters the "plug and play" mentality which liquid media formulation clearly fits into (see "Single-Use Production Systems" later in this section). A change of supplier or formulation could result in significant additional studies to demonstrate the comparability of process and product. Clearly, understanding the design space for the process through the use of quality by design principles (see Chapter 14) can greatly facilitate media interchangability, leading to a more robust secondary supply chain. In addition, there is a major company and regulatory push to move to animal-component-free or, indeed, protein-free chemically defined media (composed of sugars, amino acids, and trace elements) both to reduce the risk of animal virus contamination and to improve any batch-to-batch variation; quality by design can play a major role in understanding the impact of such a change.

Whatever the form of media used, timely supply to the upstream process group is essential to ensure continuation of the cell culture train, from small-scale seed culture to large vessel growth. Cultures often have to be kept in exponential growth phase during the seed train to maintain predictable future growth. Any delay in media supply could affect not only the viability of the culture process but also the integrity of the process if the number of cell divisions required to produce the desired cell mass is higher than that for which the process is designed.

Downstream Purification Components   Advances in recombinant technology over the last few years has pushed up yields of the target protein considerably. Depending on the type of protein, yields can now be expected to be greater than 10 g/L. Although the advantages of this are many—fewer growth batches, lower growth media consumption, reduced clean room occupation—it can put very significant pressure on "downstream" operations (so-called as these unit operations occur following the cell growth stages and are concerned with purifying the target protein from the harvest). This welcome uplift in yield also means, however, an unwelcome increase in aggregated protein, from which it is more challenging to purify and generate functional protein. The recent challenge has been how to improve throughput of the various separation and concentration steps to prevent a bottleneck from occurring. As cleaning and cleaning validation are very time-consuming activities for purification media and systems, the use of single-use systems have become more popular as a solution to this problem, to increase downstream turnaround times. Purification media, either bead, membrane, or hollow-fiber, with enhanced properties, higher flow-rate tolerances, and increased binding capacities are also being developed, with a view to reducing the number and duration of purification steps to alleviate this bottleneck issue.

Not only has the efficiency of the separation steps been a challenge, with scale-out systems composed of multiple columns sometimes used, but the use of large quantities of buffer has also been an issue. Similar to the supply of quality control tested and released growth media, a delay in delivery of buffer can also dramatically affect process success. This may be manifested as a straightforward increase in operational costs due to an increase in clean room occupancy time, through to batch rejection as a result of degradation of the target protein within the delayed upstream bulk harvest or intermediate.

Single-Use Production Systems   Single-use production systems are also referred to as *disposable systems* or *ready-to-use ware*, but all describe pre-prepared, modular process components that have been prequalified (and often presterilized) for direct use. The list of items within this supply category has grown significantly over the last few years (see Table 4.3), with several vendors now providing total packages of single-use ware for a range of process unit operations; these range from growth media and buffer preparation to bulk cell growth, clarification, chromatography, virus clearance, and indeed, final formulation. The vendor will often work with the customer to compile a disposable fluid path and scale appropriate for the product under development. Not only does this allow the developer company the luxury of "one-stop shopping" for both unit components and the connecting tubing, bags, and connecting fittings, and hence fewer supplier quality assurance and financial audits, but also peace of mind that all components are compatible and are to the same vendor standard. In addition, for smaller companies, the technical and knowledge support that can be offered by vendor companies can be a very attractive reason for developing processes with these items. Of course, the use of such systems does not remove the need for the developer company to have to construct and validate a process with such items. Even though buying plasticware off the shelf sounds very attractive from a "let someone else do the work" mindset, these systems do mean, however, that a significant amount of work is also required by the company in advance to ensure not only a steady supply of items and inventory control, but also that the incoming materials are of the correct quality. Company-specific drivers such as technical skill

TABLE 4.3   Examples of Single-Use Systems Across Upstream and Downstream Operations

Example	Unit Operation	Supplier
	Upstream	
Rocking-platform bioreactor	Cell growth	GE Healthcare (WAVE), Applikon (AppliFlex)
Stirred-tank biorector	Cell growth	Sartorius Stedim Biotech, Xcellerex, Applikon, Thermo Fisher (HyClone)
Depth membrane filtration	Gross clarification	Millipore, GE Healthcare, 3M
Tangential flow filtration	Gross clarification	Pall, GE Healthcare, Millipore
	Downstream	
Buffer preparation	Separation	Thermo Fisher (HyClone), Millipore, Satorius Stedim Biotech
Primary capture chromatography	Primary purification	GE Healthcare, Satorius Stedim Biotech, Pall
Polishing chromatography	Secondary purification	Pall, Satorius Stedim Biotech
Ultrafiltration and diafiltration membrane chromatography	Product concentration and buffer exchange	Pall, GE Healthcare, Millipore
Fluid path and storage bags	Harvest, transfer, and storage	CFlex tubing, Invitrogen, GE Healthcare

levels and economics will shape how this is manifests, such as what release testing is performed by the vendor and what by the manufacturing company.

A lot of the pros and cons of using single-use systems are similar to those described previously for liquid media in Table 4.2. Current limitations on scale may hinder adoption of this approach to all parts of the industry, especially to large-scale operations (>2000 L growth scale). Also, the environmental impact is currently a matter of hot debate. Water reduction by an exclusively single-use plant has been calculated to be over 80% lower than that of a traditional facility. Also, if total waste is calculated over the entire operation, disposable systems do not appear to be as environmentally damaging as one might think. Suffice it to say that with end-to-end manufacturing encompassing R&D, the earlier the technical, quality, and economic merits of single-use technology can enter the equation, the better.

Historically, the main drivers for the use of single-use systems has been a reduction in plant capital expenditure, increased speed to a commissioned operational state, and enhanced process flexibility, as there is often no need for stainless steel infrastructure, large equipment validation, or CIP/SIP (clean in place/steam in place) systems. The environmental grade of operational clean rooms can also be reduced for certain operations if they can be shown to be totally closed. This can also facilitate throughput, as multiple products or multiple batches can be run simultaneously within the same facility. As mentioned previously, this has to be offset against a potential increase in upfront validation workload, especially if single-use systems have not been an integral part of the manufacturing platform technology. This often means working with suppliers to ensure that the source and grade of plastic is appropriate, plus checks of their GMP process to ensure compliance. It is also likely that in addition to any data packages that can be provided by the vendor, additional extractible and leachable studies would have to be performed to ascertain the interaction between a buffer or product and disposable surfaces in contact with the fluid path. Good-quality vendors often have a baseline package covering their main plastic components and the potential extractables, and even some leachables with a standard buffer. For single-use processes, the timely supply of quality control–released plasticware is crucial to batch success. Common issues with liquid media that can impact upon this success are inventory control, quality control testing and release, quarantine, and defect-return processes.

4.11.5   Final Product Formulation, Stability, and Container Closure System

A common complaint from experienced formulation scientists, especially over cocktails at conferences, is that the biologists who typically develop the new protein-based medicines do not really think about the best way to retain product stability in the open marketplace until late in the clinical development cycle; "they just store it frozen in phosphate-buffered saline and that's it!" Of course this is a sweeping generalization, but it does often ring true, especially for small biotech companies, which often do not have the formulation experience, or indeed the budget, to address such issues; just getting the active biological into the clinic is often strain enough for them.

As mentioned previously, in an ideal world, the development scientist would have the time and resources available to develop the best possible process to generate a robust and rugged product that is of maximum potency, thus giving the biological candidate the best chance of success in the clinic. The real world, as we all know, is far less utopian. Nonetheless, the adoption of simple quality by design principles by companies can help bring formulation into the development equation earlier. For example, starting with a well-characterized target product profile will ensure that the type of formulation, administration route, packaging requirements, and temperature stability profile will be thought about to ensure that a commercially viable product is being developed which will be received favorably by clinicians and patients.

It is a pretty fundamental issue to know if a liquid of lyophilized cake is preferred, or if apparatus for liquid nitrogen vapor storage is required at clinical centers (which is often not the case). The use of multivariate experimental designs [such as design of experiment (DoE) statistics] means that a number of basic formulation parameters can be evaluated fairly quickly compared to the classic approach of changing only a single parameter and running the experiment, then repeating the process for every parameter under investigation to try to identify the optimal formulation. Of course, a balance has to be struck to avoid overdeveloping a candidate that is going to fail at phase I. However, if you are going to the expense of putting this material into a patient who trusts that it is going to be helpful to humankind, formulating to assure that it is presented in its best form should be the aim to ensure that the candidate doesn't fail as a result of an avoidable formulation issue—thus losing the baby with the bathwater.

What Instability Means for Biologicals   A range of degradative processes can affect biological molecules, all of which have the potential to have a severe impact on the potency and quality of the product and, most important, on patient safety. A nonexhaustive list of such processes follows.

- *Aggregation.* This is a big issue, generally caused when a protein becomes denatured (misshapen), so that protein molecules clump together. Not only can aggregates have reduced potency and altered pharmakokinetic profiles, they can also induce immune activation processes that have major clinical sequelae.
- *Fragmentation.* Fragmentation is often due to the hydrolysis of certain peptide bonds which link the constituent amino acids of the protein together. Shear forces can also be a cause.
- *Oxidation.* Certain amino acid residues that make up a protein are oxidized, results in changed biological activity.
- *Deamidation.* Deamidation is a degradation reaction during which the side chains of two amino acids (asparagines and glutamine) are damaged.
- *Adsorbtion.* In adsorbtion, the biological adheres to the walls of the container closure vessel in which it is stored.

Testing for Instability   The ICH guidelines (see Chapter 3) are classic regulatory documents mapping out the minimum requirement of studies that need to be performed to show the stability of a biological over a range of storage conditions and temperatures prior to human use. A key tenet is that several batches of material need to be tested, each made by the intended manufacturing process scale, contained within the representative fill volume and form. The testing needs to be performed in real time. Unfortunately for the scientist in this instance, degradation may be too slow for elongated time periods to be tested, forcing unpalatable delays to the start of clinical trials. Accelerated stability studies are therefore often used to force the biological to degrade over a shorter time frame. This approach can be extremely useful during development to identify the best formulation but also, through mathematical modeling, can be used to predict degradation rates under various storage conditions. This is useful when real-time data are scant, although the predictions will have to be confirmed in real time at some point.

Formulation Science to Reduce Instability   The gross form of a material is often dictated by restrictions identified during target product profile setting or due to stability data. To put it simply, to stabilize material is to prevent degradation processes from occurring. Main formulation options to do this are the following.

- *Temperature.* Removing energy from the system reduces the rate of biochemical activity within the formulation. Classical cold chain temperatures of 2 to 8°C are common for this reason. The amount of resources and cost not only to generate and validate such shipping systems but also to implement means that a huge amount of collective effort is being undertaken to stabilize fragile biologicals at ambient temperatures.

- *Frozen storage.* Cryostorage at temperatures such as $-20°C$ or even $-80°C$ is often common in early clinical trials, as limited formulation work has been undertaken.
- *Freeze drying (lyophilization).* Freeze drying has been the classic formulation for stabilizing biological vaccines over the years. There are three parts to generating a freeze-dried cake or powder: (1) freezing the protein with a range of addititives or excipients such as sugars to induce a protective "shell" around the protein molecules, (2) subliming the water–ice away under a vacuum to ensure that the protein remains frozen, and (3) secondary drying to force off any remaining water trapped within the solid matrix by evaporation.
- *Protectants and stabilizers.* These are molecules whose purpose is (1) to maintain the conformation of the target protein during the freezing process by minimizing interaction of the protein with ice crystals (cryoprotection), and (2) to prevent unwanted protein–protein interactions during drying (lyoprotection).
- *Solubilizers.* These additives can help prevent protein aggregation during storage or indeed during rehydration of a freeze-dried solid cake.

Sterile Fill Operations   The bulk purified liquid preparation containing a biological in its final formulation has to be fed into the final containers. Depending on whether the material is to be stored and shipped in a liquid, frozen, or lyophilized (freeze-dried) form, this generally is performed using a highly specified filling line which maintains operational sterility. Again, a number of biochemical engineering issues become apparent in maintaining product uniformity over batch sizes containing thousands of containers. Shear stresses can play a part in damaging the valuable product at the final hurdle, not only within the filling lines and dispensing head, but also during agitation of the bulk liquid.

An important difference to highlight here between classical recombinant products and cell therapies is that cells often do not have the luxury of an intermediate holding step postpurification, due to their labile nature. This puts a significant pressure on the manufacturing operation, as seamless cell harvest, preparation, filling, and storage are required.

5 Why Pharma Supply Chains Don't Perform

5.1 SUPPLY CHAIN UNDERPERFORMANCE

The first point that we make here is that many supply chains in many sectors fail to perform adequately. This is not a swipe at pharmaceuticals in isolation, and companies turning a blind eye to the better practices and linkages described in this and other books may well find themselves victims of underperforming supply chains. The plain fact is, though, that the pharmaceutical sector does seem to exhibit most of the issues of poorly performing supply chains in general and more in addition, born of the specifics of the industry's history and culture. That is where our focus will be.

5.2 IS THERE A CASE TO ANSWER?

It may seem to some readers somewhat premature to start this chapter on a presupposition of guilt. Is this a case of guilty as charged without a proper trial? Where is the evidence? The other bold presupposition is that if this is true, I actually know the reasons why they do not perform. For the sake of progress, the analysis will delay dealing with these questions until the end of the chapter. Readers who are still not convinced by that stage will certainly have access to facts that I am not in possession of and would dearly like to get hold of!

To start, then, allocation of guilt and blame will be suspended to focus on the current processes in pharmaceuticals, leading up to the creation of a supply chain for a marketed product. The drug development process covered in Chapter 3 is the major determinant of that supply chain, since the CMC section of the CTD must contain every pertinent detail, including material and product specifications, suppliers, manufacturers, process instructions, and a host of other details required for the dossier. Nothing can change after approval unless it is supported by a regulatory compliant review and action plan (either a variation or within an approved design space under a quality by design/ICH Q8 compliant registration).

The conclusion from the above is therefore that if a robust patient-supportive and cost-effective supply chain is to be achieved, all the parameters that define that supply chain must be decided within time lines demanded by the regulatory filing. We see

Supply Chain Management in the Drug Industry: Delivering Patient Value for Pharmaceuticals and Biologics, By Hedley Rees
Copyright © 2011 John Wiley & Sons, Inc.

from the CMC section in Chapter 3 that these time lines can be long and involved and often trace back to original workings and data that were generated at the preclinical stage. So this is where the story begins, starting with a helpful metaphor.

A Helpful Metaphor

Left unattended, supply chains lay around doing the human equivalent of lounging on the sofa, drinking pop (soda), eating sweets (candy), and watching TV. They behave like neglected children. No other sector seems to have neglected its (supply chain) children to the degree that pharmaceuticals have. The parents are now paying the price for all those years of neglect. The big question is: How do they get the children up off the sofa to start to become productive members of society?

For most parents faced with this dilemma, the answer will be clear: Help them change by doing something radically different. Talk to them, listen to them, guide them, encourage them, discipline them, and try to show them the error of their ways. Most of all, do something different from what you have been doing as a parent, because you are quite probably a major source of the problem.

So it is with supply chains in pharmaceuticals. In chasing massive revenues from blockbuster drugs, the industry (parent) was happy for the supply chain to stay on the sofa. Life was rosy—with both parents working and a mortgage that was tiny in comparison to the family income. Now, one parent is out of work and the other's job is under threat. The cost of soda, candy, and cable TV is rocketing—time to send the children out to work!

Through this metaphor we aim to demonstrate the importance of investing time, effort, and the occasional tears or tantrums at the earliest stages of drug development, as we go on to discuss.

5.3   BIRTH TO INFANCY: THE SUPPLY CHAIN CRITICAL STAGE

In the same way that children are all but formed for life by the age of 5, supply chains are, too. This is not specific to pharmaceuticals; the same principle applies to any supply chain. Massive steps forward have been made in supply chains in other sectors through efforts in design for manufacture and value engineering, for example. This involves bringing up supply chains working to principles that will see them set for life. This section is about what happens, in general terms, in pharmaceutical supply chains as they go through the various stages of their life cycle. The discussion is based on small molecules and is meant to be indicative of the way in which drugs are developed from the viewpoint of my personal experience. If this is not the experience of any particular reader, perhaps someone working at a center of excellence in big pharma or an undiscovered pathfinder, be assured that it is happening most of the time in most companies.

A Helpful Metaphor (continued)

Throughout this chapter, the birth of the supply chain is taken as the development candidate that emerges from the loving charge of discovery research. The tiny baby is new, exciting, and full of possibilities for a happy and successful childhood. Then it happens. A few days after the "happy" event, the parents are killed in a car crash. There are no close family members to take baby in, so foster parents are found for the tiny mite. The new parents' first priority is to make sure that they can do what is needed to sustain the baby and to understand the unique aspects of the baby's personality and physical makeup that make it tick. As they set about this task, the metaphor takes a strange twist. An angel (or is it a wicked witch?) visits their bedroom in the dead of night and whispers a chilling message in the mother's ear. The visitor informs her that they have 16 years to raise the child and then it is on its own in the big wide world—no more support for the foster parents from social services. This child is going to have to grow up in a hurry and get out and earn itself a living.

They were horrified and asked this ethereal being how she knew this. Why, my dear, she murmured, as she softly squeezed both their hands, I am the patent protection fairy!

What to make of that, then? By 16, the baby should be able to stand on its own two feet, but what if it is a slow learner? Or a bit of a scatterbrain? Or subject to the 1001 other factors that could impede one or more stages of childhood development? They promised themselves there and then not to hang about, just in case. This baby was mighty important to them.

The extension of the metaphor introduces another factor in drug development, the fact that once the patent gun has fired, time is money (or at least, that is the perception). Readers should bear this in mind as we trace through the stages of supply chain development, beginning with preclinical.

5.3.1 Preclinical Development

The development candidates selected from discovery research will typically arrive with a small quantity of the drug that has been made under laboratory conditions; there will also be a package of data relating to the molecule's progress toward becoming a physical substance in a test tube. The first stage in the supply chain is to make enough drug for the needs of preclinical testing. In particular, the quantity manufactured must satisfy the requirements of animal testing for toxicity. Someone must therefore make a batch of material in a higher quantity than that in which it has been manufactured previously. An initial route of synthesis (manufacturing method) will be determined to produce the molecule at the larger scale, and all this will be documented. There is no real attempt to make the compound overly pure at this stage. Since the initial toxicology will be carried out on this batch, maximum cover will be provided for all subsequent batches if the purity is worst case. This is often termed producing a "dirty batch."

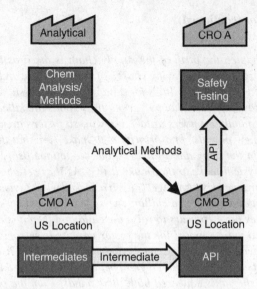

FIGURE 5.1   Typical supply chain for preclinical testing.

Sufficient API will be produced to satisfy the needs of in vitro and in vivo testing. The vast majority is used for in vivo testing in animals. There is no requirement for the compound to be in any particular dosage form at this stage since it can be administered into animals in the API natural form (as humanely as possible).

Figure 5.1 shows the simple supply chain. All the relevant data relating to the compound and its manufacture are collected as part of base information to be included in any application to run a clinical trial in humans (an IND or CTA). This is the stage where the least is known about the manufacturability of the compound.

The patent protection fairy will be taking a keen interest in progressing to the next stage of development.

5.3.2   Preparing for Phase I of Clinical Trials: Is the Drug Safe in Humans?

A successful preclinical evaluation normally results in the decision to apply to run a phase I clinical study. This requires an investigational new drug (IND) or clinical trial application (CTA). Figure 5.2 shows a supply chain for a drug for humans. In addition to API manufacture, it is necessary to convert the API into a dosage form suitable to administer to trial subjects. This is where pharmaceutical technology must be employed to determine a method of manufacture that will allow a safety study to be conducted. It could be any one of the dosage forms listed in Chapter 4. Unfortunately, not all compounds behave in ways that suit any dosage form. Often, because of this, compromises are made to get the trial under way. For example, if a compound did not form into a tablet satisfactorily, the API may be delivered by encasing it in a

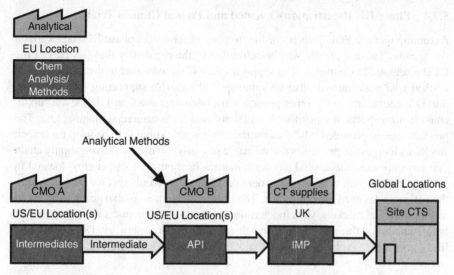

FIGURE 5.2   Typical current-state supply chain for studies in humans.

hard gelatin capsule for the sake of expediency. The patent protection fairy would have wanted that. She would have explained that establishing why the compound was not performing as a tablet and rectifying (or even finding a similar, less problematic alternative) would have caused an unacceptable delay to the program. The CMC data for the process to produce clinical trial supplies for humans will then be lodged with the regulator for approval. On approval, the trial supplies can be released, subject to all other approvals.

5.3.3   Moving into Phase II and Proof of Concept

A successful safety study at phase I will mean progression to the next stage, with a view to proving that the drug has sufficient efficacy for potential approval. Changing anything at this stage is often regarded to be somewhat risky. The regulator is perceived to be satisfied with the existing methods and process of manufacture. It is still uncertain whether the drug will proceed beyond this next stage. What would be the benefit to the sponsoring company of changing anything, such as the dosage form or the chemical or physical properties of any of the constituent materials? This could bring significant benefits in commercial manufacture, but will we be doing that? Even if we are, the margins are immense, so excess cost can be absorbed. A final consultation with the patent protection fairy confirms that progress "as is" makes sense. In practice, the only aspect that changes is the clinical trial pack that is sent to patients. The hard gel capsules may now be packaged in blisters rather than in plastic bottles. If this stage is successful, the process moves on to phase III.

5.3.4   Phase III: Registration-Oriented and Pivotal Clinical Trials

Assuming that the POC goes according to plan, much larger phase III studies are on the agenda. These typically will be submitted in the regulatory filing as part of the CTD discussed in Chapter 3. The supporting CMC data relating to the manufactured clinical trial material will also be submitted, along with supporting data collected during manufacture in the other phases. This, once approved, will define the supply chain in all respects, not just for phase III but also for commercial manufacture. The product used to provide CMC data for the filing is also suitable to be used for launch stocks, as long as the processes are validated properly. So now we have a supply chain that has only ever made products for hundreds or thousands of patients, located in well-defined clinical trial centers, where the clinical protocols specify almost exactly the patients who need to be supplied. The same supply chain is also going to be asked to supply global markets, with indeterminate quantities of products in volumes never before attempted through a totally new distribution channel network. Does that sound like a good idea? Probably not, but that is what happens just the same.

5.3.5   Commercial Launch and Supply and Phase IV: Clinical Trials After Launch

Commercial supply after launch is, of course, a postapproval activity, as are phase IV clinical trials. Focusing on commercial supply for the moment, it should be enlightening to compare the clinical to the commercial supply chain. Table 5.1 summarizes the comparison. On reviewing the table it should become clear how much more challenging the commercial supply chain is than a clinical trial chain. If those developing the supply chain had realized this, they might well have behaved differently.

1. *Inventory holding.* Through development all manufactured materials are regarded as an expense and written off against the profit-and-loss account in the year they are incurred. This means that although the inventory exists physically, it is not recorded anywhere in the accounts. Accountants like it this way because it is the more prudent way of dealing with materials that may never have any value. When a product is launched, the entire usable inventory suddenly has a value. It has to be included on the balance sheet as an asset to the business. This may sound like a minor issue, but in fact it means that any inventory that is lost, wasted, or unaccounted for must be written off the books. This can have a significant impact on company finances. Inventory control methods that had been used previously may not stand up.

2. *Demand.* There is a degree of uncertainty in clinical trial demand from unknown patient recruitment patterns. However, that pales into insignificance compared to the uncertainty of sales forecasts in global markets. If that is not obvious, remember that clinical trials support defined protocols that stipulate the number of patients to be supplied, their exact location, and their usage profile. Contrast that with worldwide sales of a product, possibly involving third-party licensees and co-promotion partners, where there are no bounds to demand, up or down. Damned if you do (put excess

TABLE 5.1 Differences Between Commercial and Clinical Supply Chains

Value-Chain Parameter	Development Value Chain	Commercial Value Chain
Inventory	Expensed	Balance sheet asset
Demand/capacity	Determinate (set by clinic protocols)	Uncertain (driven by patient markets)
Working capital	Low	High
Agreements	Investigator, CROs, development, quality/technical	Licensing, distribution, quality/technical, and commercial supply
Compliance	Increasing cGxP applies	Validation, change control, traceability, preapproval inspections
Insurance	Limited	Product liability, marine insurance, etc.
Supply base caliber	Support needs of specific studies	Able to cope with long-term market supply
Cost of goods	High: immature processes and low volume	Need to manage cost reduction to leverage higher volumes/ process maturity
Distribution logistics	Mainly express couriers to sites	Complex channel networks to wholesalers, clinics, hospitals and pharmacies
International movements	Shipped as research materials	Liable to stringent assessment because of implications for duty, tax, etc.
Packaging	Mainly regulatory driven, simple design and origination	Many stakeholders for approval and complex reprographics/ origination

inventory on the shelf) and damned if you don't (lose up to $1 million a day from being out of stock).

3. *Working capital.* The inventory investment (working capital) for commercial requirements is likely to be a significant number in the company accounts. Those responsible for this supply chain will receive close attention from business and financial management so that the investment is minimized; also, corporate responsibility will kick-in in the form of the Sarbanes–Oxley legislation. This means that controls must be in place and auditable from a financial perspective. The clinical trials supply chain will have been under this particular radar screen.

4. *Agreements.* Typically in clinical trials, the agreements relate to development projects and technical/quality agreements to meet competent authority expectations. These are either *Relatively* short term with modest cost exposure in the case of development agreements, or *Relatively* limited in scope and well prescribed by regulations. In commercial supply chains, the stakes are much higher across a multitude of

exposures, as license, supply, and service-level agreements must be drafted to manage these risks (see the contribution of in Section 9.6).

5. *Batch traceability*. Commercial supply involves the volume and complexity of batch numbers, interacting supply sources, and customer destinations hitherto unheard of in the clinical trial supply chain. The demand is therefore great for ongoing and proper tracing of pedigree. For clinical trials it is often possible to keep manual records. Commercial supply chain complexity demands computerized assistance across numbers of interfacing companies in the supply base and distribution channel.

6. *Scale of manufacture*. The consequences of producing suboptimal quality or quantity on a commercial scale can be severe. The amount of material consumed is of high value, and the scope of those receiving the material is potentially wide and much more difficult to contain should things go awry.

7. *Compliance*. The complexity of the commercial supply chain makes it much more difficult to ensure that compliance is held ongoing. There are typically multiple parties handing over between stages and working across interfacing quality systems.

8. *Insurance*. Values and exposure to loss are far higher in commercial supply chains, together with the product liability issues of a potential global customer base.

9. *Supply base caliber*. The caliber of the supply base needs to be vetted to a much higher degree in commercial supply chains. If failure of a link in the chain prevents initiation of a clinical study, that is an unsatisfactory outcome, but rectification in a simpler chain is likely to be more straightforward. A weak link in a commercial supply chain can mean disruption of an entire range of suppliers, partners, licensees, distributors, and most crucially, paying customers.

10. *Cost of goods*. The main emphasis in clinical trial supply chains is on delivering compliant test material to a site so that a study can be initiated without delay. There is little pressure to demonstrate processes designed to drive cost out. In commercial supply chains, the cost of goods receives intense attention from the financial and selling fraternities, with consequent pressure on reduction wherever possible.

11. *Distribution logistics*. The route to market in commercial supply chains is a complex network of wholesalers, clinics, specialist providers, and pharmacies. There are commercial implications that must be considered and dealt with. In clinical trials, the routes tend to be simpler and handled by specialist providers or express couriers.

12. *Packaging*. Commercial packaging involves hundreds, if not thousands, of items of artwork to be controlled and maintained. The processes of origination and reprographics need to be of high quality to meet customer expectations. Approvals can also be involved, as various sign-offs for legal, medical, marketing, supply chain, and manufacturing aspects are required. This can result in extended lead times and complexity.

13. *Change control*. The requirement for impact assessments and verification and validation of changes for marketed products, especially through the end-to-end supply chain, is demanding. In clinical trial supply chains, the process is simpler, by virtue of the reduced scope.

These are significant differences in demand in the supply chain. In terms of the metaphor above, the child has been parented to live in a smart Manhattan apartment block and actually finds itself in the back streets of one of New York's most deprived areas.

A *Helpful Metaphor* (continued)

The baby moved from infant to toddler to young child to teenager. The cosseted upbringing meant that this youngster was not streetwise, so life could be tough. What if it were to fall victim to those around who would take advantage?

As luck would have it, though, the patent protection fairy arrived on time to save the day. She gives the nervous teenager a telling piece of advice. "You have a huge inheritance," she says. "You will be able to draw on that whenever you need to. So you must share and share alike with those around you and life should be fine. There will be no need to learn the tricks of the trade in back-street New York." So that's what happened. The inheritance was there and life was fine for the adolescent—for a period of time, at least.

The metaphor describes the patent protection that drugs enjoy after approval. This is a period where the competition of back-street New York (generics or biosimilars) is held at bay. Little competition means little change. Little change means little improvement.

5.4 COMMERCIAL SUPPLY UNDER THE PATENT PROTECTION UMBRELLA

The analysis that follows relates to branded pharmaceuticals while the drug is covered by patent protection. The issues discussed relate to the special competitive environment that exists during this period.

5.4.1 Limited Competitive Alternatives

The threat of meaningful alternative products is low under patent protection compared with almost any other sector. There are two main factors at work here. First, the long development lead times means that the first to market can gain a huge lead against follow-on products from competitors. Second, even when another product is close behind, the medical components of the label claim can act as a differentiator in the eyes of medical practitioners, patients, and payers. So with strong promotional marketing behind a persuasive scientific and medical rationale for differentiation, substitutes can be kept from having any meaningful impact on revenues.

5.4.2 Fragmentation

Pharmaceuticals is a highly fragmented industrial sector, with no single company holding more than 8% of market share (it was 5% in the mid-1990s). Entrants arrive (e.g., fast-growing companies such as Shire and Cephalon), but their overall contribution to competitive pressures in such a fragmented environment has had little impact. In general, therefore, new entrants to the market make little difference to the level of competitive activity that pervades the sector. Although the rise of virtual drug developers threatened to turn this around somewhat, in practice none have got to market unaided by big pharma partners. Most don't even get beyond phase I clinical trials.

5.4.3 Supplier Power

At this stage of development, things start to become interesting in relation to supply chains. By virtue of historical development, the power within the supply base is significant. In Chapter 9 we delve into this in more detail. For the sake of understanding the issue at a high level, it is this: Few strategic procurement competencies are exercised through drug development. Just by studying the typical composition of a project team in pharma, it becomes clear that no representatives are engaged with those competencies. This can lead to a number of issues.

Adverse Supplier Selection   Volumes tend to be low, and the development fraternity generally find themselves with little supplier choice in markets where the spending they have to offer is relatively minor. For example, some of raw and starting materials will have high volume futures for the potential interest of a raft of qualified suppliers, creating meaningful competition. Commercial-scale APIs and drug products are always likely to be of key importance, as there is a strong need for mutual buyer–seller relationships. The time to identify appropriate suppliers (CMOs) and to build this relationship is in the development stage. The groundwork required to do this is seldom, if ever, carried out. Often, there is capitulation on key factors such as price and delivery—and sometimes even quality.

Lock-In   Chosen supplier(s) have to be registered in the regulatory filing, so they acquire power instantly by virtue of either total or partial exclusivity. Suppliers are keenly aware of this. In my experience, many fine chemical suppliers will know the exact requirements for their chemical intermediates or APIs in the products of prospective customers. They do this by researching financial analysts' reports of projected sales revenues for a compound. From the estimated selling price per unit, they work out how many units of product these projections convert to. Knowing how much of their product is contained in the final product, they can work out the total requirement. Therefore, when negotiating for the supply business, they can tell if they are likely to be the sole source or will be sharing with others. Very often they make the welcome discovery that they are going to be the sole source. It does not take a genius to predict their stance on key factors such as price in the upcoming negotiation.

Outsourcing of Drug Product Manufacture   Outsourced arrangements for drug product (now a widespread reality) is another potential issue. The development of a dosage form is often based on the CMO's long-term experience of processing and regulatory filing preparation for similar products for other customers. More often than not, it can be impossible to find a second source (even if it had been considered) able to replicate the product performance and supporting data of the primary supplier. Even if it were the case, time scales to bring a second source on board often extend beyond the filing submission date, so they have to be left behind as a possible variation in the future. In the procurement mindset, this screams out "strategic relationship" with the CMO. If the buying company cannot go anywhere else, how is it going to incentivize the CMO to share aims and objectives in the market? The horrible truth is that this is not going to happen. The potential for the buying company to engage the CMO in costly activities to grow their market, for no added benefit to them, is remote.

Drug developers may argue that they build strong, sharing relationships with their CMOs, and I am certain that this belief is genuinely held. However, the vast majority of supply contracts signed with CMOs contain disclaimers (in capital letters) against any liability over and above giving customers their money back should things go wrong. There will also probably be an annual price escalation clause in their contract as well as a limit on access to the CMO's premises for audit inspection and a whole raft of risk-averse clauses that the client must accept to clinch the deal. I have personal experience of a key account executive at one of the world's largest manufacturing and packing CMOs who warned that there was no possibility of a contract being signed by their lawyers until the drug launch was completed. Again, what would be the power position of the buying company if that were the case? How would they contain their cost base for the product as the market matured?

Let's conclude this section with one final example.

Observations, Views, and Experiences of the Author

A few years ago I undertook a request for proposal (RFP) exercise on behalf of a UK-based biotech client. It was for packaging and labeling of blister cards into cartons with a patient information leaflet included. There was nothing remarkable in the requirement. The RFP detailed our work requirements, projected volumes, and the key suggested heads of terms for the business arrangement. I selected a short list of candidates to receive the RFP. Two were well-known pharma specialists who were used throughout the industry across all phases of development into commercial manufacture. The third was a specialist packaging company that operated mainly in generics, medical devices, and food. This third company was a preferred supplier to the UK arm of the largest generics company in the world at the time (now number two), so I knew they had been successful on audit with a big pharma. They had also been approved by the MHRA, the UK's licensing authority.

The responses I received back were surprising, to say the least. The established CMOs sent proposals that were based on assumptions made to fit the simplest case for them. One of them assumed that an identical carton could be used for the three difference blister sizes. This would give them a single setup and maximum volume throughput. The other has stipulations on running all three products together just four times a year, again to make life simpler for them. Both also declared that the costs were indicative only, subject to confirmation. In other words, they did not want to commit until we were closer to becoming captive. There were also quite sizable costs in there for various add-on activities, such as receiving and releasing product, validation of equipment, auditing the input supplier, and developing protocols. So from these two bidders I received proposals that I couldn't rely on unless I stuck to limiting assumptions. There was no breakdown of cost as requested in the RFP document; and in execution, I would be charged for anything on top of the basic requirement of putting blisters in boxes.

The third proposer was different in a pleasing way. There was a complete breakdown of cost for the exercise. It detailed, to four decimal places, the cost of labor, carton, leaflet, outer packaging, and even the transport costs to have those items delivered. It also gave the cost of packaging origination, which the other bidders had failed to provide.

The price comparison calculation showed the first two bids to be in a similar ballpark (once the first bidder had recalculated his pricing on three different carton sizes). The third bid was nearly 2.5 times lower. Yes, just to repeat, it was 2.5 times lower! When I asked the second bidder to confirm the cost of a carton, it came back as approximately 30 cents. The equivalent in the third bidder quote was 10 cents.

There were also no add-on costs from the third bidder. Let's be honest, those "costs" the others were quoting for are basically fixed costs over the short to medium term. No new quality control person, for example, would have to be hired to cope with my extra activities. So although at some time in the future, the extra activity from me may lead to an extra recruit, that was going to be more than compensated for by the revenues generated by my business in the meantime.

The third bidder's proposed packaging method (from the choices available) was to use a semiautomatic setup. This was more labor intensive than the fully automatic proposals from the other two bidders, since machinery was used only to open and close the carton, while the operators hand-fed the blisters into the carton. It was, however, more than adequate to cope with the launch volumes and did not have the changeover capacity leakages associated with fully automatic lines. This meant that they could be flexible on run sizes and make deliveries within days. I knew they could do that because I had worked as interim purchasing manager at a large Generics company and had sourced product from them in practice.

This tale is meant to illustrate the challenge ahead in transitioning to supply chains where meaningful improvements in cost, quality, and delivery performance can take place. The third bidder, of course, was used to dealing with customers in competitive markets. These customers needed transparency of cost so that they could understand what could be done to improve their cost base. This is what the Japanese were so successful at and it was they who drove the open-book costing relationships that exist today in other sectors.

As an addendum to the case, it should be reported that there was, in the end, no requirement for a packaging contractor. The phase III study that would have called for commercial packaging failed to meet its endpoint, and there was no launch. If that had not happened, however, an interesting situation would have emerged. By far the most effective solution provider was a relatively small outfit without the "big player" compliance accoutrements of the other two bidders. Convincing the client that this third bidder was a suitable candidate to do the job would have been an uphill task, probably with less than a 50% chance of success. Hopefully, mindsets will open in the future. Certainly today, this mindset is a major inhibitor to learning and progress in our supply base.

5.4.4   The Position of Those Buying Pharmaceutical Products

In the branded pharmaceuticals market, the buyer is in a weak position, as we all know. This is reflected in the selling price, as the product will be greatly differentiated by virtue of the fact that no other producer has it to sell. The rationale for the price is that the company must recover the costs of research and development of the product. This is principally the cost of all the failures (see Chapter 1) that the company has to endure in the course of bringing this and other drugs through their pipeline.

Another complicating factor is that it is not normally the patient that actually foots the bill, nor is it the pharma manufacturer that sells the product to whoever is paying—it is an intermediary in the distribution channel. The wholesaler typically purchases product from the pharmaceutical manufacturers according to arrangements based on wholesale acquisition cost or average wholesale price. It is at this point that ownership transfers from pharma to the wholesale channel. The wholesaler will be keen to get the product into their hands since it will be a guaranteed seller. Historically, wholesaler dealer margins have been relatively contained. One counterbalance to this historical situation is the increase in "me-too" generics and niche-indication drugs. In these situations, the pharma company would never be able to get its product to patients without the wholesalers. There is no threat of those smaller companies setting up alternative facilities (that is, at least, a theoretical possibility for the big pharmas). The net result is that the entire distribution network is in the hands of third parties; none of it is owned by the pharmas, not even the ability to collect cash from customers. That is all embedded in the channel network. Increasingly, pharmas need the wholesaler to get their products to customers and receive cash in return.

This has started to place wholesalers in a more powerful position. Consolidation over recent years now means that the three largest wholesalers (McKesson, Cardinal Health, and Amerisource-Bergen) account for 80% of the channel traffic in the United States—which is power concentrated in very few hands. Again, then, any company that does not have the alternative of delivering a service itself, and the service is a necessity, is in a weaker position when it comes to bargaining. In the United

States, wholesalers routinely deliver to approximately 55,000 outlets for prescription medicines on a daily basis.[1] No one is going to believe even the biggest big pharma company if they said they could achieve it themselves.

This highlights a developing dynamic that readers should bear in mind, discussed in the next section. The net result of all this is a market where competition is weak. Since this is not a treatise on competitive strategy, however, the discussion will end here, to focus on the consequences for the supply chain.

5.5 WHAT THIS MEANS FOR THE PHARMACEUTICAL SUPPLY CHAIN

5.5.1 The Regulators Attempt to Help

However the causal links are traced, we are left with supply chains dogged by issues arising from a lifetime of neglect in the competitive environment described above. In the absence of industry attention on the supply chain, the regulators have attempted to take a lead. At times, this has done more harm than good. Our next guest contributor, Chris Oldenhof, explains.

GUEST CONTRIBUTOR SLOT: CHRIS OLDENHOF

The Regulatory Paradox

Regulations aimed at protecting patient safety are achieving the opposite. Developing and subsequently amending pharma regulations usually has one major objective: optimal protection of patient safety. However, in an increasing number of cases, the results have been exactly the opposite of what was aimed for.

In striving to improve the protection of patient safety, regulators have adhered to the following principle: "The more, and stricter, the pharma regulations, the better." The choice of developing ever stricter regulations can be made and can be defended: It implies that society is willing to pay the higher prices for medicines that result from the ever-increasing costs of compliance with the regulations. However, several implications of such an approach should not be overlooked:

1. The regulations should remain workable. When regulations become overly complex, making compliance at times impossible, the entire regulatory system will gradually lose its credibility.
2. Ever-increasing costs of compliance continually increase the gap between the manufacturing costs of compliant and noncompliant products.
3. Therefore, compliant manufacturers should be protected against having to compete against noncompliant producers because such competition will push compliant manufacturers out of business.
4. The only means of preventing illicit competition is a system of adequate, strict authority oversight and enforcement.

Examples of the Regulatory Paradox   Examples of API-related regulations that have resulted in significantly decreased patient safety are:

- Regulations requiring compliance with ICH Q7 GMP
- EU variations regulations and related procedures
- U.S. post approval change authorization regulations and related procedures

The procedures relating to these strict regulations are highly complex, and in the latter two cases even frequently unworkable. But they have one other important thing in common: the almost complete lack of authority oversight and enforcement.

As a result of the implementation of these regulations, the "competitive advantage of noncompliance" has increased dramatically. Players choosing noncompliance as their strategy find themselves operating in a competitive Walhalla: Market leaders with high ethics began to lose their competitiveness, for one API product after the other, in a market of cutthroat competition where a few dollars of price difference per kilogram of API is decisive. As a result, more and more noncompliant, unsafe APIs are being included in our medicines. Today in the off-patent pharmaceutical market segment the safety of APIs has decreased to a level that constitutes a large, growing, and often unknown risk—this in stark contrast to a regulatory API environment that has formally become much stricter but in which players easily get away with noncompliance and even with fraudulent practices.

Awareness of these issues is gradually increasing. Serious health scares, such as the 2008 heparin affair, have started to show that undermining API safety leads to fatal health incidents and may ultimately lead to large health catastrophes.

The United States and the European Union have set in motion legislative trajectories that should ultimately reinforce the pharma supply chain in an adequate manner. But the road toward that goal is still long and winding and progress is slow. It must be hoped that it will not require a full-blown health catastrophe to occur to motivate health authorities sufficiently to fix this serious problem once and for all with the very highest priority.

These are sobering words from Chris, given his standing in the industry. The puzzling thing for me when I first read this piece was why companies were looking to cut back on costs and take risks on input materials. These should always be a relatively minor component of total cost. The author believes that two factors are operating here. First, savings in API purchase cost are relatively easy to chase down compared with addressing some of the more substantive changes needed in the supply chain (discussed throughout the book). *Offshoring,* as it has come to be known, is operating widely in the pharmaceuticals market.

The market for out-of-patent products is completely different from that for branded products. This *is* a competitive market, to the extent where it is diametrically opposed to branded pharma. It is gloves-off time. At this stage, the selling price of the drug is dramatically less than that of the branded version, and the innovator company normally drops the drug, allowing the out-of-patent folks to fight over the remnants. Every penny counts, so savings in API costs are all worth having, to bulk up those scant margins.

The second cost-cutting factor is where the trouble starts for people like Chris and for his company. The barriers are down for many suppliers to enter the market, all pitching for business. The name of the game is "price," and this is where temptation must exist to compete "unfairly," as Chris describes it. There is no way to ensure that suppliers have remained compliant in the production processes—unless, of course, the manufacturer of the original branded product had stayed in the market, operating the well-established, compliant, and mature processes that had been working previously over the life of supply patients. For that to happen, the manufacturer would need to have a cost-effective supply chain running in order to accommodate the reduced selling price. The out-of-patent guys can do it—why can't branded pharma?

There is another important issue for pharma supply chains: Should regulators hold sole responsibility for influencing industrial practices? Can it be done through regulations and guidelines alone? Chris argues not and even suggests that regulations can make matters worse, in the way he describes.

We leave this point for the time being and return to it in Chapter 17. Next, we pick up on issues involved in the development process itself. Again we hear from Chris as he recounts his previous experiences in explaining some of these issues to the FDA. I learned of this through an email exchange with Chris that arose when trying to understand how sponsor companies could obtain access to information contained in a drug master file (DMF). Chris confirmed that perhaps they I couldn't. The entire content of a U.S. DMF is strictly confidential, so information from the holder will only be provided voluntarily. Even though my supplier of API was scaling the process up 2.5 times and outsourcing a key intermediate offshore, I might not be allowed to know anything about that. How I was to maintain control over the supply chain pedigree puzzled me then and it puzzles me now. It seemed to be a case of supplier confidentiality being more important than patient safety.

Anyway, that aside, Chris explained that I might not succeed in getting detailed information from the DMF and also explained how the system worked. As the exchange continued and we explored these issues further, Chris laid it out in an email message.

GUEST CONTRIBUTOR SLOT (*continued*)

The FDA should (hopefully) be aware of the big problem of change control in complex supply chains. The first time I confronted them with it was through a presentation I gave in 1997(!) at an FDA/AAPS organized event in Arlington called the "BACPAC Workshop" for an audience of about 400, including some 70 FDA staff. I remember having made an overhead sheet showing an incredibly complex supply structure of intermediates and APIs in the beta-lactam antibiotics segment; it looked like a spider web with all the producers and the many supplier–customer relationships at the API level and at intermediate levels. I then mentioned that the picture was a simplification of what the supply looked like in reality. Then I described a situation of a process change to be implemented upstream somewhere in the center of that spider web and asked the audience for advice on how to get that approved through the current FDA regulatory system. A deep silence followed that I left to continue for perhaps 10 seconds. It was wonderful. Then I concluded that we all had a problem—and I don't think anybody disagreed with that.

The head of CDER's Office of Pharmaceutical Science in those days looked quite shocked and spoke with me afterward. If I'm not mistaken, this was perhaps one of the first sparks that may ultimately have ignited FDA's 21st Century Initiative (through something began in 2000 called the FDA CMC Risk-Based Review project).

It did not end there. As he explained the DMF regulations in some more detail, he made some comments and suggestions that made absolute sense. He was talking about strategic relationships between customers and suppliers. Below is the piece in full.

GUEST CONTRIBUTOR SLOT (*continued*)

The entire DMF system (first in the United States, later in Europe) was developed in the first place specifically to enable the API manufacturer to submit confidential information to the authorities without having to share this "company core know-how" on process details with the (A)NDA or MA holders! Certain process details may be critical for the continuity of an API manufacturer because they determine his competitive advantage. So there may be very good reasons for not disclosing information in the closed part to the (A)NDA or MA holder. I know, for example, of situations in which the MA holder is also a direct competitor of the DMF holder in the API market.

Also note that when there is no DMF at all (but instead, e.g., only a CEP), the companies still need to find appropriate ways of handling change together. I think it is a false assumption that postapproval change can be managed through the regulatory submission system: It should, instead, be managed by the companies together.

"Closed parts" and "open parts" of DMFs exist only in Europe (officially called "AIM restricted part" and "applicant's part"); the U.S. DMF is entirely "closed," but of course the dosage form manufacturer will need certain parts of the included information, and API manufacturers and dosage form manufacturers should arrange for that in good cooperation. Optimal cooperation on upstream postapproval changes should be the aim. The quality agreement also plays a role in this.

It will also have to come from two sides: Sharing important, possibly confidential information with your API supplier is also something you should consider seriously. It will create better mutual understanding of how upstream changes could have an impact on downstream operations. So the closer you can get to having the two companies cooperate on postapproval change as if they were in fact one company, the better you will together be managing change.

On the other hand: Suppose that you are a generic company sourcing 900 different APIs from 300 different suppliers. It will be a huge challenge to manage all these relationships in this way.

Last but not least: A supplier who doesn't inform customers about changes that require supplements (or even annual reporting) or variations is a supplier who doesn't comply with the regulations: Only his customers can submit supplements and variations

It should be noted that the underlying message here does not relate to the merits of regulatory changes per se. It is about the difficulty of predicting the impact of positively motivated amendments when they are incorporated into complex interrelated systems. Who would have thought that raising quality standards could actually lead to inferior quality! This is the "systemic" world we live in. However, we recall from earlier in the book that there is no such thing as a quick fix in the world of supply chain improvement. It requires only(!) continuation of the search for longer-term answers. This will form the basis for some recommendations that we save for Chapter 17.

5.5.2   Quality and Resources in Perspective

In the next section, Marla Phillips lends her wealth of expertise to discuss some of the misperceptions of the role of quality and resource allocation that can severely affect supply chain performance.

GUEST CONTRIBUTOR SLOT: MARLA PHILLIPS

Resources: Why Do Regulators Care?

Thank you for the introduction Hedley. It is such a pleasure to work with a supply chain expert who is passionate in describing the criticality of quality involvement throughout the supply chain, across functional roles, and during the entire product/process life cycle. As Hedley indicated previously, ICH Q8 requires quality by design, which in turn requires ownership of quality by all professionals in our industry—quality control staff are no longer the police. So it is important to note here that my discussion about resources is not an attempt to build a monstrous quality organization but, rather, to ensure that those affecting the safety, efficacy, and quality of the final product have enough time and training to protect us all (let's face it, we and our friends and family members all take these drugs!).

One issue with the police role of a quality organization is that there is virtually no way for the organization to have enough employees to do the job they are charged with. To do that you would need one quality professional for every person in the process. This is why ICH Q8 has to be embraced by the entire organization rather than simply listing the principles of ICH Q8 in an SOP.

I have audited many firms, even recently, including big pharma, where the role of quality was the traditional role of policing the operations, and have often found myself raising my eyebrows as the quality professional describes all the daily activities that he or she (for simplicity, let's go with "he") has to perform. As he describes his daily duties, I find myself wondering how thorough a job he is doing and how it is possible that one person can be an expert in so many things. I quickly identify some key areas to delve into to assess the work he is doing: How is he protecting the safety of my friends and family? It is this eyebrow-raising experience that bothers most regulators and results in accusations that the quality organization is understaffed.

Here are a few examples of the problems associated with a traditional Quality Organization that is overworked and undertrained:

1. *From big pharma.* I took a tour of a fully enclosed nonsterile tablet manufacturing facility and had to gown in a full bunny suit with an oxygen mask and boots. The process involved took us 15 minutes, which was followed by wiping our gloves and suit with wipes (I was never clear on the purpose of this step). I looked around in disbelief, and actually wondered if I was being televised as some part of a practical joke. But I wasn't—and remember, this was a nonsterile facility. At the end of the tour, the employees were smiling as they talked about the cleanliness of their facility, but then I asked how often quality assurance representatives go out into production, since I couldn't imagine them going through the gowning process very often. The employees proudly said that quality staff is required to go out into production once each week, and they document this in a log book. Of course, I was thinking "Yikes!" Later when I reviewed investigations, it was clear that the quality staff didn't understand the process very well, and didn't have a presence in the manufacturing areas to observe real-time operations. The investigations were poor and rarely identified true root causes. But the facility was clean. This obviously is not a good use of financial or personnel resources.

2. *From virtual pharma.* A quality assurance professional explained all the responsibilities she had on a daily basis, which were too numerous to count. Again, my concern was with what level of thoroughness she doing any of her job responsibilities. She was proud that all the complaints were up to date and closed. However, when I reviewed the complaint system, I was very concerned that she felt her main role was to ensure that complainants received their complimentary bottle of drugs. There was never an investigation as to why the issue occurred, where it occurred (at the facility or in the hands of the consumer, etc.), how many other lots were affected, or the severity of the complaint. And, of course, you can imagine that a trend analysis was never conducted. Again, her responsibilities were too numerous to count, so there was no way that she was going to be able to do most of them properly, or have time to be trained in how to do them.

3. *Contract operations.* I am still amazed at how many organizations are designed to rely on the quality control systems of their contract facility, without having quality systems themselves. A proper quality agreement might be established between the sponsor company and the contract organization, but that agreement is treated as a piece of paper rather than a living document. When a deeper inspection is taken of the elements of the quality agreement, it becomes apparent that the system is built like a house of cards. The sponsor company often has SOPs to describe the

oversight of the contract operations, but in fact, the sponsor company accepts at face value what is given to them. There is no investigation, verification, or effort put into understanding what is occurring at the contract facility. Often, the sponsor company feels that resources for the quality organization can be cut drastically, because the contract facility has its own quality organization. As a result, I have seen case after case of investigations being approved that have no root cause identified. It was interesting when one contract organization told me that they don't get paid if the root cause is assigned to something they did wrong. We had this discussion when every investigation I reviewed listed the root cause as "No laboratory error." The data were being accepted as valid when there was no possible scientific way that the data could be real. [As an example, a dissolution value of 150% was accepted for a capsule product, where 150% of the material couldn't even fit inside the capsule; it wasn't scientifically possible that this could be a valid number.] It does not take long before the data and trends associated with the data become meaningless. What could be more out of control than that? Organizations involved in contract operations need to have sufficient staff members of proper expertise overseeing the operations.

4. *Across the board*. The reader might find it interesting that I am also concerned when companies use fully compliant manual systems—yes, fully compliant. The reason I am concerned is that it is rare that those companies are able to accurately track open and closed occurrences, or to conduct a trend analysis. A good example of this is the CAPA (corrective and preventative action) system. CAPAs are especially difficult to track manually, because they can remain open for extended periods of time. In concept, the process for tracking might be compliant, but I have never seen a manual system that is in a state of control. In addition, I am concerned with the personnel resources being expended to manage the manual system. Employees need to focus their time on ensuring product safety and efficacy, not on managing a manual system.

The examples above would result in increasing the resources within the quality organization, because the firms have chosen to continue with the traditional role of quality personnel policing the operations. Regulators are concerned with the use of resources in this way for many reasons: (1) the employees cannot possibly perform all the job functions they are charged with; (2) the employees are not experts in the functions they are asked to perform (quality professionals given authority over process validation when they are not engineers, over laboratory operations when they don't understand the laboratory, etc.); (3) the presence of overworked employees typically means that even less training is provided since there is no time to stop; and (4) the organization as a whole moves further and further from truly understanding and embracing the expectations for quality throughout the process. On the contrary, Hedley will continue the argument of how modernization principles result in an overall reduction in head count when properly put into practice. Not easy at first, but completely necessary.

Once again, an experienced practitioner and consultant such as Marla has a surprising tale to tell.

5.5.3   Supply Chain Management Processes and Competencies in Pharma

The final point to raise in the performance issues in pharma supply chains relates to the lack of supply chain management processes and competencies in pharmaceuticals through the product life cycle. Below I synthesize a typical illustrative job from the various recruitment sites operating on the Internet. It is framed around a requirement for a person to assume management of an outsourced pharmaceutical supply chain. This role would typically hold responsibility for end-to-end forecasting of requirements, supplier appraisal and contract negotiation, issue of production schedules, cost of goods improvement, coordination of storage and transportation providers, and so on. There would, of course, be technical requirements alongside these competencies.

This is a typical candidate profile:

- The person has experience in pharmaceutical development and manufacturing.
- The candidate has an excellent understanding and hands-on working knowledge of cGMP, quality, and regulatory requirements for clinical and commercial material.
- The person has demonstrated an ability to manage outsourced manufacturing and quality control contractors successfully.
- The position requires a degree in a relevant scientific discipline.

Scarce/custom-made materials specified Limited sourcing options Inappropriate dosage forms Contractors with insufficient capacity or capability Poor process yields Weak compliance with technical agreements	Inadequate transfer of analytical methods Shipping/storage conditions poorly specified Incorrect value customs declarations Weak contractor relationships Little knowledge of customer requirements Complex/overlapping channels ...the list goes on...

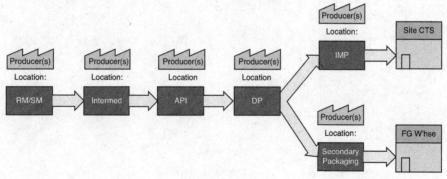

FIGURE 5.3   What is typically found when preparing for commercial launch.

No mention of any SCM competencies!

It should be mentioned that some of the big pharmas have made it a requirement for their supply chain management teams to study a formal qualification (APICS[2]–CPIM). Although this is a help, the issues we are discussing go much deeper than one group extending already existing competencies. Awareness and understanding need to be spread outside the SCM groups in the area we have discovered throughout this book that need to be on board. The position above, for example, does not stipulate any standard of competence in building and managing an outsourced supply chain. The impact of not having these people on board is demonstrated in Figure 5.3. This shows the type of issues in the clinical trial supply chain to be prepared for commercial launch which I encounter regularly.

At this point, hopefully a conclusive case has been presented and a verdict of guilty returned. There is much more evidence out there for readers to find if they are prepared to look. For those who are still not convinced, the case is adjourned for the time being as we start to build a knowledge base.

PART II
Building a Knowledge Foundation in SCM

6 Supply Chain Management as a Competitive Weapon

6.1 COMPETITION AND BUSINESS STRATEGY

Routes to success in business competition have been explored for many years by a whole host of economic and financial pundits and business schools around the globe. Plumbing to the depths typically reached in those learned analyzes cannot be contemplated within the scope of this book. That should not, however, be reason to ignore the topic, especially in relation to the role of SCM in business competition and competitive strategy. The driver for this is the idea that SCM rarely, if ever, creeps onto the radar of most business schools. Given the messages on customer value in Chapter 2 and the critical link between the supply chain and realization of customer value, isn't that something of a puzzle to be solved? Hopefully, the puzzle can begin to be unraveled through discussion here, and some underlying principles established.

To begin, some of the business basics should be covered. Companies compete to achieve their objectives. Readers will be familiar with profit, turnover, and market share objectives, for example. There is a plethora of others that can be added to the pot, and the majority of companies will have some mechanism to record, articulate, and monitor progress against their agreed objectives. From this, a company must decide how it is going to deliver against the objectives. This is, of course, the business strategy—the means by which the objectives will be met, or not, as the case may be. Strategy in business is a much used term and often means different things to different people. The definition used here is: *Strategy is the general plan or direction selected to accomplish objectives.*[1] This chapter is about how supply chain management can contribute in the fight to execute business strategies.

This vital link between the holistic of supply chain management and organizational success will be a repeating theme explored throughout the remaining text. Before moving forward, it may be helpful to introduce some well-used models relating to competitive success in business. Much of this draws on the work of Michael Porter,[2] and the limited scope in this book in relation to business strategy has prevented inclusion or analysis of many other models. The aim here has been to include enough general frameworks to drive home the SCM messages, and Porter's seem to do that admirably. We start with a non-Porter but equally well-used model, the marketing mix.

6.2 THE MARKETING MIX

Often called the "four P's," the marketing mix identifies four variables that can influence the purchase decision and hence competitive advantage: product (or service), price, promotion, and place. Clearly, the performance and characteristics of the *product* are important, but not to the exclusion of all else. Customers may be willing to forgo some additional benefits for the sake of a more affordable price. Equally, a well-promoted and positioned product may win customers over, and for some customers, having convenient access to the product may be a clincher.

SCM has a role to play in all four of these areas. The product is the output from the supply chain. The way it is designed must be interpreted in terms of processes joined together to deliver according to the final concept. Designers and their supply chain partners must operate in unison to consistently produce a differentiated product.

Even though *price* is not always based on the cost to produce, without proper control over the cost to manufacture and supply, a business has limited scope to compete on price with more cost-effective competitors. The areas where effective SCM can affect costs are wide and various. These include procurement of input materials that perform up to improved standards, building relationships with suppliers that deliver long-term benefits, scheduling of plant and equipment to get the most out of them, reducing working capital investment in inventory, and driving out costs associated with the movement of product around the globe. This is just a small sample of the impact that SCM can have on cost, which has an impact on price, which has an impact on competitive advantage. In Chapters 7 to 13 we expand significantly on this.

Promotion of a product may seem totally unconnected with the supply chain. However, a little thought reveals that presentation of the advantages of any competitive offering requires a supply chain to manufacture promotional materials and aids which in themselves must be better than those of the competition.

Finally, the *place* where the offering is made available often requires SCM support. If the product is readily available exactly where the customer wants it, this may prompt a purchase in preference to a competitive product that cannot be made available in the same way. This makes the point that SCM is a vital component of business strategy formulation. No business would consider forming a strategy without involving the finance team. Some options may be completely unaffordable. Others may seem out of reach, but some creative funding vehicle might be available to bridge a gap. The discussion must always involve the financial aspect. Similarly, the supply chain should be represented in a coherent fashion.

6.3 PORTER'S FIVE FORCES

The five-forces model has competitive rivalry in any sector as a central force acted on by four other influencing forces: the threat of new entrants (or conversely, barriers to entry), the power of buyers, the power of suppliers, and the threat of substitutes. The take-home point from this model is that in markets or sectors where entry is relatively easy, where substitutes threaten, and where power is in the hands of either suppliers or buyers, competition for customers is likely to be strong and sustainable profits hard to find. If the reverse is the case, competition will be much less in evidence and the possibility of earning substantial profits much more likely.

An important term here is *sustainable*. In the short term, clever entrepreneurs may discover a novel new product that cannot be matched at that time. There will be a window of opportunity to be seized and capitalized upon. The length and scale of that window is largely influenced by the nature of competition within that industry sector. In some markets, that window is typically relatively short-lived as competitors learn to replicate the offering and create their own competitive advantage to build market share. In other markets, competition may find it difficult to gain a foothold, for reasons that exist in that particular sector. The factors influencing this propensity toward competitive rivalry are those in the five-forces model.

6.4   PORTER'S GENERIC COMPETITIVE STRATEGIES

Porter defined three basic generic strategies: cost leadership, differentiation, and focus. The first two he identifies as the main alternative approaches: low cost to give the option to compete on lowest price, against a more differentiated offering that may be more expensive. The third strategy of focus relates to the provision of a very specialized offering to a narrow, niche-type market.

As with all general approaches, there are shades of gray and caveats that operate. For example, Porter emphasizes that cost leadership must also meet certain minimum criteria for equivalence with differentiators in the sector. The point is that lowest price must also conform to the fit-for-purpose expectations of the customer. This leads to the thought that perhaps these strategies are not, and should not be, mutually exclusive and, in fact, that a business must differentiate itself from the competition through a unique mixture of cost (price) and added value (differentiation), a mix known as *competitive advantage*. More will be said about this later, but for now it is time to consider the practical evidence. The final Porter model is his value chain.

6.5   PORTER'S VALUE CHAIN

The next and final model to be included is probably the most informative for SCM. As a unifying vehicle for dialogue on principles, Porter's work[3] contains valuable insights. The text was probably not aimed specifically at the supply chain management practitioner, since the book is accepted almost universally as a seminal text focused on business strategy. However, careful reading unearths a wealth of observations that speak volumes for the potential of professional SCM practices to substantially influence competitive edge. The message in his book is clear although not spelled out explicitly. That is, the supply chain contains the primary activities that drive value and cost in the search for competitive advantage. That advantage generates sales that, net of cost, deliver a profit margin.

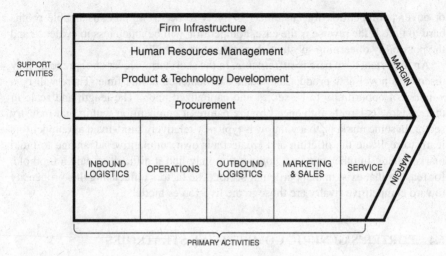

FIGURE 6.1   Generic value chain. (From Michael Porter, *Competitive Advantage: Creating and Sustaining Superior Performance*, Free Press, New York, 1985.)

Figure 6.1 depicts the model as described in the book. In very basic terms, the model asserts that firms must engage in multiple *activities* to create *value* that ultimately must be greater than the *cost* of those activities, so that a firm can generate a profit *margin* to allow it to survive and, potentially, grow. *Value* less *cost* equals *margin*. Value is nothing other than the money that customers are willing to pay—it is a "sharp end" measure. No amount of alleged value-adding activity can be claimed unless a paying customer nods her head. Similarly, cost is the hard expenditure of cash incurred when running a business. These two parameters must move in opposing directions to deliver and maintain competitive advantage consistently.

The model categorizes a firm's activities into two types: primary and support. This does not imply any hierarchy in the activities. Rather, it distinguishes those activities involved directly in conversion, demand generation, and placement of physical goods into customers' hands from those activities necessary to support, indirectly, value generation and delivery to the customer. Both sets of activities have the potential to create competitive advantage.

The main elements of the model can be summarized as follows:

- *Primary activities:* all the activities required to produce, deliver, sell, and service the final product:
  - *Inbound logistics:* activities associated with receiving, storing, and making available all the inputs required for operations.
  - *Operations:* activities necessary to transform inputs into outputs. These include operations such as machining, blending, filtering, freeze drying, packaging, and testing. The implicit assumption is that the transformation creates outputs that are more valuable than the sum of the inputs.

- *Outbound logistics:* activities related to shipping, sales order processing, and warehousing, for example. Although the Porter model refers to finished-goods warehousing, it should be borne in mind that at lower tiers in the supply chain, outbound logistics would be concerned with partly finished products that are not intended for consumers.
- *Marketing and sales:* activities focused on providing a means for purchasers to buy products and providing a stimulus to purchase. These activities link closely with the four P's above and include pricing, promotion, channel selection, and channel relations.
- *After-sales service:* activities that include provision of service and spare parts, installation, and customer training.
- *Support activities:* activities that support the primary activities and help differentiate the offering. They are categorized under the following headings:
  - *Firm infrastructure:* activities defined as supporting the entire chain rather than individual activities. Included here are general management, finance and accounting, information systems, quality management, and government affairs (in the case of pharmaceuticals, presumably including regulatory affairs). Porter uses the example of a telephone operating company gaining significant competitive advantage by maintaining effective relationships with regulatory bodies.
  - *Human resources:* activities such as recruiting, training, motivating, and rewarding staff are included. Competitive advantage can be gained here by attracting talent and developing critical skill sets that are needed to perform in the particular industry sector. This is an area where the Japanese, particularly, have excelled by focusing heavily on "cultural" employee induction program and continual mentoring on the job.
  - *Technology development:* broadly, activities such as the means of preparing documents and transporting goods, and also aspects related to the product itself. This raises an interesting parallel with improvement in general, because the implication is that almost all activities utilize "technology," even though it may be very simple. To take the preparing documents example, a typewriter, word processor, photocopier, and computer printer are all technologies that can develop competitive advantage. This is a concept to be considered further in our exploration of improvement as a key SCM activity.
  - *Procurement:* an activity set that relates to the purchase of input materials by a business. It includes primary inputs such as raw materials, machinery and equipment, and production consumables, for example, and also supports activities such as laboratory and office supplies, computer hardware, and consultancy services. An important point made is that procurement occurs across the business and does not always receive due attention from those involved. In the book the case is made for improved procurement practices to strongly affect cost, quality, and other important business benefits.

A major assertion in the model is that competitive advantage can be enhanced through effective linkages. Porter expresses linkages as "the relationship between the way one value activity is performed and the *cost* or *performance* of another." That refers principally to individuals and groups working mutually to help them and others deliver the competitive advantage proposition. He defined two types of linkage, those within the value chain of a firm, and vertical linkages (between upstream and downstream firms). Within a firm's value chain, and vertically, linkages can be primary–primary, primary–secondary, and secondary–secondary. This is of profound significance to the relevance of SCM in business strategy. Why is that the case? It is because SCM is principally about creating linkages in product and information flow. These linkages can and should operate on value and cost along with the rest of the constituents in the organization carrying out the activities in Porter's value chain.

Once a reader understands the concept of linkages, it should begin to get easier to identify situations where these is risk of destroying competitive advantage by making certain business changes. Consider the following personal observation.

Observations, Views, and Experiences of the Author

This example relates to a period when I was supply chain head of a diagnostics plant in the UK. The site was supplying products to the U.S. and EU markets. The parent company was a well-known U.S. big pharma firm. The plant was operating in an extremely competitive environment and had fairly recently been acquired by the big pharma company. One of the early decisions made by the new parent company was to shut down the UK product development section and move it to the United States as a cost-saving measure. This seemed to be a sensible idea on the face of it, given that there was already a group in the United States. What they overlooked, of course, were the strong linkages that had been formed between the UK development scientists and the manufacturing plant. The company's ability to develop new products was impaired dramatically by this action over a significant period, as fresh but lower-quality linkages were formed painstakingly with an ocean in between. This was at a time when strategically, the company was under strong pressure from competitors that had broader range product offerings. It seems unlikely that anyone actually calculated the impact of the "cost saving" on sales revenue, but they might have had a shock if they had!

This example should hold deep significance at the highest management levels when decisions are taken "for the better," normally to reduce cost. The impact of this action on the supply chain set things back years, as the departing part of the shared know-how was no longer available to impart their pearls of wisdom on the nuances of materials and specifications. Joined-up thinking at the decision-making table would surely have recognized this as an issue and managed any transition accordingly; and this is what the author believes that Porter means, in essence, by linkages. It is what we colloquially call *joined-up thinking* (along with joined-up action).

This principle also applies to the practice of outsourcing. The outsourcing epidemic in pharma that has been spreading since the 1980s has a similar potential to obstruct competitive advantage. If it is not thought out and executed carefully, it can lead to *important* linkages being severed that materially affect the power to perform. This is because an internal linkage is different from an external one. The level of engagement and commitment and a company's ability to influence those things is much higher for an internal linkage. For example, take the case of a person working in product development for a company. Such a person is likely to be far more involved personally and with others in the product's future. Even if not, the organizational structures around the person will operate to keep things on track. There is more opportunity to control events. An externally linked provider of services may be equally concerned with success, but the future of the provider and the provider's company is unlikely to hang on it.

This is not normally an issue in the less strategic activities of a business, because standards of work can be specified and monitored. Whether the activity of product development falls in this category is doubtful in my opinion. Readers are requested to hold that thought—it will be explored more fully in later chapters.

Having now set the scene with models and examples, it is time to look more closely at some of the elements of building competitive strategies.

6.6   COMPETITIVE STRATEGY AND CUSTOMERS

There will be others operating in markets where your company has objectives set (unless it is a complete monopoly). This leads to competition for customers and determines the need for competitive positioning in relation to customer markets. We now examine a structured and powerful way to go about this: strategic marketing. Strategy is the "how" for businesses wishing to deliver on their objectives. Strategic marketing is therefore about how companies relate to their markets to achieve objectives such as penetration, increased market share, and sales growth. It is described here by a world-leading expert, Malcolm McDonald, a prolific writer on this subject and practicer of his own preaching, evidenced by his successes in the business world. The language used in his contribution is the language of business schools. This is important because one of the key aims of this book is to fit SCM squarely into the world of business and those who influence it.

GUEST CONTRIBUTOR SLOT: MALCOLM MCDONALD

The Essence of Strategic Marketing

Success in commercial markets today is measured in terms of shareholder value added, having taken account of the risks associated with declared future strategies, the time value of money, and the cost of capital. The only way in which sustainable shareholder value can be created is by making offers to target markets that utilize the entire organizational asset base and take account of the needs of all stakeholder groups. Although this obviously does not apply to the public sector, the basic principle is exactly the same Fundamental to success defined in this way is:

- A deep understanding of the market
- Correct needs-based segmentation
- Differential offers targeted at these segments
- Integrated strategic marketing plans

Many of the gurus over the past 50 years, including Kotler, Tom Peters and the chairman of Unilever, agree that these four items are the pillars of successful corporate performance. Market segmentation is one of the most fundamental concepts of marketing and is the key to successful business performance. It's fairly obvious that there is no such thing as an average customer or consumer—it's a bit like saying "my head is in the oven and my feet are in the fridge, so on average I am quite comfortable." Let's also get rid of nonsensical myths about market segmentation, such as the a priori nonsense about socioeconomics, demographics, geodemographics, and the like. Let me explain. Socioeconomic classifications such as A, B, C1, C2, D, and E are useful generic descriptions which I shall refer to later, but in themselves they can only be useful at a very general level. For example, the Archbishop of Canterbury and Boy George are both As because of their spending power, but their behavior is almost certainly very different. Similarly, demographics such as young women between the ages of 18 and 24 can only ever be useful as a very high and general indication of patterns of behavior because it is clear that not all 18- to 24-year-olds behave in the same way.

In a similar way, geodemographic classifications such as ACORN, which stands for a classification of regional neighborhoods, although useful for indicating very general patterns of spending power, do not reveal the absurd assumption that everyone in one street drives the same car, reads the same newspapers, eats the same food, and so on. Yet real segmentation remains the most difficult of all marketing methodologies to implement, which is why very few organizations do it properly. Indeed, a recent *Harvard Business Review* article revealed that the main reason for the failure of 30,000 new product launches in 2006 in the United States was inadequate market segmentation. So let us set out in a very straightforward way what market segmentation is and how it can be done properly.

6.6.1   The Market Segmentation Process

The process chart shown in Figure 6.2 describes a number of steps that need to be followed for successful segmentation. From this, you will see that the process begins with market mapping, which corresponds to a deep understanding of the market.

6.6.2   Market Mapping

Essentially market mapping entails drawing a map of the flows of goods and services from producers through to end use; including a number of junctions that have an

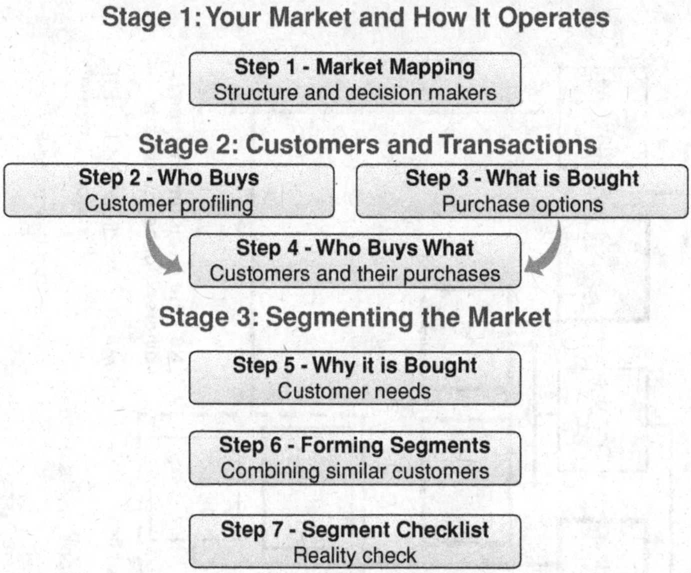

Stage 1: Your Market and How It Operates
Step 1 - Market Mapping
Structure and decision makers
Stage 2: Customers and Transactions
Step 2 - Who Buys
Customer profiling
Step 3 - What is Bought
Purchase options
Step 4 - Who Buys What
Customers and their purchases
Stage 3: Segmenting the Market
Step 5 - Why it is Bought
Customer needs
Step 6 - Forming Segments
Combining similar customers
Step 7 - Segment Checklist
Reality check

FIGURE 6.2 Market segmentation process.

influence on what is bought even though such influencers don't actually buy themselves. An example of this is architects, who don't buy radiators but who decide which type of radiator will go into which kind of building. The example of a generic market map in Figure 6.3 shows four major types of junctions, from suppliers through to end use. Where percentages and volumes or values are shown against junctions, it

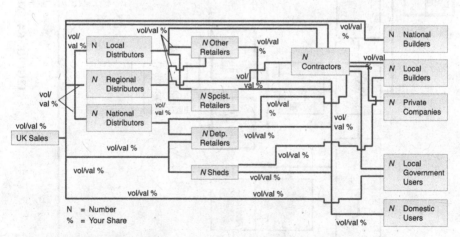

UK Sales
N Local Distributors
N Regional Distributors
N National Distributors
N Other Retailers
N Spcist. Retailers
N Detp. Retailers
N Sheds
N Contractors
N National Builders
N Local Builders
N Private Companies
N Local Government Users
N Domestic Users
vol/val %
N = Number
% = Your Share
NB. Sketch out complex junctions separately. Alternatively, build an outline map, applying details at the junctions to be segmented.

FIGURE 6.3 Generic market map, including the number of each customer type.

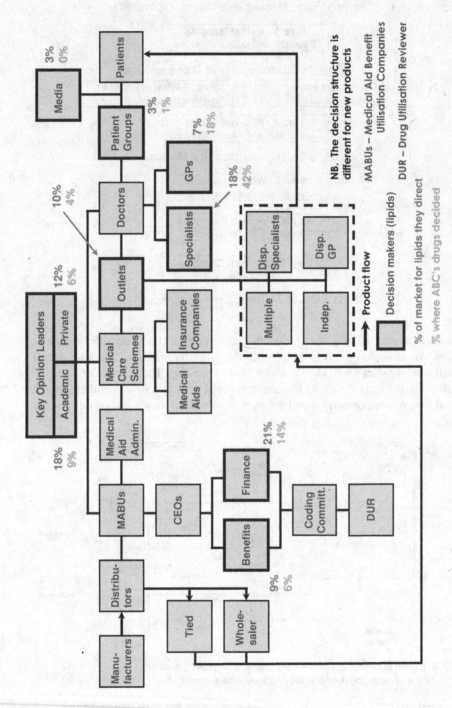

FIGURE 6.4 Market map: ethical drugs. (From S. A. Partners.)

NB. The decision structure is different for new products

MABUs – Medical Aid Benefit Utilisation Companies

DUR – Drug Utilisation Reviewer

Decision makers (lipids)

Product flow

% of market for lipids they direct

% where ABC's drugs decided

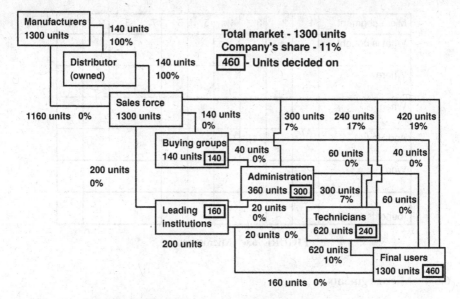

FIGURE 6.5   Market map: medical equipment.

is useful if the organization drawing the map can list its own share at each junction. This is extremely valuable in showing whether the organization matches the pattern of the general market. If not, are there opportunities for us or threats from, say, new distribution channels? In a sense, the market map is somewhat like a balance sheet in that 100% of goods and services made clearly have to balance with the number of goods and services bought at the end of the chain.

Two pharma marketing maps are shown in Figures 6.4 and 6.5. One is for lipids in South Africa. There isn't space here for a detailed case history, but it is clear that the company (ABC) just wasn't putting its marketing effort into where the real decisions were being made, as the percentages clearly show. The other map is for medical equipment, which shows that the sales force, being former technicians themselves, were targeting technicians, and they felt uncomfortable with the growing decision groups, such as buying groups and administrators.

The entire point of market mapping is to answer the question: Who is the customer? Without this knowledge of where the 80/20 rule applies in terms of where real decisions are made, market segmentation just isn't possible.

6.6.3   Return to the Market Segmentation Process

We can now return to the process shown in Figure 6.2 and move to steps 2, 3, 4, and 5, although it must be pointed out that segmentation can and should be carried out at all major junctions on the market map, not just at the far right-hand side.

Micro-segment	1	2	3	4	5	6	7	8	9	10
What is bought										
Where										
When										
And How										
Who										
Why (benefits sought)										

FIGURE 6.6   Microsegments.

6.6.4 Microsegments

Essentially, these time-consuming steps involve listing all purchase combinations that take place in the market, including different applications for the product or service. Principal forms such as size, color, and branded or unbranded are the principal channels used. When? Perhaps weekly, or once a year. How? Perhaps cash, or credit. Next, it is important to describe who behaves in each particular way using relevant descriptors such as demographics. For industrial purchases this might be standard industrial classification, or size of firm. Whereas for consumer purchases, this might be socioeconomic groups such as A, B, C1, C2, D, and E; stage in the life cycle; or age, gender, geography, lifestyle, or psychographics.

Finally, and most difficult, each purchase combination has to have a brief explanation of the reason for the particular type of behavior. In other words, we need to list the benefits sought, and it is often at this stage that an organization needs to pause and either commission market research or refer to its extant database of previous market research studies.

Although there are only 10 microsegments in Figure 6.6, it is normal in most markets for companies to identify between 30 and 50 microsegments. Remember that these microsegments are actual purchase combinations that take place in the market.

6.6.5 An Undifferentiated Market

To summarize what's been said so far, it is clear that no market is totally homogeneous (see Figure 6.7). The reality is that actual markets consist of a large number of different purchase combinations (see Figure 6.8). However, as it is impracticable to deal with more than seven to 10 market segments, a process has to be found to bring together, or cluster, all microsegments that share similar or approximately similar needs (see Figure 6.9).

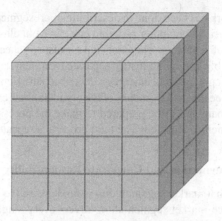

FIGURE 6.7   Undifferentiated market, but one with many different purchase combinations.

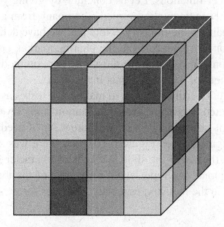

FIGURE 6.8   Different needs in a market.

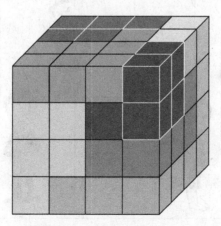

FIGURE 6.9   Segments in a market.

Once the basic work has been done in describing microsegments (i.e., steps 2, 3, 4, and 5), any good statistical computer program can carry out cluster analysis to arrive at a smaller number of segments. The final step consists of checking whether the resulting segments are big enough to justify separate treatment, are indeed sufficiently different from other segments, and have been described sufficiently well to enable the customers in them to be reached by means of the organization's communication methods; finally, the company has to be prepared to make the necessary changes to meet the needs of the segments identified. The total process is repeated from Figure 6.2.

6.6.6   Market Segmentation and Corporate Responsibility

It will now be clear that market segmentation is fundamental to corporate strategy. It is also clear that since market segmentation affects every single corporate activity, it should not just be an exercise that takes place within the marketing department and has to involve other functions. Let us conclude by giving you just one example of how sensible market segmentation turned a company from a loss maker into the most profitable company in the industry. (Note that we have deliberately selected an example from a sector far removed from the pharma market, because it shows how powerful segmentation can be, even in a loss-making commodity market, one that does not have the benefit of lots of personal interaction).

In the late 1980s, ICI Fertiliser began to make huge losses as the market matured and as prices plummeted. However, the segmentation study revealed that there were seven distinct types of farmer, each with a different set of needs. To give just three examples of these segments (see Figure 6.10), first there was a segment we called Arthur—the figure at the top of the slide, a television character known for his deals. He bought on price alone, but represented only 10% of the market, not the 100% claimed by everyone in the industry, especially the sales force.

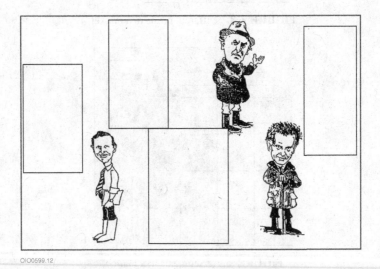

OIO0599.12

FIGURE 6.10   Personalizing segments.

Another type of farmer we called Oliver, the figure at the bottom right of the slide. Oliver would drive around his fields on his tractor with an aerial linked to a satellite and an onboard computer. He did this to analyze the soil type and would then mix P, N, and K, the principal ingredients of fertilizer, solely to get the maximum yield out of his farm. In other words, Oliver was a scientific farmer, but the supply industry believed that he was buying on price, because he bought his own ingredients as cheaply as possible. He did this, however, only because none of the suppliers bothered to understand his needs.

Another type of farmer we called David, the figure at the bottom left of the slide. David was a show-off farmer and liked his crops to look nice and healthy. He also liked his cows to have nice healthy skins. Clearly, if a sales representative had talked to David in a technical way, David would quickly switch off. To talk about the appearance of crops and livestock would also have switched Oliver off. But this is the whole point. Every single supplier in the industry totally ignored the real needs of these farmers, and the only thing anyone ever talked about was price. The result is a market driven by price discount, accompanied by substantial losses to suppliers.

Armed with this newfound information, ICI launched new products and new promotional approaches aimed at these different farmer types and got immediate results, becoming the most profitable subsidiary of ICI and the only profitable fertilizer company in the country.

Finally, apropos of the pharmaceutical industry, there is clearly no such person as a "doctor" or an "administrator." There are certainly no such faceless, average persons as "patients," all to be treated in exactly the same way. Doctors, nurses, and other professional staff recognize this intuitively and treat them as individuals. Surely it is not beyond the wit of this sector to institutionalize this process through effective segmentation. At a stroke, there would be a massive improvement on the part of the public in how they think about this much-criticized (unjustly) sector. All the segmentation work that has been done in this sector proves beyond doubt that just as in any other business, correct market definition and needs-based segmentation are the keys to long-term success and customer–patient satisfaction.

Those are mighty words that strike at the heart of the "one-size-fits-all" approach that is often taken in this sector. The words also dispel the myth of marketing as the "gin-and-tonic brigade." The analysis and attention to detail required to segment a market properly should be appreciated from the case studies above—it is immense. I am eternally grateful to Professor McDonald[4] for that contribution. His Web site is provided here for those who may want to pursue marketing further.

Observations, Views, and Experiences of the Author

There are developing predictions that a more personalized approach to medicines is trending into the sector and PricewaterhouseCoopers has produced a series of excellent reports—Pharma 2020[5]—that look at the future possibilities and this is one aspect covered. In my opinion, though, this is something that is not going to happen at an acceptable pace until pharma drives a stake into the heart of the "find it and sell it" approach that exists currently. This will first require radical rethinking of the "find" piece to be sure that what is "found" is what is needed by the market. There are huge implications here for the interface between discovery research and product development, discussed in more detail later.

As explained by Professor McDonald, identifying customer groups and then providing products and services to beat the competition is complex. This is not an easy undertaking, but the example of ICI showed that when done properly and in depth, the results can be spectacular. We saw how it turned an apparently barren land in the world of agriculture into an oasis of opportunity. This was achieved by competing on the specific mix of offerings that appealed to customers' specific needs. That mix, as explained by McDonald, was different for the various customer segments.

In Pharmaceuticals, patients are the end customers, or consumers, of products and services. Much has been written on how businesses should go about marketing their wares to consumers, and curious readers could spend the next few decades scanning all the available material. For the purposes of this book, the specifics of customer engagement are studied in relation to production systems.

I believe that SCM should sit squarely at the table of competitive strategy because how can a plan or direction to bring products to customers be "selected" without understanding and designing the associated supply chain? Let us consider the example of Japan's forage into the realms of competitive strategy in a search for supporting evidence.

6.7   THE JAPANESE EXPERIENCE

What Japanese companies achieved in the world of business and competitive strategy through the 1960s, 1970s, 1980s, and to this day, has been nothing short of miraculous. They proved that it was possible to be the lowest-cost producer by an order of magnitude compared to the competition, but at the same time, to differentiate their products. The motorcycle industry is a case in point. Not only did they have a significant price advantage but the performance was also superior to that of most of the competing products at the time. We don't see many British motorbikes around these days—nor cars, or watches—the list goes on.

None of this is new, and some may wish to argue that the gap has narrowed significantly in more recent years. That may or may not be the case—the point for discussion here is that the Japanese did not just offer extra value or lower price, they offered what we commonly call *value for money*—more value for less money—the holy grail of competition. In the next section the search for customer value as emanating from the Japanese example is examined.

6.8   TOTAL QUALITY MANAGEMENT

The total quality management (TQM) movement, which is discussed in later chapters, recognized the prime importance of consumers, but in very roundabout ways. The rise and fall of TQM is tricky to follow because although many gurus did excellent work on the topic (e.g., Deming, Juran, Crosby, Ishikawa), nothing seems to integrate it into a single, consistent set of guiding principles. There are, nonetheless, wise words on the topic that can be found in various TQM texts if the reader is prepared to search. Let's look next at something I picked up from a textbook by Bank.[6]

The first chapter, titled "Focus on the Customer," begins with a section titled "The Customer as King." It describes a popular poster for display in shops, offices, and factories to drive the message home. It reads as follows:

Customers are:

- The most important people in any business.
- Not dependent on us. We are dependent on them.
- Not an interruption to our work. They are the purpose of it.
- Doing us a favor when they come in. We are not doing them a favor by serving them.
- A part of our business, not outsiders.
- Not just a statistic. They are flesh and blood human beings with feelings and emotions, like ourselves.
- People come to us with their needs and wants. It is our job to fill them.
- Deserving of the most courteous and attentive treatment we can give them.
- The lifeblood of this and every other business. Without them we would have to close our doors.

It finishes with these words in parentheses: "Don't ever forget it!"

These are words most people would identify with, but TQM is light on ways to get to the core of a market compared to the earlier market segmentation approach. It does, however, add much to the challenge of converting good intensions into customer value. Understanding your customers' needs is irrelevant if there is no way of delivering on them as an organization. To this extent, TQM is an excellent way of extending customer needs into the delivery organization. We have more to say on TQM in later chapters; for now, we move on to lean thinking.

6.9   LEAN THINKING

Again, lean thinking is covered later in the book. For this section, however, it is useful to examine customer value from the lean perspective. It is, after all, the first principle of lean, as defined by Womack and coauthors[7]: "The critical starting point for lean thinking is value. Value can only be defined by the ultimate customer. And it's only meaningful when expressed in terms of a specific product (a good or a service, and often both at once) which meets the customer's needs at a specific price at a specific time." It goes on to say: "Value is created by the producer."

The producer is, of course, the end-to-end supply chain that converts a customer need into a physical entity (product and service). This is the critical link to SCM. To talk on the practicalities of developing customer value propositions, the UK-based consultancy S. A. Partners has agreed to make a contribution through Richard Harrison, a former managing consultant at S. A. Partners.

GUEST CONTRIBUTOR SLOT: RICHARD HARRISON

The First Principle of Almost Everything: Customer Value

Many suppliers I speak to on first meeting usually tell me when asked about their customers: "Oh, I know what my customers value." No problems here, then!

My experience is that whereas a supplier might have a good idea about how satisfied (or not) customers are with their overall product or service offering at a given moment in time, more often than not, they won't have a really crystal clear idea about the key criteria through which their customers actually measure value from a supplier—and these are the real factors that affect growth and profitability in a customer–supplier relationship. Although satisfaction is a mandatory essential element in the value equation, you ignore at your peril gaining upfront clarity and depth of understanding around the value criteria of the influencers within your customer—at different touch points within the business.

Value criteria are not a group or team phenomenon—they are part of the makeup of an individual person. We all have them and use them to measure and gauge what's important to us in our everyday lives—work and play. In a business context they are often related directly to the role a person has within the business and are often influenced by how a person is measured. In turn, these measures drive a particular type of behavior.

Value criteria are the "must have" factors which reflect what a customer values in a product or service offering and which the customer uses to "measure" and calibrate levels of satisfaction with a product or service offering and which, in turn, are linked inextricably to expectations. If our basic expectations are met, we are satisfied; if they are not met, we are disappointed; and if they are exceeded, we are delighted. We are all customers who have experienced these emotions. They help form our experiences upon which future buying decisions are based (see Figure 6.11).

To be able to explore these value criteria with a person and come away with an in-depth insight and understanding into what they mean for that person and "what good looks or feels like" for each criterion is a very powerful concept and one that is absolutely attainable in any sector or type of business. Once the value criteria are established, and recognizing that all the criteria are important to the customer, it is important to delve deeper to establish a hierarchy of criteria from their perspective. Gathering this type of information requires great communication and recording skills, an ability to listen to the language used by the customer and to play back the words used until the true meaning and understanding are established. I always do this through one-to-one face-to-face interviews (it can't be done by letter or by phone), supported by one or two people skilled in observation and recording data. Over the past eight years that we have been using this technique, I have developed a standard, repeatable, measurable process tool specifically designed to help facilitate this work, called *insight*, to help us achieve really outstanding results for our clients and their customers.

If you really listen and hear what customers are saying, they will tell you what needs to change to keep you ahead of the competition. The output from the interview

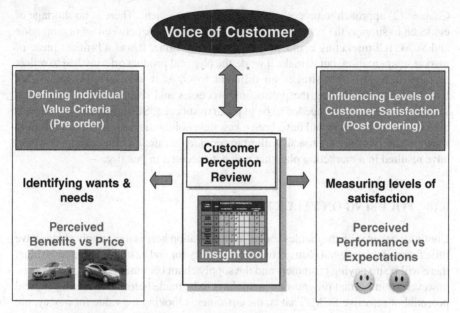

FIGURE 6.11   Customer value: what you don't know you don't know.

is a detailed understanding of the customers' value criteria across key influencers within the business, which helps suppliers align their resources more directly to the needs of their key customers.

Values can and do change over time (often very quickly) and it will be necessary to ensure that you recognize this and build in periodic account reviews with key customers to offset this risk of misalignment. The key thing is to feed back to your customers and involve them in the continuous improvement process as quickly as you are able. Doing nothing is not an option and is, indeed, a recipe for disaster. You will not be able to achieve everything they have requested, but by involving them in the improvement process from the start, they will see that you are serious about growing with them in true partnership. The result is greatly improved relationships, increased account profitability and sales growth, real differentiation from the competition, and above all, true achievement of the first principle of lean—to understand the voice of the customer.

Again, more evidence that the starting point for any business intending to supply markets is the customer. This piece also reinforces the message that customers are diverse and can differ greatly. The methods required to get at the core of a customer need must be focused and skillfully applied. Then, of course, the vital piece: alignment of the organization tasked with meeting that need. Called *strategy* or *policy deployment* by the lean fraternity, this is considered further in Chapter 12.

Reference to the other great preoccupation at the moment, six sigma, will reveal the concept of voice of the customer as the starting point of the DMAIIC (see

Chapter 12) approach to process performance improvement. There is no shortage of evidence to support the principle. This leads to a vital link between an organization and SCM. ICI marketing could not have done that alone. It was a brilliant piece of market segmentation, but to make it work, the physical product offering had to reflect the approach. Different strokes for different folks, as it were, would have meant tailoring and customizing the production processes and related supply lines. That vital piece of the jigsaw needed to be in place to succeed. SCM did not determine or drive the strategy but would have been a key stakeholder in alignment and validating the practicality of the approach. Failure to provide that underpinning support would have resulted in a marketing plan that was not executed in practice.

6.10   FOCUSING ON VALUE FOR MONEY

Continuing then with the themes above, the declaration here is that supply chains have little future if they are not focused on value delivery for end customers. Without value, there will be no paying customers and the supply chain becomes redundant. There is, however, an important progression in thinking to be made before discovering the real potential of effective SCM. That is, the customer is looking for value for money, not value in isolation. Price is a vital component of any value proposition and relatively lower costs of manufacture provide a company with far greater flexibility to compete on price.

A Helpful Metaphor

I would like a Rolls-Royce but can't afford one. Rolls-Royce as a company can pack their cars to the gunnels with valuable bits and pieces, but it's academic to me and millions of others. I'm looking for something that I can afford and then figuring out how I can get the most value for the money I have to spend, so I am interested in price as well as value. The automaker getting my business will offer me the right blend to differentiate them, in my eyes, from the competition. That means producing at a cost that allows them to meet my price and value expectations, all else being equal.

So we are talking here about the four P's, really, aren't we? The product must be right—basically, it should meet (or exceed) my expectations for that class of vehicle. The price also has to be right. I will probably have a cutoff price and a band of acceptable prices. Traveling to another country to make the purchase would probably not be acceptable, so place is defined. It may even be that I want it delivered to my home. I may not have access to the Internet to find whether the product even exists, so maybe the way the product is promoted will affect my purchase decision.

The metaphor is, of course, about creating competitive advantage in target markets. The value proposition for targeted segments can vary significantly; it not only resides in the product itself, but is also made up of other factors. These are the remaining three P's as well as, potentially, others. Companies that restrict themselves from competing on any of those criteria may exclude certain categories of customer. That is not a problem as long as the business proposition works: Value (revenue) minus cost equals margin sufficient to meet company objectives. This has certainly been the case, and more, with branded pharmaceuticals. The differentiation has, however, normally been based on products that cannot be matched (those fulfilling an unmet medical need—blockbusters). The question is: How well would it go if branded pharmaceuticals had to compete on cost as well? Not very well, we suspect. The following is a little personal cameo on the industry's attitude toward cost.

Observations, Views, and Experiences of the Author

Several years ago I presented a workshop at a conference focusing on logistics in pharmaceuticals. In one of the plenary sessions where the chairman and a few of the session speakers were taking questions, I raised my hand and asked a question relating to achieving cost transparency (open-book costing) from suppliers. The chairman reacted as if I had said that Martians had invaded New York and were eating everything in their path. He said words to the effect that this was a conference about value, not cost, and hurriedly moved on to the next question with an uncomfortable look on his face.

I felt equally embarrassed, mainly because the audience seemed to share his view. Maybe I am flattering myself, but I believe that they had all missed the real thrust behind the question—that suppliers willing to open their books to customers were demonstrating a willingness to enter into longer-term, more strategic relationships. Other sectors, encouraged by the Japanese example, had proved that to truly drive cost out of supply chains, the supply base had to partake through mutual sharing of information, including costs. This concept is anathema in many pharmaceutical supply markets, which in my opinion does not benefit either supplier or customer in the longer term; it just builds unnecessary costs into products and materials that the end customer has to pick up.

That episode set me thinking that this sector (notwithstanding generics) has been cosseted from the realities of business in competitive markets for many, many years. Whenever I mention this to industry colleagues, the example of Tagamet (a Smith-KlineBeecham product) and Zantac (a Glaxo product) raises its ugly head. The retort is: What about that for competition, then? For readers unfamiliar with this case study, Tagamet was first to market but was quickly overtaken by Zantac. The reason for this was reported by many as superior competitive positioning by the Zantac marketing team. That was probably correct, but the competition was heavily around promotion of perceived product value differences. From the accounts I've heard, there appeared to be little evidence of competition on price.

This all then made me realise what a huge potential there was for proper SCM to make performance improvements, but a mindset change was essential to progress.

This is the mindset that considers SCM as being merely about moving boxes around. In upcoming chapters we aim to put that myth to the sword. We begin the dual with a very brief description of SCM processes, aiming to whet the readers' appetite to the potential of SCM.

6.11 SCM PROCESSES IN COMPETITIVE STRATEGY

It will be helpful to remind ourselves of two extracts from Chapter 1. The first is a comment from Nick Rich:

> If you look around you, you will probably find that the world's most successful businesses have integrated supply chains. These supply chains, value networks—call them what you will—are the result of design. The best product in the world can easily be eroded when it is matched by a poorly designed supply chain.

This is the link between competitive success and the supply chain. The second is the definition of SCM, which describes the scope that must be covered to deliver the integrated supply chains that lead to competitive success:

> SCM covers the design, management, and improvement of end-to-end supply (value) chains. This includes all the stages and activities involved in moving raw materials through progressive stages to become products in customers' hands. All aspects of stewardship to achieve the above are included.

We go into these in a lot more detail in Chapters 7 to 13, but to get the most out of the present chapter, it is important to provide some summary information. The five areas that I believe make up SCM as a competitive weapon are:

1. *Production and inventory control:* managing supply, demand, and inventory levels to meet customer requirements.
2. *Strategic procurement:* acquisition of goods and services from third parties.
3. *Storage, transportation, and distribution:* stewardship of products and materials during transfer between trading partners.
4. *Information systems:* managing flows of information associated with the activities above.
5. *Improvement:* search for better ways of doing things from an end-user perspective.

These make up the SCM armory and are activities that appear either expressly or implicitly in Porter's value chain model. We explain it here by adapting the model to suit.

As firms join together to create supply lines, a physical, interconnected value chain forms. This is the sum total of all steps—operation, store, transport, hold, inspect—from digging material out of the ground to getting a product in the hands of a consumer. These are, in effect, the primary activities of the various firms in the chain, linking them together. Similarly, to achieve an integrated supply chain, the support activities need to link up in a complementary way.

Some illustrative examples should help:

- *SCM-to-SCM internal linkages.* Production and inventory control (P&IC) must link effectively with strategic procurement to establish the demand load on the supply chain and define a supply base that is capable of providing a suitable capacity range to cope. Procurement must ensure that P&IC is serviced by suppliers, providing materials that are fit for purpose so that schedules are not disrupted.
- *SCM to other internal support activities.* Strategic procurement must work effectively with product development to identify and screen new technologies within the supply base that could provide innovative solutions for customers. Product development should, accordingly, include procurement in its early stage work on possible new designs.
- *SCM to other internal primary activities.* Marketing staff and those responsible for storage, transportation, and distribution need to work together to ensure that products (especially those that are temperature- or time-critical) are delivered to customers as and when required, to meet or match competitors' performance.
- *SCM to upstream activities.* Goods receiving activities at the downstream firm should be matched with dispatch activities at the supplying firm.
- *SCM to downstream activities.* Order and forecasting systems at the downstream firm should be linked with production scheduling at the upstream firm.

This list can be continued as the reader imagines the multitude of linkages that can and need to be in place for maximum advantage. All these will potentially have a positive impact on the quality, cost, and delivery performance of a firm competing in the world of supplying to paying customers. This is what the Japanese were masters of: creating collaborative linkages internally, with their suppliers and with their customers.

Where it may be helpful to make the case more forcefully is in a world that is not instantly identified with paying customers: such as the world of drug development. Why should the point be made more explicit in this world? Because there is virtually no interest or awareness of the relevance of proper SCM in the corridors of many of these enterprises, as I have found at my cost.

Observations, Views, and Experiences of the Author

As mentioned previously, I left permanent employment mid-2005 to try and make it as an independent consultant, using my hard-won SCM competency in biotech. Having made a success of it working with the larger biotech firms, it seemed like a good idea at the time. What I had failed to realize was that these relatively larger companies had invited me in because they had gotten to the stage (phase III) where executives with commercial exposure had joined. As very few biotech companies ever got to that stage, there was a very limited prospective client base—to say the least.

I then set about developing persuasive (I hoped) arguments based on the logic of early-stage supply chain thinking. After speaking to what seemed like a million people at biotech companies, a stark conclusion started to form. No one was interested in considering the future supply chain, and hence work would be difficult to find. The rationale was always this. Why would a CEO or senior manager of a company wishing to exit via an initial public offering or trade sale worry about the condition of their supply chain—that will be someone else's problem. What they were making and selling was a package of intellectual property and data, not a supply chain. Those statements, or words to that effect, I heard uttered many, many times.

Did I give up? No, but nearly. Through the next section and the remainder of the book will weave exactly the same logical arguments as to why even the smallest biotech firm should invest time (and a modest amount of money as a prerequisite to doing business) in learning and applying the principles of SCM (as embodied in the principles of twenty-first-century modernization) as they relate to the future needs of successful businesses.

6.12   SCM IN BIOTECH AND VIRTUAL COMPANIES

In this section we consider an example that hopefully will drive the message home to a stakeholder group that rarely associates itself with the benefits of effective SCM. This is the example of a small drug development company taking a compound through the various stages of development. At the preclinical stage there will be suppliers to select (e.g., API manufacturer, safety testing CRO, storage and transport provider). There will need to be simple systems of recording where drug is located and its quantity and status; the drug will need to get to the CRO in good time and in good condition through careful planning; and most important of all, there should be an emerging focus on improvement opportunities, as this is the point where problems are easy to fix but difficult to spot unless people are sensitized to the importance of looking and acting.

From this stage onward, the supply chain elements grow in terms of risk and complexity. Proper SCM can make a huge contribution to the strategic needs of this business, as we explain below. The business is likely to have the aim of selling itself or the compound before marketing. It could happen at any stage of development, or it could not happen at all if the compound is found wanting in any way (which is the predominant outcome based on the reported rates of attrition). The customer for this company or its product is likely to be another company. The strategic imperatives are different for companies with marketed products, but the potential of SCM support is the same. Next we discuss the strategic factors for this business.

6.12.1   Investor Confidence

Small drug development companies depend on a flow of funds from investors to operate and survive; hence they need to be attractive as investment opportunities. The investors' hard-earned money will be ploughed into capital equipment and inventory procured from third parties. They will require a respectable return on their money, so test drugs must be produced and delivered to investigator sites in a timely fashion so that the necessary clinical and nonclinical data can be derived. Along the way, there will be a minefield of possible accidents waiting to happen, and it takes an experienced eye to spot these risks ahead of time. If things are not managed properly, investors may be reluctant to provide additional funds to continue the business.

6.12.2   Cash Runaway

There is always a finite pot of money provided by investors that will not, in the short term, be topped up by sales revenues. The supply chain is a major source of cash burn, involving procurement of expensive materials and high expenditures on CRO and CMO services. Clinical trials themselves are expensive to run, and any delay in drug arriving at a site will affect time lines and cost. SCM can conserve cash runaway if engaged with effect.

This view is supported by a comment from an experienced biotech executive, Peter Worrall, CEO of Pharminox in the UK (previously CFO of Vernalis). This is what Peter said in his contribution to a *Biotech PharmaFlow Newsletter*[8]: "There can be a huge disparity in the cost of identical outsourced services provided by different CROs. For small companies who rely heavily on outsourcing, effective procurement is absolutely essential to maximize the cash runway and to get the best value for money." Peter is a person who fully appreciates the potential for SCM processes and the way in which they can be harnessed for the benefit of a small company. Hopefully, his sentiments will hit home to the financial backers of such companies.

6.12.3   Partner Credibility

Big pharma is always eyeing up biotechs and their promising compounds. If any of the compounds happen to be licensed by a big pharma company, that company will demand compliance with supply chain processes that are commonly place in the big pharma world. Knowledge and demonstrated application of these processes by the biotech firm can be extremely valuable in building credibility. A biotech group that can demonstrate a working knowledge of big pharma commercial systems and processes can earn a firm checkmark in the due-diligence box. The converse is equally true (see the contribution by James Ryan in Section 9.6).

Meeting or exceeding these needs can mean that credibility goes sky high, along with the business relationship and potential for opportunities in the future.

6.12.4 Asset Valuation

The value proposition that small drug development companies have is to increase the value of the asset (compound) between acquisition (or discovery) and divestment. This is achieved by compiling a dossier of data that proves that the asset can be advanced to at least the next stage of development by showing an appropriate degree of quality, safety, and efficacy. The acquiring company will then review that dossier and perform a due-diligence exercise to decide whether or not to license the compound. If they do make an offer, the financial terms to the biotech firm will reflect the overall package they are taking on.

The point to bear in mind is that weakness in the supply chain and the associated processes not only affect credibility, they can affect valuations positively or negatively. A well-presented dossier with a clear sourcing strategy, capable suppliers, and strong agreements in place can make all the difference. Conversely, a fragile supply chain that needs to be rebuilt or does not reach an appropriate standard can knock millions of dollars off asset valuations and affect exit strategies for the company and its investors.

6.12.5 Risk Management

The final point to consider is that risk abounds in development supply chains. It takes only one temperature excursion that is not properly investigated, documented, and corrected by the sponsor to bring an entire study to its knees; and remember that it is the sponsor's ultimate responsibility, of course, not that of the contractors involved. In fact, so many other things can go wrong in the supply chain that it is lunacy not to perform a structured risk assessment of the end-to-end supply chain. This is a real opportunity for biotech firms to protect their investment, but rarely is it done, let alone executed properly.

6.13   COMPETITION IN PHARMACEUTICALS

To finish this chapter we should look briefly at some specifics of competition in the pharmaceutical sector. This is a topic in itself, and the intention is not to go any further than to inform the supply chain practitioner of some key influencing factors. This extends the discussion above on the nature of competition, exemplified by the Tagamet–Zantac case (Section 6.10). These battles seem always be based principally on two of the four P's: product and promotion. Battling over price, or cost from the buyer's perspective, is rarely on offer. There are also some classes of compounds where the market is crowded with only mildly differentiated products: for example, triptans.

Triptans are vasoconstrictor drugs (they aim to shrink blood vessels in the brain) developed for migraine. The first of these (sumatriptan) was launched by Glaxo in 1983 and is still by far the market leader. Over the years, another six triptans have been launched with various degrees of efficacy. None could really argue a powerful and unassailable case to say that any of them is any better than sumatriptan, which has now been out of patent for a number of years. It is difficult to see how the development of all these similar versions has added anything to patients' experience of the condition.

Price does become the subject of competition, of course, when a branded drug exits the patent protection umbrella. The product then attains the status often termed *generic* or *biosimilar* (biologically derived product outside patent protection). At this point, the change in competitive behavior is dramatic. Prices can tumble up to tenfold in the space of a few days following loss of protection. Those in at the start can make a killing [e.g., one of the world's largest generic companies was reputed to have been making £1 million a day in the UK when the SSRI (antidepressant) brand Cipramil (citalopram) went generic]. The profit opportunity was short lived as the competition caught up, but that company still benefited significantly from that opportunistic maneuvre; and that is probably the word to describe competition in generics—*opportunistic*.

Aside from these speculative opportunities, making a living in generics is difficult, to say the least. The full-service providers often buy inventory from competitors just to remain in stock, so that customers do not abandon them. This commonly means selling at a loss! It is almost the opposite extreme of branded pharma. If only there were a halfway house, where companies could make sensible margins throughout the product life cycle; is that such an impossible dream? More on this topic later.

7 Supply Chain Management Holistic

7.1 THE RELEVANCE OF SCM TO PHARMACEUTICALS

The remaining five chapters in Part II cover the basic disciplines of SCM. Those who have spent their lives immersed in other areas of pharmaceuticals, with different challenges, should have a brief introduction to why these chapters will be important to them.

Almost everyone operating in this industry is both an influencer of and is influenced by SCM. For example, research chemists depend on a supply of laboratory reagents to carry out their experiments. These must be sourced and paid for appropriately, be transported and available on-time, be stored properly, and be improved to meet increasingly rigorous standards. Records must be kept to identify what is available for current and future use. The outcome of a research chemist's work may be a new molecular structure that could form the basis of a medical breakthrough—the starting point for a clinical trial supply chain that could eventually lead to a commercial supply to patients in the same way that chemical reagents were supplied to the chemists. Surely, therefore, on that basis, there is an important obligation on us all to have heightened levels of understanding, no matter where the current level of understanding.

As we have already discussed, supply chains are about delivering value to end customers. This value is created through a series of value-adding stages (production) that are built up progressively: Raw materials become partially finished materials become finished products. The story therefore begins with production.

7.2 PRODUCTION SYSTEMS AND THE SCM HOLISTIC

What do we mean in this book by the term *production system*? In simple terms, we refer to all those activities involved in designing, building, and managing systems of people and resources working in concert to supply finished product to end customers. Within the overall production system for a product there will be hundreds or thousands of subproduction systems that take place through the production journey. Many of

Supply Chain Management in the Drug Industry: Delivering Patient Value for Pharmaceuticals and Biologics, By Hedley Rees
Copyright © 2011 John Wiley & Sons, Inc.

these may not seem obviously to be production, but production is the conversion of an object from one form to another (higher value) form. This could therefore include creating a master cell bank, filtering a bulk liquid, and making up a test reagent, among many others. Then there are all the support activities required for these production stages to take place. Not all of it is about making widgets!

SCM is therefore regarded throughout this book in terms of the total interrelationships that exist within the production system, both physical and information based. Where processes of SCM are discussed, it is an implicit assumption that they refer to production systems. The two are inextricably linked.

7.3   THE CORE OF SCM

To recap earlier concepts, the core mission of SCM is to support the continual delivery of competitive advantage in target markets. Achieving this involves work on customer value and cost simultaneously (supporting Porter's value chain concept). This then helps a business generate a profit margin to invest, grow, and reward stakeholders. This must remain the central theme in designing and operating supply chain processes. All too often, companies drive down costs only to destroy customer value and the associated competitive advantage. Similarly, it is possible to create costs that do not deliver customer value and therefore reduce margin and the potential to invest and grow. In my view, the discipline of SCM has been evolving in recognition of this concept. This has resulted in organic development of the linkages that are increasingly recognized as the processes of SCM (or whatever it makes sense to call it). The discipline is still, however, relatively young and continuously developing. There is much to be done to establish SCM properly as a key business process in the same way as, say, marketing, accounting, and human resource management are recognized.

For SCM to succeed there must be complete integration of the processes. There can only be one supply chain (value stream in "lean" parlance) for a particular product, in the same way that a human has only one body. It may be complex, involved, and joined in peculiar ways, but it is still only one. The same product may be produced by a different company, but that will then be a different supply chain. The heart, lungs, brain, and nervous system must know their role and work in concert with all other organs of that one body.

7.4   FIRST PRINCIPLE OF SCM

Through the chapters on the nuts and bolts of SCM (Chapters 8 to 13), the focus will be on maintaining a level that is understandable to a nonspecialist. The bias will be toward stating the obvious, so as to avoid missing a fundamental principle. In the main, hopefully, the result will be a book that does not contravene the received knowledge of SCM experts nor baffle the pharmaceutical scientist wishing to dip litmus paper into the test tube that is SCM.

To summarize the principles raised in earlier chapters, if we could pick whatever we needed from self-sustaining trees in our back gardens, supply chains would not exist. For most people these days, this is not the case. The products and services we demand must be produced and delivered through stages. As the stages progress, value builds into something called inventory. Increasingly, valuable inventory is passed along the line until it eventually reaches an end customer. Hopefully, the end customer will reward all our efforts with a handful of cash that can then be passed back down the line.

The journey to cash starts with the *production* of a raw material. This may seem a strange word to use for raw materials because typically we think of them as being *sourced*. They are, of course, sourced by the next stage, but they still have to be produced: dug out of the ground and converted into something usable. If the raw material is, for example, iron ore, it is produced by the diggers, shovels, and picks breaking it out of the ground and piling it in mounds on the floor. So in the text, *production* will be the name applied to the physical value-changing activities throughout the supply chain. This will be termed the *production stage*.

The next stage is *delivery*, moving the product produced from point A to point B. There is not an intended transformation or change of value here. The intent is merely to move the material to the next stage of production and on to the eventual end customer. Although this is not strictly a value-adding activity set, it is essential; otherwise, the customer will not get the product. The only case where delivery would not be essential is where the product grows on trees in our backyard. This does not happen often these days.

The third stage is *limbo*. In fact, it is not actually the third stage because it occurs before, during, and after both production and delivery (e.g., raw materials lay in the ground waiting to be produced). It is highlighted as the third stage since to mention it first would probably have been unfamiliar or confusing for the reader.

Observations, Views, and Experiences of the Author

The description above represents the way that I have come to regard the supply chain, breaking it down into the simplest possible terms. The first two stages are pretty well known. Production is the event or series of events that add value to inventory through physical activities. Again, delivery is pretty universally accepted as moving inventory between locations. I was trying to think of a term that could describe that third state of going nowhere, doing nothing that I find (am I alone?) happens along the way, and limbo seemed an appropriate title. Inventory spends most of its time in limbo. Between every production stage and delivery stage, there is a limbo stage. Very often, there is more than one, quite often a lot more than one. We give names to the limbo stage, such as queuing, a temporary stoppage, a blockage, waiting time, delay, downtime, idle time, changeover, machine malfunction, and underutilization. The more innovative reader may have better, even more expressive terms. Whatever it is called, the stage is about waiting for something to happen.

From this, then, any supply chain can be described simply as a series of three possible stages—production, delivery, and limbo—joined together. Readers may be relieved to know that I am not going to carry this last term forward in the book, since this is meant to be a serious text. It may, however, help to bear in mind that inventory in supply chains spends the vast majority of time "waiting in limbo" or waiting as it is from here on.

This leads to what we regard as the first principle of SCM: that materials and products (inventory) can only ever be in one of three stages: production, delivery or waiting. These stages account for *time* spent in the supply chain, a *pivotal* concept in supply chains. What is the evidence for this statement? This will emerge throughout the book, as will many other concepts of SCM. For now, it must suffice to include some words from Taiichi Ohno's original definition of *lean*: "All we are doing is looking at the time line from the moment the customer gives us an order to the point when we collect the cash. And we are reducing that time line by removing the non-value-added wastes."[1] That was it. In the desperate post–World War II era, the race was on to get cash in the door. In pursuing that objective, Taiichi Ohno demonstrated that an unwavering focus on lead-time reduction had miraculous results in the supply chain. This insight clicked with me while I was listening to another speaker at the ManuPharma 2005 Summit. His name is Ian Glenday, a close associate of Dan Jones. What struck me about Ian, aside from the fact that he was a riveting speaker with a powerful message, was his scientific qualification in microbiology. (He is the recipient of the 2010 Shingo Prize.) So there is hope for all you scientists out there!

In his presentation, Ian described how he had been fortunate enough to visit Japan in the 1980s to study under Sensei Yoshiki Iwata from Toyota Gosei, one of the first suppliers to be taught the Toyota production system. His learning was amazing and is described more fully in Chapter 15, but the concept is noted here briefly because it is such an important aspect but one that I believe is consistently missed, although it is undeniably a founding principle of the lean philosophy (and SCM). The teaching message was that by progressively shortening the time interval allowed for the cycle of production, radical improvement had to be made to achieve it. For example, assume that a production process had been producing a range of products every month that was reduced to produce the same range every two weeks. Then the time was reduced to every week and ultimately to every day. That required solving such problems as extended changeover times, defects, and supplier issues. We won't say too much about this at the moment, but it is food for thought for those who believe that lean is merely about removing wasted activity.

7.5   SUPPLY CHAINS AS A SERIES OF INTERCONNECTED SYSTEMS

To aid the discussion from here on, readers should find it helpful to return to Porter's value chain model, but with some modification. Figure 7.1 shows the primary activities drawn down into the physical supply chain covered by the firm in question. That will then link up with the other physical supply chains, from other firms, into an

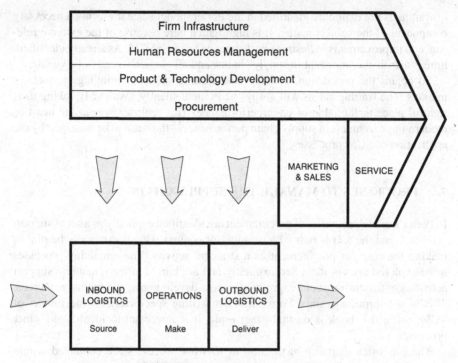

FIGURE 7.1 Adapted Porter model.

end-to-end supply chain, beginning with raw materials and ending with patients. The primary activities will occur in the supply chain, which will be regarded as a series of physical production, delivery, and waiting stages. Figure 7.2 shows a simplified schematic of how firms must join together in the route to market.

This remains totally consistent with the Porter model, except that in- and outbound logistics have been combined and termed delivery, since they are both fundamentally activities concerned with the movement of goods from one point to another. Operations has been renamed production but represent the same conversion activities as operations (the name change is made because support activities also often have responsibilities under the title *operations*: e.g., clinical operations). The final stage

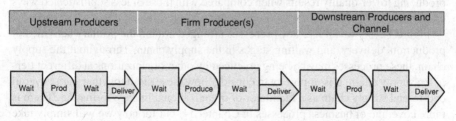

FIGURE 7.2 Firms joining up en route to market.

of waiting is not explicitly identified in the Porter model since it was not a necessary component of the subject matter. It is highlighted here because of the extreme relevance to improvements in business performance through SCM. As already identified, time is a critical component in supply chains, and all elements need to be visible.

So begins the production, delivery, and waiting stages of bringing products to markets. The waiting stages will always be in there silently, insidiously, taking their rightful place at the table of underperformance. This realization is at the heart of modern improvements in supply chain performance—the beast to be managed by the application of SCM processes.

7.6 PROCESSES TO MANAGE THE SUPPLY CHAIN

In Porter's model, activities of procurement are identified explicitly as a set of support activities, and the text is rich with meaningful content. This is extremely helpful in making the case for procurement as a strategic activity. The remaining processes to be explored are not identified explicitly and are buried in the remaining support activities of firm infrastructure, product/process development, and human resources. This is not surprising, since Porter was not writing specifically on the subject of SCM. Since this book is on that exact topic, it is important to identify the other processes.

There is often disparity of opinion as to what processes are contained within SCM. Terms such as *procurement, purchasing, materials management, supply management, logistics, inventory management, production planning, capacity planning, customer services, distribution management*, even *operations management* are used interchangeably. Similarly, organization structures often look very confused where roles and responsibilities are ill defined. In one organization, supply chain managers report to logistics managers, and in others, the reverse is the case. Attempts have been made to define standard terminology and approaches, such as the *SCOR model*[2], but in no way do these have the same universal acceptance as can be seen, for example, in accounting standards.

The version here is my own particular blend based on working experience. The important point to remember is that each process has the potential to operate in powerful ways. However, it is the manner in which they are integrated (through linkages) that is the vital ingredient. Without a clear understanding of the mission and purpose of each process set, strong individual processes can actually work against each other, producing lower-quality results when compared with those of less sophisticated ways of working.

Figure 7.3 shows all five key processes arranged around the primary activities of production, delivery, and waiting stages in the supply chain. Throughout the supply chain, these processes may be being practiced by other organizations at different tiers in the supply chain. It is important to consider how these mesh together in the overall end-to-end supply chain as a facilitator of organizational linkage formation. There is more coverage of business processes in Chapter 11, but for now we will simply take an initial view.

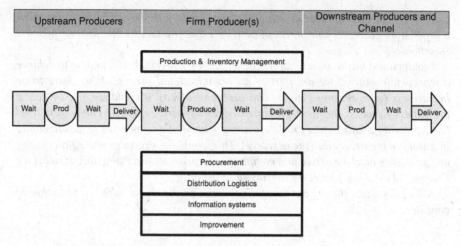

FIGURE 7.3   Processes around firms joining up en route to market.

7.7   A WORD ABOUT PROCESSES

Observations, Views, and Experiences of the Author

This section is included because I seem to have spent a large portion of my working life semiconfused about the descriptions and treatment of processes; similarly, I find myself in conversation where the word crops up frequently and I wonder, deep down, if I share a common understanding with my fellow conversationalists. Readers may wonder why that is important, and the reason is this. We have terms such as key processes *and* core processes *(both of which the theory says we shouldn't have too may of) and then there are* business processes *and* manufacturing processes *(of which there appear to be vast numbers). Then we have business process reengineering (BPR), process improvement, business process management (BPM), process control, process (this), and (that) process.*

The problem is that we try to understand what each of these terms means and to discover which one will do the trick for us. So I resolved a few years ago to have a clear understanding what relevance such processes have in the business world. My conclusion is that in general, a process converts something (object, material, situation, piece of paper, person) from one state to another, more valuable (by implication) state. So the first essential is a change from a precursor state to a target state. By this definition, a machine turning out widgets is a production process and the machine operator is a process operator. However, to qualify properly as a process by the definition most commonly subscribed to, there must be a second essential aspect: collaborative activity to achieve the desired change of state. The definition below is taken from Ould.[3] "The goal (target state) normally involves collaborative activity to convert an object or situation from one state into another state. The change of state could refer to a material (including documents) or a person receiving a service." An even simpler definition is suggested by BPTrends,[4] *which describes a process as "a repeatable series of activities that produces value for one or more stakeholders."*

    I understand this to mean that whenever we work together with people to achieve a worthwhile output, we are part of an organizational process. If we were to be in business (with revenues, costs, and profits involved), it could equally be called a business process. Business processes occur at various levels. The lowest level (e.g., entering a sales order) rolls up, along with similar processes (e.g., allocating inventory to the order) into the next level. This would be, say, sales order processing; and so it goes until we arrive at a complete enterprise resource planning system (see Chapter 11). All are processes varying in scope only.

    Not to overguild the lily but hopefully to build on the above, here is a metaphor to consider:

A Helpful Metaphor

By writing and placing a stamp on a letter, a process takes place. The component parts of the finished letter—paper, envelope, stamp—are transformed, using tools—pen, ink, tongue to lick stamp—into a document ready for the postal system. Taking and mailing the letter is another process. Up to this point, the process will normally involve only one person. This level of process is not typically regarded as requiring process skills and methods, but nonetheless, it is a process. So when is a process considered worthy of process management?

    When the mailbox is opened, a second person is involved in the processing; the mailman. In emptying the mailbox and taking the letters to the depot, a business process starts to emerge. These processes build up until the state of the letter moves to "delivered." The important point to remember is that business processes require collaborative activity, structure, and flow to achieve an end result.

    The message in the metaphor is that processes are everywhere, and the term can mean many things to many people. A person working alone carrying out an activity (such as stamping the letter) is not regarded as forming part of a process until a certain amount of collaboration and value flow is involved. This means that a process operator in a chemical company working on a "conversion" process—a chemical reaction to produce an end product—is not yet part of the business process. However, once the operator needs to record and move production and downgrade the inventory quantity consumed, the business process starts. The person ordering that chemical for further use will use a work order or purchase order process, which is part of a larger procurement process where the relevant supplier is identified and selected. Thus, it is important to be precise when defining processes; otherwise, there is scope for confusion and error. We must clearly define the starting point, the endpoint, and all stages in between.

7.8   HOW THE SCM PROCESSES SHOULD MESH TOGETHER

The raison d'être of a supply chain is to pass value along the line until it reaches the customer. In the line could be factories, people, machines, equipment, differing modes of transport, warehouses, and retail outlets. Inventory is produced, stored, and waiting and moving between locations. People are picking materials, working on them, inspecting them, scrapping some, sending some for rework, but in the main, are producing goods fit for customer purposes. The role of SCM is to facilitate all of this in a manner whereby the customer's expectations of value delivered is aligned with experience at the point of delivery.

As we further explore processes meshing together, there will emerge some critical, make-or-break interfaces, where the greater good of the business needs to override organizational boundaries. At these interfaces, a co-dependence exists that must be respected. The various organizational entities involved must understand that very clearly. For example, production facilities can run well or poorly, depending on the way the schedules are defined and managed. In the same way, customers can be pleased or disappointed according to how well production meets their schedules. Successful SCM involves developing realistic production schedules that take account of operating constraints and real-world issues. Production departments underpin and share that success by being honest about capabilities and delivering on properly agreed commitments. This is often where things can go wrong in supply chains. This is a key area that will be examined in later chapters. For now, a brief overview of the processes is appropriate.

7.9   PRODUCTION AND INVENTORY CONTROL

This process set is purposely shown at the top of the supply chain stack since to manage flow properly requires a clear view of the customer on the one hand and the supply chain on the other. To do this, the best vantage point must be selected, and this is obviously on top of the building! This is a highly reactive responsibility area because so many things can happen in the supply chain to affect the flow of materials. Machines break down, suppliers fail, operators get sick, people do dumb things, and rejects are produced. Whenever any of these things happens it has the potential to let the customer down unless adjustments are made. This means that P&IC must be strongly linked with the producers (those with responsibility to produce the physical inventory), so that agreement can be reached on appropriate action. It also means that the business needs producers to work with P&IC to find solutions, even if that sometimes involves taking the more difficult route. This is one of the critical interfaces mentioned in Section 7.4.

7.10   STRATEGIC PROCUREMENT

The second of the business process set to consider is procurement. In his model, Porter defines procurement as a discrete set of support activities, basically describing it as the "function of purchasing inputs used in the firm's value chain." Whereas Porter uses the term *function*, we make it very clear here that procurement is not necessarily the domain of any particular organizational function within a business. The emphasis is on the activities being carried out within the organization, but the important thing is that the process be defined and followed. There are examples of exemplary procurements being carried out by nonprocurement personnel and pretty disastrous ones being spearheaded by procurement functional staff. There are also many examples of the converse. Hopefully, readers of this book will be able to contribute to tipping the balance toward successful procurements for both groups.

It should also be noted that there is a very clear role of facilitation that needs to be carried out, the stewardship of which can be well invested in a specialist function. The process does not happen naturally, and organizational approaches can be ad hoc unless there is clearly identified ownership. The important point to remember is that ownership relates to definition and application of the correct processes, not necessarily to carrying out the processes themselves.

7.11 TRANSPORTATION, STORAGE, AND DISTRIBUTION

Sometimes called distribution logistics, this is the third of the businesses processes. The role of transportation, storage, and distribution is to store and move goods with integrity and to deal with the associated issues of local, national, and international trade and commerce. This aspect of SCM is often mistakenly regarded as the entirety of the discipline, leading to SCM being regarded at a much reduced scope in the business world. Unhelpful as this is to development of proper SCM organizations and strategies, it is a widespread misconception.

The responsibility set is highly specialized and focused on transferring and maintaining the invested value between two defined locations. It is not intended that any value-adding activity occur. The starting point is to define the goods to be transported and/or stored in as much detail as will satisfy customers and all the various national and international competent authorities involved. Whatever paperwork or documentation required must be raised, checked for accuracy, and monitored through the passage. The entire physical transfer process and receipt by the customer must be tracked closely and confirmation of successful outcomes achieved.

7.12 INFORMATION SYSTEMS AND TECHNOLOGY

SCM needs information to be able to operate effectively and often is dependent on others to generate that information. For example, the latest version of material specifications may need to accompany purchase orders issued by the team responsible for purchases. Those specifications are likely to have been drown up by another group (e.g., design) and without the ability to share databases, this would involve manually transferring information from one set of records to another; and this is how it used to be in the days of precomputer technology. The tremendous advances in technology and business process management over the years resulted in great new opportunities to share and manipulate data. This has in some ways been a two-edged sword. There is so much information available now and it is so easy to connect, it is difficult to truly identify the core of what is needed.

7.13 IMPROVEMENT

Improvement is the last set of processes to be included but is arguably the most influential and enduring. Improvement seems to be a natural component of the human condition. For whatever reason, people on the whole attempt to influence their environment for the better, either for themselves or for those around them. In Japan this was given the name *kaizen, kai* meaning "change" and *zen* meaning "for the better." This analysis does not attempt to clarify the reasoning. It is taken for granted, and the focus is on how improvement activities have progressed over the years and what has been learned from them to build a body of knowledge to help create sustainable improvement.

A critical point to mention here is that end-to-end supply chains are systemic entities, made up of independencies whereby seemingly innocuous events can have complex knock-on effects in apparently unrelated areas. These interdependencies involve people as individuals interacting in complex ways. People influence the system, and the system influences the people. Improvement is therefore elusive, transitory, and often short-lived. Those are the facts. Anyone offering improvement "out of the box" or a "do it yourself" tool kit is deluding himself or herself and attempting to delude you. Improvement is change, and we all accept the fact that change is difficult. So, by inference, improvement is difficult.

8 Production and Inventory Control

8.1 CORE MISSION

In Chapter 7 we considered an end-to-end supply chain as a continuum of connected production, delivery, and waiting stages. The fundamental role of P&IC is to orchestrate activities so that those stages work in accord with end-customer requirements for product. To achieve this, it must be the conductor of primary activities as they affect quantity and timing. This is not meant to bestow power or prestige on the process. It is merely recognition that the customer calls the tune in terms of demand for the product and there must be an allocated responsibility to remain engaged with that demand and to arrange supply to support.

It starts with demand for a product (or service) from an end customer (a patient in pharmaceuticals). Clearly, the finished product must be produced so that it is available to be consumed when the patient requires it. That production must be planned, executed, and result in consumption in the form of a sale. This is the core mission of P&IC: to manage and balance demand and supply optimally through the physical supply chain using the specific tools and levers at its disposal. It is likely that other firms' supply chains will be feeding into the finished product supply chain and P&IC activities carried out within firms in those supply chains (lower-tier suppliers). The mission is exactly the same. Each company in the supply chain must understand the consumption requirement of their customers and plan production and inventory accordingly. This is, again, an example of the critical need to establish organizational linkages in the management of supply chains. Readers may wish to take some time to consider these linkages from their own personal understanding of organizational life.

8.2 FIRST PRINCIPLES OF PRODUCTION AND INVENTORY CONTROL

The following metaphor, based on making cake in a kitchen, is intended to draw out the first principles of P&IC. Through the metaphor, the basics of P&IC can be explored and, hopefully, understood. The main objective is to demonstrate that none of this is anything more than common sense and simple mathematics applied to fit the particular circumstances at hand. What we cover here are the basic principles that underpin all the complex systems' jargon, such as enterprise resource planning (ERP),

Supply Chain Management in the Drug Industry: Delivering Patient Value for Pharmaceuticals and Biologics, By Hedley Rees
Copyright © 2011 John Wiley & Sons, Inc.

materials requirements planning (MRP I), manufacturing resource planning (MRP II), sales and operations planning (S&OP), advanced planning and optimization (APO), and all the others so often bandied about in SCM circles (those not familiar with these terms will find them explained later in the chapter). So on with the metaphor.

A Helpful Metaphor

Imagine that your spouse or partner has asked you to help make cakes. Your job is to produce the "mix" that will be piped into the individual baking pans. The ingredients are in a kitchen cupboard and you have the recipe and all the equipment, including the mixer. You set about the task, reading the recipe (at least the men will!), grabbing the ingredients, weighing them out where necessary, setting up the mixer, mixing it all up, filling up a bowl, and covering it with cling wrap—job done!

This part of the metaphor aims to highlight how easy it is to be working in a supply chain but not realize the importance of SCM because the demands on the supply chain are not particularly onerous; it also introduces some key elements of SCM. There are basic elements of SCM within the metaphor and even though there will be no formal consideration of them, you will almost certainly make a subconscious, commonsense assessment. There was a plentiful supply of the necessary ingredients in the cupboard, the mixer could easily produce the one mix needed to feed the family, and there was no great desire to eat the cake in any particular, set time frame. The mixture just had to be ready by the end of the day, when the spouse arrives home to complete the job.

Next, the cake metaphor is restated using the language of SCM. There was sufficient starting *inventory* and *capacity* to meet the order *lead time*; or stated a little more fully: The aim is to produce *output inventory* (a quantity of mix) from *input inventory* (ingredients). This is achieved through the production stage by using the *capacity* of the mixer to blend the mix. The total time taken to make output inventory available is the *lead time*.

Inventory is the consequence of the production of a product or material. *Starting inventory* (ingredients) is the outcome of the previous production stage. *Finishing inventory* (mix) is the outcome of the current production stage. Inventory is therefore consumed and created throughout all the production stages.

Capacity is the ability of the production-stage equipment (i.e., the mixer) to pass work through it. If, for example, the mixer was capable of making 5 kg of mix and that could be done every 20 minutes, the capacity is 15 kg per hour or 120 kg every 8 hours.

Lead time is the total time of all production, delivery, and waiting stages, beginning with the moment when the need for more inventory is identified: in this case the total time taken to read the recipe, set up the mixer, obtain the ingredients from the cupboard, collect them together, put them in the bowl, set up and work the mixing cycle, collect the mix output in a suitable container, and put cling wrap over the container ready for filling.

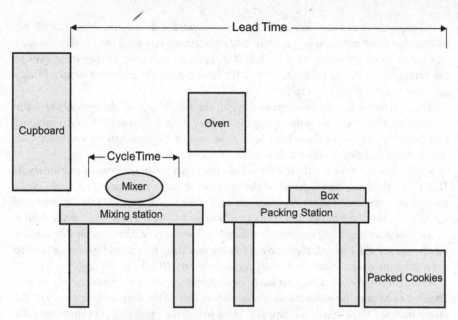

FIGURE 8.1   Lead time to make nutty noggins.

Lead time should not be confused with cycle time and a moment should be taken here to explain, because this is an important distinction that is often not well understood. The *cycle time* is the time it takes for the food mixer to pass through the cycle of setting up and producing a mix. Here, lead time and cycle time are the same. If we now look at the entire process of making the cakes (see Figure 8.1) that lead time includes machine (mixer) cycle time plus time in the oven plus delivery to the next stage, and so on. Thus, reductions in cycle time need to translate into total lead-time reductions before the full benefits accrue. If a reduction in cycle time merely results in the material waiting around longer, it is not a true benefit. Readers should keep an eye out for this principle through this and subsequent chapters.

Understanding the three variables above is critical to successful P&IC. It is now time to return to the metaphor and delve into a rather more demanding development.

A Helpful Metaphor (continued)

Imagine now that your spouse or partner arrives home and informs you that the local school has asked your family to provide cookies for their fund-raising event planned for the following weekend. The school has estimated they will need 500 of your famed home-produced nutty noggins. Suddenly, there is a supply chain on the agenda! There is now a customer for our cookies (the school) and an expectation of supply (an order to produce 500 units) to a specific time scale (by the weekend). How does the family develop a supply chain to produce the necessary inventory of cookies in the required lead time? Not a problem, says Dad. I'll do the mix, Mom can fill the baking pans and put them in the oven, and little Jimmy can pack the finished cookies into boxes to go off to the school. Then it will just be a case of driving them over to the principal's office Saturday morning. We have a plan! He arranged to take Friday off work to start the project in good time.

The day following the fund-raising event, the family are all sat around the table conducting a postmortem on the disappointment of the previous day. The nutty noggins had failed to make it to the school before the end of the fund-raising event. In fact, they were still sitting on the kitchen table. What went wrong?

As they played back events, it all became clear. This is what happened in a nutshell: Dad had calculated that if he filled the mixer to maximum capacity, he could make enough mix to produce all the cookies. By his calculations, it would take an hour and a half to do the three mixes. Each mix would need one hour in the oven, so in total it would take four and a half hours to be ready to allow the cookies to cool and be packed into boxes for the event. If they started Friday morning, that would be ample time to get it all done over the day and ready for delivery by 10:00 a.m. the following day.

Friday morning, Dad was up early and started on his job of making the mixes. To get a headstart, he made the three batches of mix to the maximum capacity of the mixer and sat them ready waiting for Mom to fill the pans and pop them into the oven. The first lot of filled pans were loaded into the oven. When Mom checked the progress of the baking, there was little evidence of the customary rising associated with successful baking. In fact, they were as flat as pancakes. When Mom checked Dad's mix, she could see the problem—it had not had the proper mixing to get air into the batter. Dad had allowed only the same amount of mixing time that he normally used for half the quantity in the bowl. How was he to know that more mix needed a longer mixing time? (What was that, Mom—he should have asked?)

Anyway, the net result was that the first lot of mix had to be thrown away, starting again with newly prepared mix. Worse yet, all the mix that Dad had already made had to be trashed as well. Add to this the fact that the oven could only manage to fit cookies from half of the mix, so that was also going to slow the entire process down.

Dad trudged off to get fresh ingredients from the cupboard to start all over again and was horrified to realize that the nuts, a vital ingredient in the noggins, were nearly all gone. There were enough nuts to make one batch of mix but no more. He shouted to Mom: Where do we get these nuts from? Mom's reply was: "I have to get them sent in from out of town. They can normally deliver the next working day, but not on weekends." When Dad got off the phone from the lady at the nut shop, his worst fears had been confirmed—no nuts until Monday!

Back in the real world, there are so many lessons in this metaphor. Those familiar with SCM will have seen the catastrophe coming and probably also felt Dad's pain! The good news is that all this could have been avoided if the principles of SCM had been applied from the start. The first and fundamental message here is that supply chain function is significantly impaired when there are defects in the process. When there are defects to the extent that Dad managed to achieve, things fall apart. There is a well-known game that lean practitioners use to drive this point home. It typically uses children's blocks to represent products to be manufactured and quickly demonstrates that defective assembly of the blocks (e.g., through not reading the instructions properly) is the fundamental inhibitor of goods leaving the factory gates. All the sophisticated supply chain tools in the world are useless without this fundamental requirement for quality.

Second, Dad needed to consider the production arrangement as a totality, not as a series of isolated steps. If he had done that, it would have been obvious that the oven was the rate-determining step or bottleneck. By making mix to the capacity of the mixer, he was stuffing the system with inventory that it couldn't handle. Third, by calculating the time required to make 500 cookies based on the mixer capacity, he was underestimating the total time needed for 500 cookies and making false promises to customers. If the nut shortage hadn't gotten him, the bottleneck with the oven probably would have.

This is now the point to review what Dad could have done to save himself from the verbal tongue lashing he eventually got from Mom. It revolves entirely around the three parameters mentioned above, which we term "The Wholesome Trinity," or TWT (Welsh for "neat, tidy, or smart"). They are explained here as a foundation for a learning opportunity for Dad.

8.2.1 Inventory

Any excess of production over consumption (usage) results in inventory. Conversely, desired consumption not supported by inventory results in a shortage. So, in very simple terms, the P&IC competency set involves balancing consumption, production, and inventory in line with consumer demand to avoid shortages or excess inventory.

Inventory is a dirty word in some quarters. It is often regarded as unnecessary waste or excessive investment in working capital and is subjected to radical inventory reduction programs (normally driven from the accounting fraternity). The just-in-time bandwagon in the 1980s added to the fervor, and lean has fueled the fire further (not purposely, but through misinterpretation of the principles).

From the metaphor above, it should become clear that inventory is the lifeblood of an organization's supply of product to customers. What wouldn't Dad have done for a usable inventory of cake mix? Imagine shopping for, say, an iPod and the salesperson remarking: "We don't have one of those for you today, sir, but we have been very successful in containing our investment in working capital."

The message is that inventory is vitally important, but it must be in the right place at the right time and in the right quantity, not just at the end customer. Inventory must exist at all tiers in the supply chain; otherwise, there will be nothing from which to make the finished product. Readers should treat the hype of just-in-time and inventory-less manufacturing systems with a very large grain of salt. In the same way that a typical adult needs eight pints of blood circulating around the body, supply systems need their eight pints' worth of inventory. Problems arise only if there is a surge or depletion of "blood" in a part of the system. Nature has found biological ways of balancing blood volume in normal, everyday circumstances. For supply chains, humans have not been as successful in designing similar self-balancing mechanisms (although the Japanese approach has helped).

In the shop cited above, inventory would be the iPod sitting on the shelf. In a pharmacy it would be the package of medicine resting in the cabinet. The package of medicine would have been produced from tablets of a certain strength and packaging materials. These would have been inventory at some point, having been made from other materials feeding into the conversion process that made them. So it goes on until the very first material required to start the whole thing is reached: chemicals, base commodities, human tissue, and so on.

Aside from inventory having a balance sheet value on which accountants focus, its primary role is to perform a function within the material or product it feeds into. This function is defined by the material or product specifications. Specifications are vitally important because they define what is required for the material or product to be "fit for purpose." This "fitness" will have been defined by those responsible for design and development and the necessary confirmations and tests will have been carried out. Each different specification is identified by a unique code number known as an item or part number.

Once set, the specifications must be documented and held securely to be used for all production activities. There is typically a formula, recipe, or bill of materials (termed *product structure*) that defines how the various inventory items are put together. The increasing complexity of dealing with the relationships between items, product structures, and the needs of supply has been addressed in some respects through the use of information systems and information technology. We expand on this in Section 11.4.

8.2.2   Capacity

In simple terms, *capacity* is the ability of any conversion process to get through work. This is measured as a volume of work (e.g., tons or bottles produced) and a time period (e.g., week or shift). The capacity of a machine can therefore be expressed as 1000 bottles per minute or 50 kg per shift. It is important to bear in mind that the common definition of capacity, as a measure of the amount that can be held or contained by something, can lead to confusion. This places the focus on input rather than output. Capacity must be measured on output, not on input. The preferred definition of *capacity* is that it is the maximum amount of work that a process or organization is capable of completing in a given period of time. It is analogous to a pipe rather than a bucket. Next we discuss important aspects of capacity.

Capacity Constraints   There is always a capacity constraint, rate-determining step, bottleneck operation—call it what you will—in any production process. The good news is that this simplifies planning immensely. The bad news is that the constraint can vary with the mix of products running through the process. Taking the good news first, in general terms, there is only a need to plan the constraint in any production process. For example, in the cake metaphor, the oven turned out to be the constraint.

If Dad had done his time estimates on the capacity of the oven (notwithstanding the mix-up in execution of the mix), he would probably have been successful. As for the bad news, if Dad had been making miniature macaroons, where lots would fit into the oven but they were labor-intentive and time consuming to fill, the baking pan filling operation might become the constraint. This brings us to production load.

Production Load   Load is determined from the products that are planned based on the capacity. In other words, load is *demand* for capacity, and *capacity availability* is the supply. The corollary to this is that sufficient capacity cannot be established until the load is known. Load is measured in the same units as those taken to measure the capacity. For example, if a machine's capacity is 200 kg per shift, the load of one product may be 25 kg, the next 40 kg, and so on. However, it is not just a case of adding up the loads to fill the capacity. There is such a thing as capacity leakage.

Capacity Leakage   *Capacity leakage* refers to all the things that steal time. It could be planned, such as a batch changeover, or unplanned, such as a machine breakdown. Either way, there must be recognition that time is lost in production and allowances must be made. Capacity leakage is often measured as a percentage of total available time and is termed *overall equipment effectiveness* (OEE). This again is a greatly misunderstood measure, as eager beavers record OEEs for every piece of equipment in a plant. Hopefully, the nutty noggin example shows that it is only the bottleneck that is important (see also Goldratt and Cox's book *The goal*[1]).

Demonstrated Capacity   There is a golden rule in P&IC that when planning load onto a production process, the assumed capacity availability should be determined "as demonstrated." *Demonstrated capacity* is the throughput net of all the possible capacity losses (leakages) that can occur. The importance of this cannot be overstated. Wishful thinking can be a sore temptation, especially when others downstream are screaming for supplies. The fact is, though, that if a process has never actually made an average of more than 100 units over a shift, planning for 120 will not make it happen. Those unfamiliar with the world of SCM may find it strange that this point is emphasized this way. The thought may be that this is obvious but in practice, it can't be obvious, because it is a very common issue that we explore further below.

8.2.3   Lead Time

Lead time is the third member of TWT and arguably the most elusive concept. Capacity and inventory are critical to control but relatively easy to see and measure. Lead time is as long as a piece of string made up of smaller pieces of string of unknown length. It represents the length of time that a consuming facility or customer has to wait from the point at which a need for supply is recognized. Typically, this involves an instruction to a source point to initiate the process of supply.

While the consuming plant is waiting for the inventory, work must continue using inventory on hand. The longer the wait, the greater the inventory that must be held in stock. There is a cash outflow associated with holding this inventory, which is, at a minimum, the interest payment on the working capital investment (not including fixed costs of storage, etc.). This is an area that accountants traditionally focus on, and sadly, they often pressurize businesses to reduce inventory without actually reducing lead times. If lead time is not reduced successfully, this is a recipe for crippling customer service levels in the longer term.

The other interesting thing about lead time is that it always seems to be orders of magnitude longer than the actual processing time. It is not uncommon for businesses to order three months (lead time) in advance something that takes 20 minutes to make (machine or process cycle time). There is therefore much potential for lead-time reduction!

8.3   THE WHOLESOME TRINITY IN P&IC

Now we are in a position to advise Dad as to what he should have done. With an order in hand, he knew exactly how many cookies he needed to make and when to deliver them. His task was therefore to manage the capacity of the system to get the cookies through in time to meet the order. This means identifying the rate-determining step by calculating the load (500 cookies) on each conversion step. He would then have recognized that the oven was the constraint that would slow him up. He would therefore had started the job earlier and, hopefully, reduced the size of the mix batch. If it was still a batch size that hadn't been processed previously, he would have checked with production (Mom) to as certain whether the mix was going to be sufficiently aerated or if it needed more time. If it needed more time, the cumulative (total) lead time would need to be adjusted again when he calculated the start date. Perhap, Dad should have taken Thursday off as well.

The next point concerns the ingredients in the cupboard. A cursory check of available starting inventory would not have been sufficient. The recipe (or bill of materials) told him how much of everything he needed to have on hand. Knowing the stakes associated with failure to supply, however, he should have reviewed his safety stock policy. Anything that he couldn't pick up quickly from the corner shop would be a candidate for safety holding. Hence, at the very least, he should have stocked up on nuts before starting.

The final point relates to satisfying his customers' expectation for the goods to arrive within the lead time allowed. It was therefore for Dad to manage the lead time by monitoring progress through the system. Dad should have planned the timings of production stages and then lay them onto some tracking device—say, a loading board. As the job was actually passing through the various stages, Dad could be ticking off compliance with the plan or identifying corrective action to get back on track. Unfortunately, the first time around there was such a catastrophe with the starting operation that nothing could have saved him. This again reinforces the importance of the low defect rates required to make SCM successful.

The discussion above covers the general requirements for the make-to-order arrangement. The two dimensions to be managed are lead time and capacity. There is now a twist on the horizon to prove that life in SCM can be further complicated by customers who are unable or unwilling to provide a firm order for a definite amount of inventory at a specific time. We start as is customary with a helpful metaphor, this time concerning a gentleman from Wales (a constituent country of the UK) named Dai.

A Helpful Metaphor

Dai has promised his children a pool party and tomorrow looks like a sunny day. He needs to go out to the local supermarket and buy one of those erect-o-pools. Once he has done that, all he needs to do is put it up and fill it with water (quite a lot of water). He would rather not spend money for a pool until he absolutely has to. Unfortunately, the kids are demanding, to say the least, and insist that if it is sunny, they must be in the pool from first light (I did say that they were demanding). Dai knows that in the morning it will take a couple of hours to erect the pool and the same again to fill it with water. By then the kids will have missed valuable "splash time." However, if the Welsh weather is true to form, the sunshine predicted could just as easily be torrential rain—and Dai's work and cash flow will be wasted. What does he do?

This is the universal dilemma of P&IC: whether to produce ahead of known customer demand. Does he risk the children leaving home in the event of blistering sunshine, or wait until he knows the weather is good, thus saving effort and cash in the event of rain? If Dai's children are as demanding as we suspect, he will go for the former. This means that he will get the pool up and running the night before. However, Dai actually works in P&IC at the local factory and did what he had been trained to do—design and control the conversion process to reflect customer demand.

The full pool represents *finished inventory*. The customers will not be satisfied until they have a "dive in and feel the flow" moment. The unerected pool will be *starting inventory* (once purchased), along with the water supply, hose, and any other bits and pieces that he needs. The lead time to produce the finished product will be the combination of setting up the hose, erecting the pool, and filling it with water. The fill time is dependent on the capacity of the hose, the rate at which water flows through it. Now we still have The Wholesome Trinity.

A Helpful Metaphor (continued)

Dai runs this through again in his mind. If the kids remain firm, he will have to produce a filled pool (hold finished inventory) before he knows what the weather is like (which drives customer demand). If he could persuade the kids that a reasonable wait was acceptable, as long as they did not have to wait longer than that, he should be in the clear (satisfied customers).

So what did Dai do following his deliberations? He negotiated a light breakfast for the kids, which gave him enough time to fill the pool he bought and erected the night before. The larger-capacity hose he borrowed from Jim next door meant he could fill the pool in super-quick time. He knew that the investment in a pool was a forgone conclusion, but at least he could save his time and the environment if the weather had turned nasty overnight. What a star you are, Dai!

This metaphor introduces the concept of the need to hold inventory in anticipation of customer demand. This is termed *make-to-stock* or *make-for-inventory* (the second term will be used here to be consistent with our use of the word *inventory*). Companies would clearly wish to wait for an order before committing working capital to production. In many cases, though, the market demands some element of risk, to retain demanding customers whose requirements could be serviced by the competition. Dai knew he couldn't afford to wait for an "order" from his kids because then the opportunity would be lost. What he actually did was to find a halfway house where he could configure-to-order by making some adjustments in the production process. That is, he could get his product close to final-stage completion, but not complete until the customer actually pressed the button. This would save all the water that would have been wasted if it had rained (and rain is a common occurrence in Wales!).

In summary, the end-to-end supply chain has a total lead time made up of all the elements that contribute to lead time (the sum of all the wait–produce–wait–deliver stages), often called the *cumulative lead time*. If plans have not been made for production of the product and the associated materials, the consumer must wait the full cumulative lead time (this can often run into years; see Dan Jones' commentary in Section 4.1). Clearly, this will not be acceptable to most paying customers. A decision therefore needs to be made based on the consumer's expectations for product availability. If the consumer is a patient requiring a prescription medicine, any wait may be unacceptable. If, on the other hand, a consumer requires a new car, a wait of weeks or even months may be acceptable. End customers for ships or major construction projects may not just need to wait the cumulative lead time of manufacture but also the time it takes for design.

This is a fundamental decision in P&IC and is always driven by customer expectations. If the customer needs it to be available on tap, inventory must be held in anticipation. The next decision is based on how long the customer is prepared to wait. If it is days up to a few weeks, *configure-to-order* may be the solution. This means holding inventory of all the components parts that may be needed and only putting them together when the order is received. Dell, the computer maker, is famous for this, although they also have clever ways of steering customers toward configurations that are popular, to reduce variety. If it is an item like furniture, the expectation may be that four to six weeks is OK, in which case it can be made to order, given that the raw materials are available. It then moves on to high-investment products that are of a standard design, such as aircraft, but where suppliers would be reluctant to invest in working capital without first having an order in hand. Finally, there is *design-* or *engineer-to-order*, where each product is designated for a specific customer and could not be offered to anyone else. Such a product must await the full design and manufacturing time line.

8.4 THE WHOLESOME TRINITY AND CUSTOMER EXPECTATIONS

The cases described above suggest that the supply chain must be managed differently according to customer expectations. In fact, there are only two broad possibilities: The customer is either willing to wait for a certain period of time or is not willing to wait. In the case of Dad and the cookies, the customer was willing and able to provide an order and wait the requisite time. Dai's pool example was initially a no-wait proposition and would have entailed Dai having the product "on the shelf" in time for the customers' arrival. Luckily, Dai was able to come up with a halfway house and prevent having to invest entirely in finished inventory.

The other case to consider is when a customer will not wait. The important principle here is that if a customer is unable to wait a certain time, a guess *must* be made as to the quantity planned to be produced, in the hope that the customer will still require the product when it is completed and available. If that guess isn't made, the customer is not going to get the product when the immediate need occurs (because of the necessary lead time). The guess is normally termed a *forecast*, the supply chain process is known as *demand forecasting*, and the P&IC activity is termed *make-for-inventory*.

Demand for products is the sum total of those collective persons' need for consumption. Since the end customer's decision to purchase a product is dependent on nothing other than personal preference or need, this is known as *independent demand*. This is the starting point for P&IC in circumstances where the customer won't wait. Independent demand is therefore a critical aspect to understand as the basis for SCM and should *always* be the starting point from which to design, build, and manage the supply chain. In the nutty noggins metaphor, this independent demand must be satisfied by the production of inventory if the family is to be successful in supplying the school event.

This adds a fourth dimension to P&IC, *independent demand*, to add to inventory, capacity, and lead time. To satisfy the former, the remaining three must be manipulated in particular ways. This is the challenge of P&IC. Independent demand forecasting typically starts with sales forecasts or projections generated by marketing staff. It is important that marketing personnel understand the need to develop figures that are fit for the intended use, since these figures will be the starting point for working capital investment in inventory. Sometimes marketers can inflate numbers provided to planning staff to ensure that sufficient supplies are produced. This can lead to obsolescence write-off and excess inventory in the supply chain.

Depending on the product and/or market dynamics, sales forecasting can be an onerous task. Various modeling tools have been devised to help in this area, and some very sophisticated computer modeling techniques are available. However, since sales forecasts will always be wrong to some degree, the emphasis should be on establishing upper and lower extremes of demand and a base rate (known as *takt* in the lean approach). This allows P&IC staff to determine schedules that optimize the balance between obsolescence and risk of failure to supply.

In practice, of course, a company will go to varying degrees of analysis to make a guess that is as close to the actual outcome as possible. The more uncertain the market, often, the greater the depth of analysis. It is beyond our scope in this book to delve into the various statistical forecasting techniques available to help with forecasting, and in my opinion it is, more often than not, unnecessary to go to great lengths to be precise.

We now return to the cookies metaphor to further examine the make-for-inventory case.

A Helpful Metaphor (continued)

The following year the family is offered a second chance by the school. This time, however, the principal has invited another cookie-maker to run a stall, just in case things go wrong a second time. The school authorities have also said that they will not commit to an order; it is up to the family to turn up with however many cookies they can sell and take their chances against the competition.

Dad is far from dull and recognizes instantly the potential difficulty in deciding how many cookies to make. Too few and they may run out of inventory on event day, too many and the family fortune may be converted into unwanted cookies in the trash. The problem is that they have to commit to production in order to source the ingredients and make the cookies in time. What they need is a sales forecast! We can't make any decisions regarding production until we know the projected demand.

Mom sets off to the school for discussions with those who should know. On her return, this is what she had discovered from the event organizers. One hundred twenty tickets had been sold so far, with a week to go. People also just turned up on the day, and in previous years this had been about the same number as those buying ahead. One year, though, when the weather was particularly good, nearly four times as many turned up.

Demand for your cookies was likely to be high given the generous sugar content in nutty noggins and the high percentage of "sweet teeth" in the area. The competition (another family in the area) was an unknown quantity when it came to cookie making, but had a good reputation as keen amateur chefs. By now, Dad is scratching his head and starting to worry. He must decide how many cookies to produce and take along to the event. There will be no second chance because there would be no option to make more in time if sales took off (he should also test the validity of that assumption). He needs an accurate forecast! There is uncertainty present at a number of levels. How many people will turn up? Of those turning up, how many will want to buy cookies? How many cookies will buyers eat, on average? Will nutty noggins steal the show, or will the competition's creations win the day? Or will it be neck-and-neck?

Whatever Dad does, the likelihood is he will get it wrong and be left with either stale cookies or disappointed customers. All he can do in the end is to make a judgment that is the best he can achieve for the "family business." Fundamentally, if the cookies are cheap and the prices are good (high margin), he can afford to write-off waste cookies and still do well. If the cookies are not cheap to make and customers won't pay inflated prices (low margins), he should err on the side of caution with his production schedule. This is the time for Dad to pull his laptop out, get his math head on, and do some simple modeling of the possible outcomes. He should spend more time on this than on forecast accuracy.

There we leave Dad for the time being, for some more investigation of the utility of TWT.

8.5   LEVERAGING THE WHOLESOME TRINITY

The above may appear a vast oversimplification of the major constituents involved in P&IC, but it *really* is that simple at the concept level. However, much as understanding what the throttle, brake, and steering wheel do on a car, it by no means makes driving an easy task. So it is in P&IC. Using all three in concert to achieve successful outcomes requires skill, knowledge and a healthy respect for the perils of dangerous driving!

Whichever is the case; there are always only three basic variables involved in the planning process: inventory, lead time, and capacity. To reiterate, in a make-for-inventory environment, lead time is set to zero (no customer wait) with capacity managed to regulate inventory. In a make-to-order environment, finished inventory is set to zero and capacity is managed to control lead time (customer waits a known mutually agreed period). In both cases, capacity must be managed. Since most modern supply chains are a series of supply stages from lower- to higher-tier suppliers, each tier must determine a policy for each item of inventory. The guiding principle should always be: What is needed to support the end customer? For example, in a configure-to-order environment, the next-lower-level suppliers must make-for-inventory, since the end customer is only willing to wait the configuration time, not the additional time to make the components. In practice, supply chains are made up of a combination of make-for-inventory and make-to-order policies.

Interestingly, lean thinking has made good use of this concept through the use of kanbans and supermarkets (see also Section 11.2.8). The concept of supermarkets works in a manner similar to supermarket shelves, whereby inventory levels are maintained at all times (as far as possible) within set levels. As inventory is drawn by customers, shelf replenishment takes place based on set rules. These are, in fact, closed-loop replenishment (sub-) systems. In simple terms (although there are sophisticated variations), they are activated by a trigger, or signal (*kanban*), to produce a fixed amount of inventory and then stop (i.e., maintain a "steady state"). The trigger point and make quantity are determined by average end-customer demand. Cleverly, these loops then become self-managing and work somewhat akin to the body's immune system. They only operate in response to an attack on the system (depletion of inventory). Similarly, antibodies "produce" only when there is a need to repel attacks on the body's steady state.

What lean thinking has not recognized so effectively in my opinion is the balance required when make-to-order *must* be employed. This then calls for active management of lead time to meet the demands of the system. For example, if materials are being sourced from faraway lands involving complex supply networks, making-to-order may be the only alternative. This can lead to customer satisfaction only if the material arrives on time and in sufficient quantity.

8.6 THE IMPACT OF VARIETY ON SUPPLY CHAINS

Readers could be forgiven at this stage for wondering what the fuss in managing supply chains is all about. There was an obvious learning-curve effect as Dad cracked the problems of setting up to supply customers, but from then on, he has it nailed, doesn't he? Now that he has the equipment set up, knows what inventory he needs to have on hand before starting, and can achieve sufficient flow through the facility, where's the problem?

The answer is that there unlikely to be a problem if our customers are happy to eat nutty noggins as their one and only cookie treat. Customers are not normally that staid in their ways, however. They like variety and soon start demanding other tasty alternatives. So it's back to the helpful metaphor.

A Helpful Metaphor (continued)

As luck would have it, the second year's event was a roaring success. Although good at creating savory foods, the family in competition was a dismal failure with their cookies, and our family cleaned up. Dad had decided to go for broke with his production volumes, and it had worked out. With the new injection of funds into the business, Dad had expansion plans on his mind. It didn't take him long to set up a little shop counter at the back of the house so he could grow some trade.

Mom and Dad then set about adding a couple more products to the portfolio by offering several noggin flavors; they decided on blueberry, cherry, and the original chocolate. When the recipes were complete, it was time to think about production. The equipment to make the cookies could be the same as before, but the mixer would need to be changed over between each flavor. This involved simply removing the bowl, washing and drying it, and replacing it on the stand. That shouldn't be a problem—it was just a case of allowing a bit of extra time on top of mixing time.

The following week, after launch of the new product lines, desperation and despair had returned to Dad's world as it did after the first school event. The family again sat in the kitchen contemplating the nightmare of the previous week. "If only I had made more of the blueberry and a lot less of that damn cherry; and sales of the original chocolate flavor didn't suffer despite the new additions."

They ran out of inventory of the blueberry noggins after the first few hours, so needed to get the equipment set up to produce more almost immediately. How many to produce now? Having seen such a good demand, Dad decided to make a full batch at mixer capacity. If they went this quickly at the start, who knows how high demand could go? Learning from his previous mistake, Dad gave the batch a lot longer mixing time. He also consulted Mom to confirm that it had been prepared properly before putting it in the oven. The oven was now a larger-capacity model able to take a full mix in one go. Fresh supplies were on their way!

As Dad orchestrated the production flow, Mom appeared from the shop to inform him that the original chocolate noggins were running low and could do with topping up. How could he do that, though, because the machinery was occupied making product for all those future customers for blueberry noggins. The extra mixing time for the large batch meant that Dad had to wait longer than he would have liked to change over to chocolate noggins. He was relieved to see the last of the blueberry mix go into the baking pans so he could set up for chocolate. As he started cleaning the bowl he was horrified to find that the residue from the blueberry was sticking like glue. He scrubbed and scrubbed, but it held firm. He searched the house to find a suitable scouring device. Eventually, one was found, and 20 minutes of hard scrubbing later, the bowl was clean.

Racing like made now, Dad thrust the bowl back onto its stand and went off to find the ingredients. He glanced at his watch on his way to the cupboard and realized that he would not have time to get a batch through and into the oven before the end of the day. He had other family commitments to meet so he had to wait until the following day before starting the chocolate mix.

Up bright and early the following day, Dad started on the mix. He decided on a smaller batch this time to cut down on time. Some of the ingredients were getting low as well. Dad cursed the cherry noggins that had used up ingredients for product that was not selling. Still, once this batch of chocolate is through, life will get less frenetic. That was when Mom appeared from the shop again. She informed Dad that the cherry noggins were starting to go stale given the lack of movement and poor air circulation on the shelves. Most of them would probably go in the trash. Although there were few customers for them, the customers there were loved them with a passion. They were also regular and profitable customers for the original noggins. He didn't need only the chocolate noggins now; he needed the cherry as well!

Dad was now in backlog big time. What can he do? Someone suggested that he should go back to making just the chocolate nutty noggins until he knew a bit more about managing supply chains. Now who was that—Mom?

The metaphor aims to bring home the supply chain difficulties that emerge when equipment and processes need to be changed over. Independent demand is prone to sudden change as customers do what customers do—make unpredictable choices. The production facility, as with the supertanker in Chapter 1, is nothing like as forgiving of change. Each time a changeover takes place, capacity leaks out of the system. The greater the number of changeovers, the greater is the leakage.

Leakages have a far larger impact than many people appreciate. Often, a machine may need to run suboptimally for a period after a change to "get back into the swing of it." There is nothing more detrimental to machine efficiency than stopping and starting. It is not unusual to see blister packaging lines in Europe running at overall equipment effectiveness in the middle 20%. The number of variants required for a range of different languages, run on high-speed lines with time-consuming changeover times, means that these machines spend more that 70% of the time idle.

Observations, Views, and Experiences of the Author

This story is a personal favorite of mine! As an industrial engineer earlier in my career, it was my job to set standard times for machine operations. In the secondary packaging facility, there were two lines that labeled, cartoned, inserted a package leaflet, and overwrapped the product that was being fed through to them in unlabeled filled and capped bottles.

The lines were what I would call "mature" (i.e., quite old) and ran at 80 bottles per minute nominal machine speed. When all capacity leakages were taken into account, the demonstrated output was about 40 bottles per minute. The project engineers had decided in previous budgeting rounds that a new, higher-speed line was required. (Rhetorical question: If you have a budget, why not use it?) One of the drivers for this decision was that the project engineers had been criticized on a similar project in the previous year for purchasing a machine that was not "quick" enough. They were not going to suffer the same indignity again. This time they went for a high-tech machine to run at 220 bottles per minute nominal speed. After all the calculations were done, this new machine was going to be able to get through all the product that was to go through the existing lines, plus another range of products on top of that—and all that would take just six weeks of the year! What would they do with all that spare time!

Some readers may have guessed what is coming next—a "dad in the kitchen the following day" moment. When the new machine was installed, the plant suffered the most horrendous backorder situation it had ever encountered. It was an order of magnitude worse that anything that had happened before. The markets were in an uproar. The site leader was in despair. The engineers were in hiding. There was only one group not totally shocked by the events as they unfolded—the operators.

They knew that the two "mature" lines were workhorses: The setups were pretty straightforward—there was little to go wrong when they were running. If one line did go down for any reason, they could prioritize and channel work through the other line while repairs were made. Repairs were normally mechanical adjustments and technology-free. When the line was back up, the queue that had formed could be worked back down to an acceptable level of wait time for customers.

With the single new line, there was only one channel in, and in all cases where there is only one door, an orderly (at least initially) queue forms. Since the feeder department was making to forecast, that queue contained product that was only a guess at what customers needed. As actual sales differed from to the guess, customers wished to change their requirements. This meant reshuffling the queue to put the most urgent first. In doing this, those orders that were reshuffled back in the queue once and then twice and then a third time eventually became dire emergencies. Even though they were small quantities for infrequent customers, some were influential and soon the company reputation was going down the drain. The supply chain was branded a total failure.

8.7   DESIGNING APPROPRIATE PRODUCTION SYSTEMS

Hopefully, the metaphor has set the reader thinking about a supply chain that has to produce a variety product and the need for that to be accommodated properly. The other realization should be that managing a supply chain is not just about information related to supply and demand. It is also heavily influenced by the arrangement of machinery and equipment within the physical supply chain. Inappropriately designed systems can leave P&IC in impossible situations. The converse is also true, but is less common.

It was at the time when customers started to become more demanding of variety that the concept of mass production began to fail. The traditional manner of arranging facilities had been based on the concept of division of labor (or effort) proposed by Adam Smith and F. W. Taylor: that is, to separate the various production stages so that they could become increasingly productive in terms of output per time period based on the learning-curve effect. In those days, machines were replacing labor and making big savings. Since there was little variety (hence few change overs), machine utilization could be kept high. Machinery became far more productive than manual labor.

To maintain this advantage, machines and equipment were organized around their specific types. That is, grinding machines would be separate from milling machines, which would be separate from lathes, which would be separate from polishers, for example. The aim was then to run the maximum volume through the machinery to drive unit costs down. If they had capacity problems and needed to buy a new machine, it would be installed with all the others of a similar class.

The aim was then to run the machines (maximize utilization) for as long a possible to get the most from economies of scale, which made for very low cost per unit. Although there was little variety, this concept held true for total cost as well. High volumes meant that as well as labor costs being low, material costs could be held low (large buying quantities), and overheads were not inflated by complex requirements needing to be managed by supervisory and auxiliary staff. Variety blew a hole in all that, or more accurately, the requirements for multiple machine and process changeovers spoiled the show. Changeovers meant that people were at a standstill waiting for things to get going again. When this stage was reached, the third element of time in the supply chain suddenly began to grow almost exponentially. This is the waiting stage—and it was only going to get worse.

The lean fraternity christened this outcome a *process village* and the scheduling was termed *batch and queue*. Each machine in the production sequence would run off a batch of product (similar to a pharma batch but not necessarily controlled by lot number) to last a period of time and then move onto the next product. Batches were typically large to achieve the desired (perceived) economies of scale. If more than one component was to be produced on the machine, a changeover would be required. Batch sizes would be maximized to minimize the number of changeovers within the constraint of the total demand for each component. To hit those high volumes, producers had become accustomed to making a product and then testing it afterward. Presumably this was because management focus was on "meeting the numbers." Any problem then found therefore resulted in an entire batch having to be reworked or even scrapped, with a consequent disruption of production activities and the formation of fresh queues. Given the focus on volume at the expense of other quality-based factors, the chances of defects being found at inspection were also relatively high.

This was the point at which complications started to set in for mass production. Although machines were much faster than human beings, changeover between jobs took much longer. The larger and faster the machine, the longer it took. Product variety brought with it lower volumes, more changeovers, and hence increased machine downtime (capacity leakage); also, of course, forecasting became even less accurate, as it was more difficult to predict the exact breakdown of customer preferences for various options within a class (e.g., blueberry vs. cherry vs. chocolate noggins.). This made it more likely that what was produced in the batch was not what the customer wanted, so it was set aside while the product that the customer apparently really wanted was rushed into production. The net result of this was massive queues in our plants—and not just one but queues all over the place, at almost every stage, as production ran to the highest volumes they could set (to achieve those essential economies of scale), and they guessed at customer needs.

Readers may now be forgiven for thinking that if these queues were so prevalent, why didn't someone do something about them? The answer is simple—they were invisible. The queues—"paper" queues as it were—existed in the backlog of orders waiting to pass through the production process. Lines of orders in the scheduling process waited for their turn on the machine. Increasingly in larger companies, these orders were sitting in the materials management systems that had become popular to help manage the increasing complexity. The logic used (see Chapter 11) was based on forecasts, batches of production, and economic order quantities for component purchases—the logic of batch and queue.

At this point some commentators were suggesting that enough was enough. Mass producers were stuffing plants with component parts at the input end and waiting for products to pop out the other end, with huge and unpredictable lead times and varying levels of quality. Why were the lead times so long and varied and quality so poor? The answer is that if mass production had remained at the level of the Model T Ford, there probably wouldn't have been an issue. With a product that could be "any color as long as it is black," customers could turn up at Ford's door with barely any wait—a flow of identical cars left the assembly line every day. But when the external environment changed without any adjustment in the thinking patterns of those engaged in production, the result was as described above.

As the issues of dealing with variety became increasingly apparent, however, initiatives to address the problems began to emerge.

- *Variety reduction.* This solution looked at ways of reducing the number of finished products and component parts through two broad approaches: standardization and simplification. An example of this in pharmaceuticals was the attempt to move to multilingual packaging in Europe, so that a single pack could be supplied to three, four, or more markets. The author was involved in these initiatives in the early 1990s, and initial gains were made in customer service and costs. However, a set of regulations known as the *blue box regulations*, introduced in the late 1990s, effectively meant that only one language could be accommodated on a package. Those gains were reversed instantly. To this day, the author is not sure if regulators really appreciate the impact this reversal had on productivity levels in packaging plants. Whether it is beyond the wit of technology and modern man ever to make an impact in this area remains to be seen.

- *Value engineering and value analysis.* This approach involved questioning and challenging the function of every component in a product so that (1) it is proved to be necessary and (2) it is not over- or underspecified. Whatever is unnecessary or specified improperly is removed or amended. The activity is called *value engineering* when it is performed at the design stage and *value analysis* when carried out on designs already in production.

- *Group technology.* This method attempted to group products together into families similar enough to be able to pass through machines and equipment arranged in sequence. Instead of each machine making batches, the product would flow from one machine to the next until it got to the end. This significantly reduced work in progress. Following from this principle, cellular production became an extension of the approach.

- *Cellular production.* This technique involved not only the machines and their operators grouped together, but some of the indirect functions that had previously been spread over the entire plant were allocated to production cells to provide more focused support: typically consisting of line engineers, P&IC staff, materials handlers, and others. Reporting relationships were changed as well, so that a single cell manager would take overall responsibility for achieving production and quality objectives. One of the key aims was to increase functional identification with and commitment to the products and markets they were supplying.

- *Runners, repeaters, and strangers.* This approach is a personal favorite of mine. I first came across it in the early 1990s while completing the Cranfield Development Program. It is a potentially powerful approach to proper design of production systems and is part of the lean tool box. The concept behind it is to place products into one of three categories:
  - *Runners.* These are higher-volume products that typically follow the *Patero principle*: approximately 80% of the volume is accounted for by 20% of the

products. (Ian Glenday, through his work on the Glenday sieve, has refined that further through experience. He estimates that 50% of volume is concentrated in only 6% of products.) The machinery and equipment arrangement to produce the runners would be geared up for speed and high throughput. By limiting the mix to a reduced number of products, the variety and hence the need for changeover are very much reduced. As a consequence, production will tend to run at high OEEs.

- *Repeaters.* These are the products that form the vast bulk of variants. They therefore require more careful scheduling to prevent the associated greater propensity for demand fluctuation, creating instability and wasteful changeovers. The machinery and equipment arrangement needs to incorporate greater mix flexibility through shorter, simpler setups. It would not make sense to run these products on high-capacity lines with elongated changeover times. The capacity leakages are likely to be huge, as are the consequent queues. Often, semiautomatic (mix of operators and machinery) rather than fully automated methods are more appropriate.

- *Strangers.* Strangers may only pop up occasionally, and no one really welcomes trying to incorporate these products into their well-laid plans. Strangers are a fact of life, however, in terms of spares or replacement parts, for example. They can sometimes be accommodated into the repeater facility, but this can also be disruptive for regular customers. It may be more cost-effective to have a totally different but very flexible setup for these. In pharmaceutical terms, it may merely be the ability to provide hand-packing facilities when the need arises.

The exact way in which categorization is determined is less important than achievement of a successful result: that is, a production system that prevents variation and changeovers from interfering with overall throughput efficiency.

P&IC is covered further in Chapter 11. Readers expecting to hear about computer-based support available to SCM will find that in Chapter 11. The reason for delaying until then is to divorce the principles of SCM from the current plethora of computerized "solutions" available to companies and SCM practitioners. In my view we are at the stage where the packaging of "best practices" in predetermined "black boxes" relieves those involved of the need to understand the underlying principles. Consequently, proper thinking regarding these issues does not take place, and the supply chain suffers accordingly.

Finally, for those readers who are still concerned about the plight of Dad and the noggin debacle, there is good news. He did actually book himself into a course in lean thinking at Dan Jones' Lean Academy at Ross-on-Wye. More on this in Chapter 12, but why not learn about the rest of SCM first? This takes us to strategic procurement.

9 Strategic Procurement

9.1 CORE MISSION

In the chapter title we placed the word *strategic* before *procurement* to emphasize the importance of taking a long-term, business-supportive view of the procurement process when dealing with supply chains. It involves identifying the materials, services, machinery, and equipment engaged specifically in taking products to market; then operating procurement processes focused on those supply chains. All organizations need to source externally to some extent: perhaps in a limited range of goods and services or as a major proportion of the organization's spending. Whatever the span, a measured approach to procurement can yield tremendous benefits to an organization.

Procurement as a business process relates to the acquisition of goods and services from third parties as necessary inputs to a business. This entails creating and cultivating competencies, services, agreements, and actions within the supply base to help build the desired competitive advantage in the target market. A supply base consists of all the third-party organizations, firms, and businesses that provide goods and services in both primary and support activities.

Procurement can be carried out anywhere in a business with absolutely no involvement of a procurement or purchasing organizational function. Most organizations, however, establish a functional department with responsibility for buying goods and services from third parities. These departments can be named variously: sourcing, purchasing, buying, procurement, supplies management, or something similar. The important point to bear in mind is that procurement is a concern for every business, and functional responsibilities must be defined with that in mind. It should also be recognized that the process can be made infinitely more powerful by investing *stewardship* of the process into one function. The entirety of a firm's basket of purchased goods and services forms what is known as the *purchasing portfolio* of the business. Proper understanding and management of the purchasing portfolio is an absolute prerequisite for effective procurement, and this is to be covered next.

One final point to consider before moving on is the fact that the terms *procurement* and *purchasing* are often used interchangeably. For the sake of clarity, we will consider procurement to be the set of process activities required to make third-party goods and services available to an organization. This involves the complete cycle from the initiation of an organizational desire to procure goods and services through to their being available for use. Purchasing is a subset of procurement which involves

---

Supply Chain Management in the Drug Industry: Delivering Patient Value for Pharmaceuticals and Biologics, By Hedley Rees
Copyright © 2011 John Wiley & Sons, Inc.

certain competencies related to dealings with third parties, such as the terms and conditions of purchase, supply contracts, and supply market intelligence. Although the next section deals with the *purchasing portfolio*, it could equally be dealing with the *procurement portfolio*.

9.2 THE PURCHASING PORTFOLIO

Many supply arrangements will have minimal impact on an organization, whereas others may be of fundamental significance. Understanding of this concept was transformed in the 1980s by Peter Kraljic and his Kraljic matrix. Peter Kraljic (pronounced "Kra-litch"), an ex-McKinsey consultant, devised a 2 × 2 matrix that probably did for procurement what the Boston matrix did for marketing. It informed the profession on where and how to focus valuable resources and more important, where not to. Kraljic's ideas were first publicized in 1983 in the *Harvard Business Review*.[1] His article recognized that purchasing had been pigeonholed too narrowly and was not meeting the needs of strategic supply management. That is, it was not contributing properly to the generation of competitive advantage from the supply base. A basic outline of the model is described below.

9.2.1 The Kraljic Matrix

Kraljic defined two dimensions for the matrix:

1. *Profit impact:* the potential for an item or items in the portfolio to affect the profit margin of a business. As value minus cost equals margin, these items may be adding to the top (innovation) or the bottom (cost improvement) line.
2. *Supply risk:* the likelihood of failure to secure the requisite supply when required. This can relate to internal (e.g., overly tight specification) or external (e.g., scarcity) factors.

Armed with this model it was possible to segment the purchasing portfolio such that items or groups of items could be treated according to the respective positioning within the matrix. The four possible segments are explained below.

1. *Leverage.* This segment is often identified with the traditional role of the purchasing function and has been dubbed the "adversarial" approach. This is not fair, however, because it is a legitimate approach in the appropriate circumstances. This item class represents relatively high expenditures where there is an adequate base of prospective suppliers able to meet requirements: for example, a fleet of cars for a sales force, or office refurbishment. The buyer is in a strong position to exploit the opportunity by seeking the best deal through competitive bidding.
2. *Noncritical.* These are the 80% of purchases that typically account for approximately 5% of the total portfolio value. They are the multitude of small

purchases that must be made to keep a business supplied with routine materials. The user knows what is required and can find it easily at a price that could not possibly damage the business. Emphasis should be on reducing functional effort using efficient processes by automating transactions and engaging users more directly; also, buyers should look for opportunities to move to leverage by consolidating purchases.

3. *Strategic.* This segment, which is critical to the competitive advantage generated from within the supply base, can relate to goods and services supplied to primary or support activities. The common theme is that the category of items contributes to profit margins (revenue up or cost down), and security of supply is in doubt. It could be specialist machinery or processing of a novel ingredient in a flagship product. The focus in this segment is on long-term commitment to relationships for mutual benefit. This means building partnerships or alliances that keep driving toward sustained competitive advantage in the marketplace. This is not just a job for a purchasing function; the requirement is for a team working across the relevant functional boundaries, often led by a technology expert.

4. *Bottleneck.* These are items that have the potential, if not managed properly, to bring proceedings to a halt. Being of relatively low value, they are likely to be off the radar screen if not given proper attention. If, for example, a small amount of a particular reagent is necessary to run a manufacturing process, even though it may be cheap to acquire, it should receive close attention given its criticality.

The model outlined above is very simple but powerful. It is difficult to overestimate its value, particularly as a means of winning over sceptical colleagues who are wary of functional involvement with a specialist area. I have used this numerous times with clinical and nonclinical leaders to explain that in the strategic box, they take the lead. The role of procurement is to facilitate the process. They will not get an inappropriate CRO thrust upon them to save a few pennies here and there. They will, however, be urged to define their requirements very specifically, spread the net wide for potential providers, and produce a professional document to provide to prospective suppliers so that they can bid with confidence and to help them understand the commercial terms by which they will be bound.

It is now time to hear from Peter Evans, an expert in the field of procurement and strategic sourcing, for an account of his adaption of the model in everyday practice.

GUEST CONTRIBUTOR SLOT: PETER EVANS

Segmenting Expenditure: The Need for a Portfolio-Based Approach[2]

Whatever the detailed goals and objectives of any purchasing group, one of its key activities relates to the successful selection of sources of supply. However, in most companies the range of goods, materials, and services to be sourced is enormous.

There will be important differences between the approaches required to select suppliers for office supplies, for example, compared to the sourcing of important raw materials or components or the selection of a market research provider.

A well-proven way of helping to determine the best approach is by segmenting the total expenditure using a technique called *portfolio analysis*, a purchasing planning and decision support tool adapted from several strategic marketing models. Portfolio analysis helps to manage and control the list of everything for which purchasing has responsibility; we call this the *purchased portfolio*. First, the total portfolio is sorted into a small number of *categories* of expenditure (sometimes referred to as "commodities," a term that can lead to confusion and misunderstanding). This reduces the initial challenge of purchasing—being overwhelmed by the sheer number of individual line items or part numbers under management. In most situations the number of categories will be small and quite manageable (typically between 10 and 30 categories in a large manufacturing and marketing organization). It is quite feasible to contemplate developing sourcing for 30 categories, whereas 10,000 line items seems impossible.

Once the total expenditure has been identified and sorted into categories, we can move forward into segmentation. This will enable us, initially, to determine the best approaches for source selection and, over the longer term, to the ongoing processes of supplier management. The method of carrying out portfolio analysis is very straightforward and requires little in the way of special training. All that is needed is an assessment of two factors for each category of expenditure, which is usually carried out by the individuals or teams who are responsible for sourcing each category.

Approach to Portfolio Analysis   The first assessment factor is the *financial importance* (sometimes called the *profit impact*) to the business of the expenditure for the category concerned. This is usually based on the relative amount being expended for the specific category compared to the total for expenditure, rated as high or low.

The second factor to be assessed is the degree of *market difficulty* of the category: how many potential alternative suppliers are available in the marketplace, and how easy it would be to move from one to another. Market difficulty is influenced by things and practices internal to the company and by external forces in the supply chain and supply market. Internal factors include the ways in which specifications and performance testing criteria are written, the supplier quality approvals and certifications required, lead-time and forecasting issues, delivery requirements and shipping needs, customer or end-user direction, and of course, the preferences of our colleagues inside the company [these opinions (sometimes subjective and anecdotal) are often the major influencing factor in deciding sourcing arrangements].

The degree of market difficulty is also affected by external factors. These will be concerned with the number of suppliers and potential suppliers with the capability to meet the demands; the availability of capacity; technological factors, including access to patented and proprietary processes; the investment required to turn a potential supplier into a real sourcing option; the degree of collusion among suppliers in

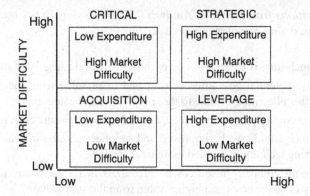

FIGURE 9.1   Portfolio analysis.

the marketplace; and legal, environmental, health and safety, and other external or governmental requirements. The degree of market difficulty is rated in the same way that financial importance was rated, either high or low.

From these two ratings we are now in a position to segment each category of expenditure using a simple four-box matrix, shown in Figure 9.1.[3] Each of the four segments has been given a descriptive name:

1. *Acquisition:* those categories with a low expenditure and low market difficulty. Examples include office supplies, stationery, and some classes of MRO (maintenance, repair, and operating supplies).
2. *Critical:* those categories with a low expenditure but high market difficulty. Examples include spare parts required from manufacturers of equipment, software and its support, and flavors, colors, fragrances, minor ingredients, and additives.
3. *Leverage:* those categories with a high expenditure and low market difficulty. Examples include packaging components, standard materials or components, and services such as cleaning, security, and catering.
4. *Strategic:* those categories with a high expenditure and high market difficulty. Examples include special components or materials; items for which the supplier controls the process, technology, capacity, or intellectual property; and goods and services that have become single sourced.

With the initial portfolio analysis completed, it is important that it be used to review and challenge the status quo. It is possible to move categories from one segment of the portfolio to another through planned actions by the purchaser, but before doing this, it is useful to employ portfolio analysis as a framework to reconsider a number of important aspects of the ways in which sources of supply are selected.

Ten Key Questions from Portfolio Analysis   The following 10 key questions need to be considered after completing a portfolio analysis:

1. How much time is being spent on each segment and category of the portfolio?
2. Does the potential cost improvement and extra value from the supply base justify this allocation of time to these segments and categories?
3. Does the emphasis need to change, and how should resources be reallocated?
4. How much could cost be improved and supplier value be increased by better purchasing techniques applied more intensively?
5. How could company resources be organized in the best way to maximize delivery of lower costs and higher value from the supply base?
6. What is the relative balance of power between the company and its suppliers for each category of expenditure?
7. How should this balance of power be changed, and what actions are needed to make this happen?
8. What relationships exist with suppliers in each segment, and are they appropriate?
9. Which relationships need changing, and how will that be planned and implemented?
10. What are the priority areas that will maximize purchasing contribution to the business while addressing risks and vulnerabilities in the supply chain?

Guidelines for Sourcing in Each Segment   From the portfolio analysis segmentation, a number of guidelines can be developed. These relate to strategic options, allocation of purchasing resources, techniques to be applied, and relationships with suppliers. In every case we should also consider alternative portfolio analysis positions and what is needed to make a change. A few useful guidelines for each segment are provided below.

Acquisition

- *Strategy:* Automate, consolidate, and delegate to reduce complexity, administrative burden, and paperwork; supplier reduction.
- *Resources:* Minimize the amount of resources for this segment.
- *Techniques:* Supply base rationalization, purchasing cards, added value from suppliers.
- *Supplier relationships:* No requirement for close relationships.
- *Options to move:* Move to leverage by grouping and consolidation of demands.

Critical

- *Strategy:* Manage and reduce risk; introduce alternatives; work with others.
- *Resources:* May need periodic review and concentrated effort from time to time.

- *Techniques:* Risk management and contingency planning; market, technical, and supplier analysis; contracting to protect interests.
- *Supplier relationships:* May need close relationships with a few selected vendors.
- *Options to move:* Move to acquisition by introducing alternative suppliers or materials; move to strategic or leverage by consolidating with other categories.

Leverage

- *Strategy:* Maximize profit by aggressive cost management.
- *Resources:* Requires regular application and significant amounts of resource.
- *Techniques:* Competition analysis, inquiries and quotation analysis, conditioning, tactical negotiation, basic cost analysis, price list analysis, changes of suppliers.
- *Supplier relationships:* No need for close relationships with leverage suppliers since there is no expectation of continuity of business; beware of suppliers attempts to move to close relationships and drive the portfolio analysis up to strategic.
- *Options to move:* Move to strategic by working with fewer selected suppliers who have demonstrated a desire and commitment to work together for mutual benefit; there needs to be a robust process to ensure that any closer relationship remains a sustainable option over time.

Strategic

- *Strategy:* The two basic strategic options are either to remain in the strategic segment and work closely with the supplier to generate extra value or to move to leverage by lowering the market difficulty.
- *Resources:* Requires major amounts of resources, usually from purchasing and a number of functional areas to be applied consistently over time.
- *Techniques:* Market, technical, supplier and supply chain analysis, source planning, performance contracting, purchase price cost analysis, continuous improvement methods, supplier development, strategic negotiation, relationship management.
- *Supplier relationships:* Should be aiming for mutual commitment to close relationships delivering measurable extra value to both companies; should be aiming for consistency vertically in both organizations as well as across functions; objective performance indicators should underpin the relationship.
- *Options to move:* Move to leverage by developing alternative suppliers or by removing internal barriers to other options.

Summary   The use of portfolio analysis segmentation enables companies to plan the maximum competitive advantage from their supply base. Portfolio analysis also provides a conceptual framework to review sourcing strategy, to develop more appropriate supplier relationships, and to help define which categories will produce the best return for the application of purchasing resources. Finally, it is a model that forces senior managers to realize that purchasing is taking its responsibility very seriously by demonstrating the more strategic aspects of sourcing.

I suspect that many readers, having digested this account from Peter, will have revised some of their views on the power and potential of strategic procurement. As we saw in the marketing environment and as we will see in the world of production and supply chains, one size fits all is never enough. There is an unhelpful perception of procurement functions that pervades many minds in business. It tends to pigeonhole the competency area into the activity of leveraging down the purchase price (with the associated negative impact on supply relationships). The discussion above should realign that thinking. To further explain the potential for segmentation of a purchasing portfolio, we follow with a metaphor of how the model would apply to a well-known setting, the restaurant business.

A Helpful Metaphor

Imagine that Tom has inherited a significant sum of money and can indulge his life's dream of opening a fish restaurant on Long Island. He is starting from scratch but does know a lot about procurement and sets about developing a plan for his purchasing portfolio. Tom will need premises, staff, catering equipment, food and materials, and all the other thousand and one things that are needed to run a restaurant.

So what is in Tom's strategic box? Well, first, the premises needs to be in exactly the right spot, and those spots are not easy to come by. It will also be a major expenditure, and financing the deal will definitely need specialist input. (Tom's inheritance was not that significant!) Clearly, this has a huge potential to be a drain on profitability, depending on how the procurement goes. This is in the strategic box, and Tom needs to focus effort on it, involving all the key players and advisors. Get this right and there is a foundation for customers to roll in; get it wrong and the cash will soon run away. Tom must either lead this himself or use someone who understands the business need and is empowered to act.

What else is in the strategic box? Well, although it is not always recognized, appointing staff is a form of procurement. In Section 9.3 the stages in recruitment are shown to be identical to those in the table: specify requirements, select suitable candidate, sign contract of employment, and pay a salary. To make his offering tick Tom needs to get some key appointments right: namely, a head chef and maitre d'. Again, such people are in short supply and need to be attracted to a potential new employer and then looked after. However, if they produce a unique service offering in that part of Long Island, the benefit could be immense. There may be other things in the strategic box and be assured that if they are there, Tom will pick them out.

In the leverage box there will certainly be the fitting out of a fully equipped kitchen, and this will take a significant amount of cash. However, there should be no shortage of suppliers with the equipment to do a high-quality job—and at the end of the day, a kitchen is a kitchen. The quality of the food should not depend on the cooking facilities (although I am sure that there are some who would argue that point—but don't forget that this is only an illustrative metaphor!). With a clear specification of the equipment requirements, Tom can set a good leverage negotiator off to scour the market and drive a hard bargain. This could be the case for the restaurant furniture as well.

The rest of the purchasing portfolio will be a diverse multitude of many things. Tablecloths, napkins, plates, screws, nuts, glasses, decorations, pictures, cutlery, and so on—the list goes on. The vast majority of these will be easy-to-source, low-budget items. There may be some opportunity to group together certain items to make it a larger purchase and convert to leverage. Those that cannot be converted can be purchased as required either on credit cards or by using some other convenient and efficient way that meets the needs of administration. These make up the noncritical items.

Tom is keen to make a good impression on the opening night, so he decides to have special napkins made with the restaurant name and logo embossed in the corner. He only wants the best, and there is a specialist supplier on the West Coast who Tom used before who does a great job (although he is extremely popular). This could easily fall into the noncritical basket, where items are on short lead times and in relatively plentiful supply. However, Tom is a wise man and makes sure that the procurement is well planned in advance and that a longer-term schedule of requirements is agreed to with the supplier. He allocates responsibility for monitoring the supplier to someone who he knows understands the importance of having these available for the day of opening.

Tom is planning on developing a "signature dish" for the restaurant. He and the head chef put their heads together and come up with a very special lobster and crab combination they decide to call "Tom's Tasty Taste Bud Teaser" (not good, I know, but Tom didn't get everything right!). This provides the final learning point through the metaphor. To deliver consistently exacting standards for the high-quality seafood ingredients, it may be prudent for the head chef to form a close understanding with the supplier and possibly even to pay a premium. This will necessitate direct discussions between the chef and the supplier so that the correct balance of cost and value is achieved. This should provide some food for thought for those procurement personnel who believe that suppliers are their domain alone.

Readers should have some insights into the utility of the portfolio approach and how it could be applied in practical situations. The next step is to understand procurement as a process or as a series of stages that make up the full cycle of procurement.

9.3   THE PROCESS OF PROCUREMENT

Once the segmentation (or categorization) of the purchasing portfolio has been defined and agreed to by stakeholders, the stages in the process need to be identified and applied appropriately. The process involves four discrete steps for any part of the

TABLE 9.1   Stages in the Procurement Process

Stage	Activities	Key Considerations

Specification	Define category
	Identify stakeholders
	Determine portfolio positioning
	Review document requirements
	Prepare statement of work
	Review performance requirements
	Compile the appropriate tender
	  document (i.e., RFI/ITT/RFQ/RFP)
	Plan for procurement
		Leverage: Purchasing agrees to
		  specifications with users and
		  compiles an RFP for tender
		Noncritical: User determines
		  specifications (catalog/
		  Web site)
		Bottleneck: Reduce risk
		Strategic: Business led, team
		  approach, purchasing facilitates

Selection	Collect supply market intelligence List prospective candidates Prescreen to shortlist Issue tender document Carry out selection process Review stakeholder buy-in Complete selection	*Leverage:* Create competition *Noncritical:* User deals directly with supplier chosen *Bottleneck:* Look for alternatives *Strategic:* Balanced decision

Commitment	Prepare relevant documents:
	  Supply agreement
	  Service agreement
	  Purchase order
	  Memorandum of understanding
	    (risks)
	  Letter of intent (risks)
	  Appropriate contractual instrument
		Leverage: Lock in concessions
		Noncritical: As simple as possible
		Bottleneck: Mitigations in place
		Strategic: Relationship building
		  behaviors

Payment	Confirm delivery of goods or service Check as appropriate Identify deficiencies Revert to supplier and resolve Check payment terms against invoice Pay invoice	*Leverage:* Comply with negotiated terms *Noncritical:* As simple as possible *Bottleneck:* Mitigations in place *Strategic:* Integrate processes

portfolio, although the activities and involvement will differ according to the portfolio positioning. These stages are described below (refer to Table 9.1 for a summary).

9.3.1   Specification

The specification stage involves gaining clarity on the item(s) or service(s) to be procured. Sometimes termed a user requirements specification (URS), it is a stage that is so often performed poorly. For whatever reason (e.g., undue haste, ignorance, or arrogance), individuals or groups can forge ahead believing that they have a clear picture of what is required. The result is often an inappropriate solution to the business need presented to prospective suppliers and equally inappropriate proposals being presented back.

Another issue that often occurs here is that the specification is based on an existing offering in the market from a particular supplier that discounts other similar or functionally equivalent offerings. To avoid these potential issues, the approach recommended is as follows:

- Define the portfolio position.
- Identify the stakeholders.
- Engage stakeholders according to Peter Evans' presentation in Section 9.2.1.
- Document requirements appropriate to the portfolio position.
- Identify the terms of purchase proposed.
- Compile a tender document: either
  - A request for information (RFI)
  - An invitation to tender (ITT)
  - A request for quotation (RFQ)
  - A request for proposal (RFP)
- Plan for procurement.

9.3.2 Selection

Once the requirement has been specified, it is time to select the appropriate supplier(s). This involves the following:

- Scour the prospective suppliers in the market.
- List capable candidates.
- Prescreen to a short list (could be based on an RFI).
- Issue a tender document.
- Assess the responses.
- Make a selection (the involvement of stakeholders depends on portfolio positioning).

9.3.3 Commitment

The commitment stage is the point where the terms and conditions underpinning the transaction are committed to legal form. It can as simple as agreeing to pay the driver for the goods when he delivers them to your receiving bay—cash on delivery. For more enduring transactions it could involve a multipage supply agreement and anything in between. The following are the typical documents:

- Purchase order
- Supply agreement
- Service agreement
- Memorandum of understanding (risks)

- Letter of Intent (risks)
- Other contract type

The appropriate paperwork is then completed and the necessary signatures gained to signify a binding agreement.

9.3.4 Payment

Payment, the final stage, involves:

- Confirmation of delivery of goods or service
- Checking for completeness
- Reporting any deficiencies
- Resolution with supplier
- Checking of payment terms against invoice
- Payment of invoice

Payment is often regarded as the domain of financial accounts, but there is an important dimension for a purchasing practitioner because proper compliance with agreed-upon payment terms is a key factor in maintaining good relationships.

Armed with a sound understanding of the portfolio approach and the stages involved in procurement, it is now time to move on to some important and often business-critical aspects of the discipline. None of this is anything other than common sense, and I have attempted to de-jargonize the language as much as possible. Again, the all-pervading message is that SCM processes work across organizations and are organizational concerns. The aspects to be covered begin with strategic sourcing.

9.4 STRATEGIC SOURCING AND PLANNING

Sourcing is a term in common business parlance that appears to be well understood. Basically, it involves finding and engaging sources of supply for a firm. Adding the word *strategic* does not change the nature of the activity; it merely focuses on specific areas relating to procurement that may affect the strategy of the business. The fundamental requirement therefore is knowledge and engagement with business strategy in order to understand the longer-term needs from the supply base. The UK's Chartered Institute of Purchasing and Supply defines *strategic sourcing* as follows[4]: "Satisfying an organization's needs from markets via the proactive and planned analysis of supply markets and the selection of suppliers, with the objective of delivering solutions to meet pre-determined and agreed organisational needs."

This is a helpful definition, but it is important to pick up the implicit messages. Proactivity must be planned over the long term, where long term is related to the life cycle of the products concerned. For example, strategic sourcing plans for an aircraft should ideally span decades, whereas for shorter-term projects they may only need to cover the next 12 to 24 months. Readers should ask themselves where the pharmaceutical industry is positioned: Is the typical sourcing horizon consistent with the life cycle of the product?

The other implicit message is that there are a limited number of items and/or categories that warrant this type of attention. The purchasing portfolio is, as always, the starting point to set the target. The previous segmentation work should provide a rich picture of the supply base at any one point in time. Strategic sourcing then uses this picture to plan future requirements, based on the business need.

There is a potential confusion here that should be resolved before going further. It is that the word *strategic* in strategic sourcing does not correspond exactly with the *strategic quadrant* in portfolio analysis. Portfolio analysis informs a business on how to operate and behave with suppliers that occupy a particular quadrant, strategic being one of them. The aim of *strategic* sourcing is to draw up long-term plans for how the business will get the most from all quadrants of the portfolio. Invariably (if the segmentation is carried out properly), the routine quadrant can be ignored. The remaining quadrants are likely, however, to contain categories for strategic sourcing plans.

In the leverage quadrant there may be major purchases of capital equipment to be deployed across the organization. Long-term sourcing plans may deliver significant cost and operational savings for a cash-constrained business. Bottleneck items may be constraining the business from expanding or exposing it to excess risk of failure. Sourcing plans may be necessary in these areas to develop new supply sources. Finally, in the strategic quadrant, business needs may be moving into new technologies or markets where the changes need to be planned into the current supply base structure.

Let's look next at an example from my own experience.

Observations, Views, and Experiences of the Author

This relates to a manufacturing site with a cross-functional team reviewing the sourcing strategy for their portfolio of biological raw and starting materials. The team had been set up by higher management first to resolve near-term issues in manufacture and then to introduce longer-term fixes. They had been working on this for some time and had some real successes under their belt. When I joined the team, there was still a lot to be done.

The head of R&D was leading the team in a facilitative manner, all relevant functions were represented, and there was an experienced project manager working according to method and process. Several of the team members were experienced in process excellence and were either green or black belts in six sigma. The remaining magic ingredient was a burning desire to make a difference in the manufacturing processes.

Figure 9.2 depicts the segmentation that the team developed. The findings were extremely enlightening. When we examined the supply base we found tens of different

200

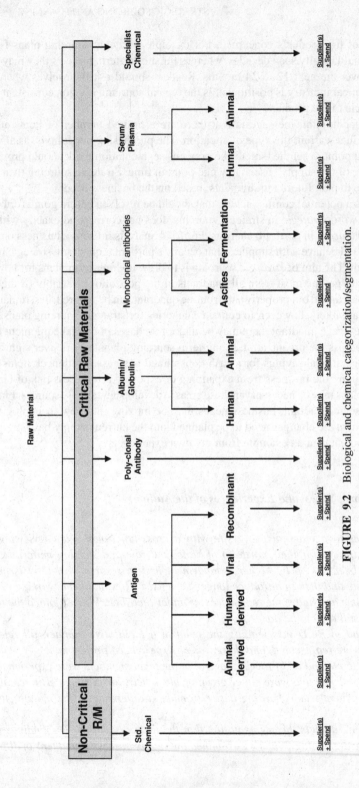

FIGURE 9.2 Biological and chemical categorization/segmentation.

suppliers for each category, with a significant amount of overlap in the manufacturing competencies they were providing. Some of the suppliers were working at their "edge of (in)competence" in some categories but were top class in others. From this we were able to identify a few strategic suppliers for each category. Some suppliers could provide cover for several categories. Now we were building a strategic approach to procurement.

Another benefit that arose from the exercise was identification of a sole-sourced, rather scarce biological. The supplier was taking advantage of our firm on price and service because of the sole-source position. The supplier was gambling on the company not being willing to undertake the resource-intensive program of supplier qualification and material validation involved. With this team in place, involving research biochemists plus quality control and manufacturing staff, it was possible to tender, qualify, and validate a high-grade second source. This resulted in a projected saving (this material was orders of magnitude more expensive than platinum per milligram) of over £1.5 million over a four-year period. The service level rose dramatically as well.

One final point relates to a comment the team leader (who was also director of development research) made to me soon after we met. He observed that the company approach to suppliers was puzzling to him. He said "we should be rolling out the red carpet to some of these guys"; and that hadn't been happening. I couldn't have agreed more!

9.5   OUTSOURCING

The next important subset of procurement activities to be examined are related to outsourcing, where a third-party organization contracts to deliver a particular service to a buying company that it cannot, or would rather not, perform for itself. It is covered here because of the tremendous dependence on outsourcing at present, both in drug development in general and in supply chain operations in particular.

9.5.1   Rationale for Outsourcing in General

There are two main rationales for outsourcing:

1. The company does not have the resources to maintain an in-house capability to perform the necessary activities.
2. The company believes that the core competencies required could be carried out more effectively by an experienced third party. This is typically called a *make vs. buy decision.*

The first rationale is obviously not always a choice. Many SMEs (biotech/virtual companies in pharma) cannot afford to set up their own facilities, other than to provide office space and pay wages to core staff. Outsourcing is a way of life in these cases, and effective procurement practices are critical to success. As learned earlier, the growth of SMEs in pharma development was facilitated by the availability of third-party service providers, which in turn drove demand for the services. This has been an ongoing spiral ever since. Below is an extract from my Biotech PharmaFlow Web site which explains further.

> For many biotech and emerging pharma companies intent on getting into the clinic, or indeed carrying on to commercial supply, outsourcing is the only feasible option given the need to conserve cash. Often and perversely, skills and experience of the laws of commercial exchange are not regarded as high priority, even though vast sums of money may be spent with third parties. Not only that, but the third parties need to be managed in a relationship where the balance of power shifts dramatically pre and post contract [see the work of Andrew Cox in Section 9.5.2]. Ignore that at your peril!
>
> It is now becoming increasingly recognised that procurement of outsourced services is a vital cross-functional process (not a function called "procurement") with a life cycle that covers definition of need, supplier selection, terms of agreement, and payment completion. Involvement of the appropriate people at each stage is of fundamental importance. This process is not rocket science, can be applied using structured tools and techniques, and can be adopted across the organisation for maximum impact on "value for money."
>
> If a company outsources major operational activities such as clinical trials, manufacture, logistics services, etc., these will likely have a significant effect on financial statements. The company's procurement processes are a large contributor to internal controls. The following questions are relevant to ask:
>
> - How are outsourced services and materials being controlled through the life cycle?
> - What controls are there on consumption and movement of inventory?
> - What controls are in place at the contractor's subcontractors?
> - Do contracts reflect the need for higher levels of audit access?
> - Do you have a register of all third parties subject to corporate governance?
> - Are legal, finance, purchasing, internal audit, and end users all on the same page?
> - Is information being supplied by third parties accurate and appropriate?
>
> You may well have this all under control, but it may be worth checking again!

It should be clear that I am sounding a warning bell to those who are not professionally prepared for outsourcing. It should also set the scene for later examination of some of the challenges of outsourcing once the second case has been identified. In the second case above, the make vs. buy decision, the buying company has a choice. Is it more beneficial to carry out the activities internally or to pass them on to more qualified companies that can spread their costs over a number of clients? This is a very important choice and, as always, should be considered in the light of *sustainable* competitive advantage. It should therefore be implicit in the analysis that competitive advantage is better served by using a third-party provider, through either lower costs or increased value. The sustainable element means that the outsourcing arrangement must *continue* to deliver the intended benefits during and following implementation. Sadly, this understanding is often absent in many cost-driven initiatives to outsource.

As an example, a company outsourcing on the basis of cost improvement must be clear that the revenue-earning potential is not affected adversely because the service becomes "commoditized." This may well have been the case in the financial services sector during the mass offshoring of call center services (certainly from the customer's viewpoint). Many of the organizations involved have reverted to previous in-house arrangements at the behest of frustrated customers. There are also examples closer to home where outsourced arrangements have not delivered the anticipated benefits.

So how should companies with a choice make decisions on outsourcing? There is a very simple answer. If the service is critical to a business's strategy toward competitive advantage in chosen markets, it should *not* be outsourced. As always, it seems to be the case that there are very clear areas at the extremes of business activities. The answer here is normally unambiguous. Janitorial services are clearly obvious candidates, and product design teams are unlikely to be outsourced. In between, the choice becomes more challenging, and only the companies themselves can decide after careful consideration of their circumstances. There is, however, one golden guideline that I would like to propose: If a practical and enforceable contract cannot be devised that allows the outsourcing company to respond flexibly and cost-effectively to business pressures for change, it is a doubtful candidate for outsourcing.

9.5.2   Nature and Challenge of Outsourced Relationships

An important consideration for outsourcing is the nature of the relationship involved compared to a traditional in-house approach. These are fundamentally contractual relationships and so are defined by preagreed terms set out in a contract. Although the supplying company may be willing to accommodate alternative arrangements, there is no obligation to do so. Any attempts at coercion would obviously be fruitless and the only avenue for resolution would be renegotiation of the contract. This could be a time-consuming process and ultimately end in the supplier not wishing to do business on the revised terms. What happens then? The competency set no longer exists in the organization, so where does a buyer of these services go for an alternative? Switching costs could be prohibitive, so there is a real dilemma here. Your business must either battle on against customer need or look for a longer-term resource, neither of which would be ideal.

This leads on to some "revealing" work carried out in the UK by Andrew Cox of Birmingham University and chairman of the advisory board of the international institute for Advanced Purchasing and Supply. Professor Cox received criticism from some sections of the purchasing fraternity, due to his forthright views on power and dependence in supply chains. At that time there was much interest in partnership sourcing and other shared relationship–based approaches. Many buying companies entered single-sourcing relationships with "partners" only to find that the benefits of "being in bed together" were not all they were cracked up to be.

Cox was, rightly in my opinion, focusing on the relative power differentials between buyer and seller as the basis for informing procurement strategy. Firms do not and cannot behave as individuals free to enter into personal arrangements and partnerships. They are distinct legal entities with boards of directors and pressures to perform and deliver shareholder value. Buyer–seller relationships are therefore certain to be formed and governed by these pressures. This reality is true throughout the procurement process, but whereas the consequences of a failed relationship in general procurement of goods are normally confined to certain transactions, poor outsourcing arrangements can cripple a business.

In a paper,[5] Cox presented some remarkably incisive observations. The first point made is that buyers should have a methodology to ensure that strategically important resources are not outsourced to suppliers. Earlier in this section it was noted that outsourcing was not recommended for activities that were critical to competitive advantage and what Cox stresses as the ability "to earn above-normal returns."

The paper then goes on to examine the potential pitfalls once a decision to outsource has been made. The next section will consider the former point; here, the pitfalls are explored. Cox defines *adverse selection* as being where the buying company or outsourcing practitioner fails to realize that their relative power positions switch once the deal is done. If they make a poor (suboptimal) selection, it is too late once the contact is signed. Inadequate due diligence and selection criteria can lead to a lifetime of regret. Believe it or not, there are suppliers out there who would claim competence in certain areas but actually possess little of it! The counter to that is to avoid the *moral hazard* by making suitable precontractual provisions in the agreement. The message in this is that buyers and suppliers must understand the fit between them. Put very simply, this means that (inexperienced) buyers can be seduced by suppliers who make promises they cannot keep.

9.5.3 Outsourcing in Pharmaceuticals

In Chapter 1 I recounted the industry's significant move toward outsourcing activities such as clinical and nonclinical development, manufacturing, and distribution logistics services. Not being party to the discussions that took place in pharma boardrooms during the 1980s and 1990s, it is difficult to say exactly what started it. The fact is that decisions were made across almost the whole of big pharma to outsource on a major scale.

The other widely held view about pharma in those times was that procurement practices were underdeveloped compared with practices in other sectors. In 1991, the *McKinsey Quarterly*[6] showed an illustration of the relative maturity of purchasing organizations in various sectors—with pharmaceuticals at the bottom of the pile. Pharmaceutical purchasers were in the lowest quadrant, basically as order placers for the factory. Purchasing in pharmaceuticals was described on an effectiveness scale:

- *Theme:* serve the factory
- *Organizational form:* at factories only, reports to plant manager or lower
- *Key skills:* clerical, logistics
- *Sample activities:* identify suppliers, expedite orders

Automotives and microcomputers (with Japan rated highest) were at the top under "strategic procurement."

- *Theme:* strategic procurement
- *Organizational form:* center-led, with execution in strategic business units (SBUs); extensive use of cross-functional teams
- *Key skills:* supplier development, cross-functional problem solving
- *Sample activities:* supplier certification, make vs. buy decisions, challenge specifications, total system cost analysis

This was a report produced in 1991, well after outsourcing had been established and was under way as the new working model. If, as suggested, procurement existed only at factories and even then it was a lower-level set of competencies, what conclusions can be drawn from the results of today? What are we to infer from this as to the quality and effectiveness of the outsourcing processes adopted at the time? Anyone familiar with the sector will know there is more than a fair amount of adverse selection and moral hazard floating around. Concerning though that is, it is not the primary issue in my opinion. The main issue relates to critical assets.

Critical assets should be kept under the control of the business. Intellectual property—yes, of course. New targets for research—another yes. What about product development? What about generation of the data to go into a regulatory filing? Determination of analytical methods? Specification of process development protocols? All these are typically outsourced. In an environment where change is on the agenda prompted by twenty-first-century modernization from the regulators, what is the incentive for contract organizations to respond? We will leave the reader with that thought and consider it further in later chapters. We'll finish with some more thoughts from my Web site.

A Typical Problem   There is general uneasiness that "best value" is not being achieved in clinical research organization relationships, evidenced by some or all of the following:

- Unavailability of key skill sets
- Frequent change orders (scope and cost changes)
- Unexpected work invoices
- Excessive pass-through costs
- Activities not adding sufficient value
- Key clinical and scientific staff tied up in areas in which they are not experienced or trained

Some points to consider:

- Were all relevant players involved in project scope generation?
- Was the original scope statement detailed enough?

- How clear were mutual expectations throughout the tendering process?
- Were the key interfaces defined?
- Were staff trained in managing outsourced relationships?

This problem case was based on practical experience of outsourced relationship with clinical research organizations. I assumed management responsibility for a contract management group and was amazed at the issues of containing cost and value delivery within reasonable bounds once projects had begun.

The next section deals with many of the issues of adverse selection and moral hazard above, and much more besides. It is presented by James Ryan of Morrison and Foerster.

GUEST CONTRIBUTOR SLOT: JAMES RYAN

9.6   BASIC PRINCIPLES IN CONTRACTING FOR SUPPLY

The negotiation and drafting of manufacturing and supply agreements for the bio-pharmaceutical sector and the explanation of the law underlying these contracts has formed the basis of entire books. The purpose of this commentary is to act as a general guide to the key principles to be considered by a purchaser when negotiating biopharmaceutical manufacturing and supply agreements. This commentary does not to go into detail on how such agreements are structured or the provisions that this type of agreement typically contains.

Lawyers Take on Supply Chain Management   To the eyes of a lawyer who advises pharmaceutical and biotechnology companies on the outsourcing of their manufacturing and supply arrangements, the supply chain consists of two things: (1) the documentation that regulates how products are produced, released, and distributed [i.e., product specifications, SOPs, manufacturing records, and the like (the "how it should be done" side of manufacture and supply)], and (2) the physical production and distribution processes (the "how it is done" side of the supply chain). The aim of the lawyer advising a company on the outsourcing of its manufacturing and supply arrangements is to help the company assure that a manufacturing and supply agreement does two things. First, the agreement should integrate the two parts of the supply chain to produce a cohesive process so that the physical manufacturing and supply activities are performed in accordance with the processes dictated in the technical documents. Second, the agreement must regulate the relationship between the purchaser and the supplier and how these parties interact. In essence, the manufacturing and supply agreement should be thought of as the document that brings the entire manufacturing arrangement together in one place: the "master" document that regulates the entire supply arrangement and the business relationship between purchaser and supplier. Remember, it is only through the terms of the manufacturing and supply agreement that the purchaser can enforce the manufacturing arrangements agreed to with the supplier and it is only by bringing a claim for breach of contract under the supply agreement that the purchaser has any ability to recover losses or damages that may have been suffered as a result of a breach of the contract.

However, the manufacturing and supply agreement should not just be seen as something that regulates the relationship between purchaser and supplier. The supply chain can be a core asset of a biopharmaceutical company whose business is focused on the development and/or commercialization of pharmaceutical products but which has outsourced the manufacture and supply of these products. Having the necessary manufacturing and supply agreements in place to cover each stage in the outsourced supply chain so as to creates a seamless process from purchase of the raw materials through to release and distribution of the finished product and properly regulates the relationship between purchaser and supplier at each step in the process can add value to a company, making it easier to raise investment capital, sell rights to the product in question, or even sell the entire company. If the agreements regulating the manufacture and supply of product are poorly drafted, if the terms agreed upon with the supplier(s) expose the purchaser to unreasonable or excess risks or liabilities, or if the chain of manufacturing and supply agreements covering the stages in the supply chain from raw material purchase through to release and distribution of finished product is incomplete, the value of the product (and the company) can plummet, making it very difficult for investors in the company to exit. This is a very real risk—as a firm we have seen product acquisitions and company acquisitions fall through or proceed at greatly reduced prices purely as a result of incomplete or poorly documented supply chains. Getting the legal documentation right is therefore very important, especially for a young company funded by venture capital.

Purpose of the Manufacturing and Supply Agreement   The purpose of the contracting exercise is to produce an agreement that protects both the purchaser and supplier. This protection is achieved through discussion of the supply arrangements and the risks associated with these arrangements, followed by clear, precise, and unambiguous drafting of the supply agreement to reflect the outcome of these discussions. Looking at the issues that should be addressed by a manufacturing and supply agreement in slightly more detail, it is possible to separate the types of provisions contained in the agreement into four discrete areas.

1. *Recording the supply arrangements.* The manufacturing and supply arrangements agreed between the purchaser and the supplier should be recorded clearly and accurately in the agreement. The agreement should clearly describe the responsibilities of each party at each step in the supply process, and the terms recorded in the agreement should reflect what is going to happen in practice. However, the agreement should not just record the process of how product is to be manufactured and/or supplied; it should also set out the legal and regulatory requirements (such as cGMP) that must be complied with during the manufacture and supply process, the specifications and other quality requirements for the product produced and supplied, how product is to be delivered and released to the purchaser, what documentation needs to accompany a delivery, how delivered product is accepted and rejected, and

the like. This is the part of the agreement that specifies the processes and procedures set out in the SOPs, specification documents, manufacturing records, and the like to be complied with (and how these processes and procedures are to be complied with) during the physical manufacturing and supply processes. This can be thought of as the mechanical side of the agreement.

2. *Integration.* If the supply chain consists of numerous separate steps with each step being performed by a different supplier, the agreement governing a particular step in the supply chain needs to dovetail with the agreements covering each of the preceding and subsequent steps in the chain so as to produce a seamless process that allows product to flow freely from one step or manufacturer to the next step or manufacturer without bottlenecks or choke points forming. In the circumstance where each step in the process is outsourced to a different manufacturer, the purchaser is dependent on each manufacturer in the chain supplying the correct material to the next manufacturer in the chain. It is therefore vital that the mechanisms governing each transition in the supply chain are integrated; otherwise, there is a risk of delay in the production process.

Getting the two steps in the contracting process described above correct requires the purchaser and its lawyer to sit down together and the purchaser to invest the time in explaining to its lawyer the entire manufacturing process, from the purchase of the raw material through to the release of finished product. It is only through going through this process that the purchaser can be sure that the agreement it ends up with will accurately reflect the supply process it requires. Getting this part of the agreement right is essential because if the supply process agreed with the supplier is not the process that the purchaser actually requires, the product produced at the end of the supply chain may not meet the necessary legal or regulatory requirements for putting the product into humans, and the intermediate product produced at one step of the supply chain may not have the correct chemical or biological profile required to progress to the next step in the manufacturing process. Further, making significant changes to the manufacturing and supply process after the relevant agreements have been signed can have knock-on (and adverse) consequences on the rest of the supply chain, especially the supply price.

3. *Stress testing.* The arrangements agreed to with a supplier prior to the drafting and negotiation of a manufacturing and supply agreement generally look at how the manufacturing or supply process is intended to work. As a general rule, the parties will not have spent a great deal of time looking at what happens if the supply chain breaks down. The manufacturing and supply agreement needs to address the question "what if?" at each stage in the supply chain and the remedy or mitigating actions to be taken to avoid or lessen the risk of a supply failure during each step. During negotiation of the manufacturing and supply agreement, the purchaser should spend as much time discussing what happens if the supply process breaks down at any particular point in the supply chain (and drafting to address this point) as it does setting down how the process works if everything goes according to plan.

The steps to be taken to avoid the occurrence of a "what if" scenario or to mitigate the consequences of a "what if" vary from agreement to agreement. However, it is at this level in the supply chain documentation, where the "what if's" are addressed and dealt with, that the supply chain goes from being just a mechanical or technical document to something that can add value to the company. It is also at this level where an SCM professional such as Hedley and the legal adviser really work together. It is probably fair to say that the SCM professional is slightly biased in his approach toward ensuring that the supply chain is optimized to meet the purchaser's requirements with as little waste in the system as possible. By contrast, the lawyer has a bias toward thinking about the potential risks in the supply arrangement and dealing with the consequences when the supply chain goes wrong for whatever reason. The roles of the two professionals really overlap where they work together to devise solutions to the "what if" scenarios that have been identified to avoid a breakdown in the supply chain. The reason that the two professionals work together at this point is that the payment of compensation to the purchaser for lost sales and/or lost product due to a supplier's failure to comply with the terms of the manufacturing and supply agreement is not really a sufficient remedy for the lack of stock in the market and loss of market share. It is far better to have contingencies in place to deal with short-term supply failures due to late or nondelivery of a batch of product than to claim damages against the defaulting supplier. The SCM adviser and the lawyer work together to see where there is risk in the supply chain and how this risk can be avoided or lessened.

The steps that can be taken to mitigate or avoid the risk of a supply failure depend on the nature of the product, the structure of the supply chain, and on the allocation of risk–reward between the parties that has been agreed to (see further below). At one end of the spectrum, supply failure can be dealt with through the purchaser keeping a stock of the finished product, and each supplier in the supply chain being required to keep a stock of the starting and finishing materials they deal with. In this type of arrangement the real issues are (a) how long stock can be kept (which is driven by shelf life), (b) how expensive it is to manufacture and store the required volumes of raw material, intermediates, and finished product, and (c) who is to bear the cost of producing and keeping these stocks at each step in the process. At the other end of the spectrum is the possibility of having backup suppliers for each step or each key step in the supply chain. How this "redundancy" of capacity can be integrated into the main supply chain arrangements and the impact this will have on cost is a complex issue, which involves looking at the cost of qualifying backup sites and putting sufficient volumes of product through these sites to keep them in a state of readiness should a supply failure happen at the lead site. Added to this is the fact that the price charged by the main supplier for a particular step may be dependent on the volume of orders placed with it and the level of exclusivity that the supplier has been awarded. The situation is further complicated, as it was on a deal that Hedley and I worked on together, where the key supplier was using a patented manufacturing process that it was not prepared to share with a third-party backup facility. The solution reached on this type of issue is a matter of cost–benefit analysis and risk allocation. In the final analysis the purchaser has to ask whether the risk of a supply failure justifies this expense of keeping the required stocks available or qualifying and maintaining backup production sites.

4. *Relationship with the supplier.* The final set of issues that a manufacturing and supply agreement deals with is the relationship between the purchaser and the

supplier, the allocation of risk between the parties, and the allocation of control over the manufacturing and supply process between the parties.

a. *Communication and change control.* As discussed previously, for a supply chain to work, the contractual provisions governing a particular step need to accurately reflect the purchaser's supply arrangements and need to integrate properly and fully with the other links in the supply chain. However, one has to accept that no system is perfect, and over time the manufacturing process and quality requirements may change, either because of the development of improvements in the manufacturing process or at the request of regulatory authorities. For this reason, most manufacturing and supply arrangements will contain a change control mechanism to allow for changes in the manufacturing and supply terms to be discussed, agreed to, and implemented in an orderly fashion. Importantly, no matter what procedure is settled on to manage the change control process, the final say on matters relating to product and the process by which it is produced must rest with the purchaser.

The forum used to discuss these changes varies from agreement to agreement. It can be dealt with through the creation of a management committee, which meets regularly to discuss the agreement, changes to the agreement, and the parties' relationship, or it can be dealt with through the appointment by each party of a contract or project manager, who meets regularly with his or her counterpart to discuss the supply arrangements. The forum at which these types of issue are discussed is irrelevant in many respects; the key point to take away is that creation of a forum for this type of regular communication between the parties is important for maintenance of the supply chain and the relationship between the parties. The supply arrangement can be a long-term arrangement, and if the arrangement is to be successful, the parties need to maintain a regular and open line of communication.

b. *Control.* When we talk about control over the manufacturing and supply process, we mean two things: (1) control over how the product is manufactured and the specifications to which the product is manufactured, and (2) control of the intellectual property and other proprietary rights in the product. Ultimately, the product and the process by which it is made should be the purchaser's assets, and the purchaser should have control over how a product is made and the specifications to which it is made. The purchaser, as the person who will hold the regulatory approvals for the product and who will be putting the product on the market, will bear the primary liability for defects in the product. It is therefore essential that the purchaser maintain control over the product and the process by which it is produced. This is also crucial should the manufacturing and supply agreement have to be terminated for any reason. In this situation the purchaser must be able to take back the right to supply from the terminated supplier and take this right elsewhere. For this transition to be possible, the product and the manufacturing process must be controlled by, and in the possession of, the purchaser. This also means that all intellectual property rights in the product and the manufacturing process created during the term of the agreement must be owned by, or at the very least licensed to, the purchaser so that the purchaser can take manufacture of the product elsewhere. As a word of caution, if the supplier itself has a proprietary process that is used for producing the product, it is vital that rights to this proprietary process are also obtained on entering into the agreement (even if the right to use this proprietary process is not exercisable unless and until the agreement is terminated due to the supplier's failure). Otherwise, the purchaser may not be able to take production away from that supplier; that is, by selecting a supplier who has a proprietary process that needs to be used to produce the product, the purchaser has given up an element of control over the product, which increases the level of difficulty that may be encountered if the purchaser wants to take back production at a later time. This is not always an avoidable risk (indeed, in some situations the only person who can manufacture product the way it needs to be manufactured is the person with the proprietary process), but a purchaser should be aware of the risk inherent in making this choice of supplier.

c. *Risk allocation.*   When we talk about risk allocation in a manufacturing and supply agreement, what we really mean is how much of the risk the supplier is going to bear (a) if it fails to supply the product ordered by the time agreed (or at all), and (b) if the product it supplies is defective in some way. Under a supply arrangement, the supplier will try to limit its financial liability to the purchaser as much as possible. This is because the return the supplier can make on its services is limited and there is a significant risk inherent in the manufacturing and supply of pharmaceuticals—death or injury to users of the product. The limitation on liability can take a number of forms, but the principal ways in which the supplier will try to limit its liability are as follows: (1) the supplier will try to exclude liability to the purchaser for loss of profits, turnover, and the like arising from its failure to supply or its supply of defective product; (2) the supplier will try to put an absolute financial cap on its liability under the agreement (the amount of the cap usually being a multiple of the amount of money that it has received under the supply agreement at the time the liability arises); (3) the supplier will try to limit the remedies available to the purchaser for certain types of breach of the supply obligation. By way of example, the supplier will try to limit it liability to the purchaser for supplying defective product to either (1) replacing the defective batch at its next available opportunity, or (2) refunding the fees paid for the defective batch of product. The effect of this type of exclusion is that if the supplier fails to supply product of the necessary quality, and this failure results in the purchaser losing sales, the purchaser cannot recover the lost profit on these sales from the supplier. This is why the risk management provisions discussed above under "Stress Testing" can be so important, as it is through these steps that the integrity of the supply chain is maintained. It is because of the financial limitations that will probably be placed on the supplier's liability for failing to supply product that meets the required specification that the purchaser and the purchaser's advisers are driven to find alternative methods for dealing with the risk of a supply failure.

The position reached on negotiation on these risk allocation points is dependent on the type of supply arrangement involved (i.e., if the agreement relates to the manufacturing process development and scale-up, the risk for failed batches will lie mostly with the purchaser). If the product to be supplied is to be manufactured pursuant to a proven and validated production process, more of the risk for the failure of a batch to meet specification lies with the supplier. Other factors that can affect the allocation of risk between the parties to a supply agreement include the payment arrangements reached between the parties. At one end of the spectrum is the situation where the supplier is paid a price for production under a straightforward contract manufacturing arrangement. In this scenario the supplier is not going to be willing to accept much risk other than for failed batches. At the other end of the spectrum is the situation where the supplier is being paid for a product supplied by being reimbursed its base cost of manufacture (with no profit margin) and/or by receiving a royalty on sales. By electing to take a greater share of the value of a product, the supplier should take a greater share of the risk (as it is going to recover far more value from the deal than it would have done on a straight contract manufacturing basis).

What This Means for the Contract Negotiations

1. There are some points on which a purchaser cannot move. When it comes to documenting the manufacturing and supply arrangements that control a supply chain, there are some provisions on which the purchaser does not have much scope to negotiate. These provisions tend to be the provisions dealing with the mechanics of how product is to be manufactured and released, the quality standards to which product must be manufactured, and the integration of one supply agreement with the next supply agreement in the supply chain. These provisions must reflect the purchaser's supply requirements. The flexibility around these terms comes through the inclusion of a change control process that allows changes to be made to these provisions when change is required.

2. There are some points on which the purchaser has latitude to negotiate. When it comes to negotiation of the provisions of the manufacturing and supply agreement that do not relate to the production process, the quality requirements, and the release arrangements, the purchaser has more scope to negotiate. For example, the price and payment terms, the contractual provisions dealing with supply failures, and the provisions capping or limiting the supplier's liability are all provisions on which the purchaser has greater freedom to negotiate. Where a purchaser can get to on these points is a matter for negotiation but is influenced by the nature of the supply services being provided and the manner in which the supplier is to be compensated for its services, but remember, where the supply agreement ends up on these points can affect the value of the purchaser's business.

There are many, many extremely important points and issues contained in the words here. The surprise that I had when working with Morrison & Foerster and James was that their advice was to steer clear of lawyers' involvement until the fundamentals of the business deal were sealed. Their role was then about delivering an agreement to underpin the true intensions of the contracting parties. Those are lawyers' words certainly worth heeding!

The chapter ends with a particular issue that often crops up in organizations.

9.7   FINALLY, TYPICAL ORGANIZATIONAL TENSION OVER PROCUREMENT

Tensions often arise between the procurement/purchasing/buying function and end users/budget holders/line managers, and so on, in terms of who has the upper hand in the process. It is not unusual for buying departments to become merely order placers that add very little value to the process, other than making it easier to clear an invoice. Conversely, users of critical materials can find themselves working with inferior materials and products, due to limitations placed on them by the buying department. This is an age-old problem that causes the buying fraternity much angst and frustration through lack of involvement; or end users anger and rage because they cannot get a *proper* supply of what they really need to do a good job.

It is my belief that much of the problem resides in two areas. First, the process is not properly understood (it is organization wide, not functional). Second, the segmentation of goods and services being procured is unclear. The solution to this problem has been addressed here. Readers should return to the beginning of this chapter and reread Sections 9.2 and 9.3. With that, we move on to the next chapter, with an invitation to readers new or less experienced in strategic procurement to search out further material on this vitally important topic.

10 Transportation, Storage, and Distribution

10.1 DEFINING THE CORE MISSION

To arrive successfully in customers' hands, goods and materials need to be moved from A to B. They must be handled, stored, transported, distributed, and administered in such a way as to meet the needs of those customers. In addition to that, there are a multitude of requirements from competent authorities around the world that must be met. These can relate to all aspects of health and safety (including hazardous, toxic, and biological materials), international trade and commerce, taxation, border security, and of course, the regulations of good distribution practice (GDP) that apply to pharmaceuticals. As discussed previously, this storage and movement of goods takes place across the entire supply chain and over global trade and country boundaries.

It has increasingly become a specialist area. Regulations are constantly being updated to keep in step with a changing world, particularly as governments pursue new and evolving agendas. There is also a significant cost component in the more networked and specialist supply chains of today. The length of supply chains in geographical terms has become a secondary consideration in pharmaceuticals compared to the pursuit of low-cost supply sources and fiscal benefits. This has led to supply chains that can span the globe several times, with the associated cost and complexity. Biologicals have also injected significant growth in the need for cold chain transport and storage, which again has added to the cost burden.

The final aspect associated with this is the high risk of failure in the absence of proper transport and storage. This is a dimension beyond cost, extending potentially into the survival and growth of a business. One lost shipment of a key compound, due to improper storage, transport, or administration, can lead to an entire phase of a clinical trial being delayed or even aborted. For a small cash-constrained biotech firm, this could have major business implications if replenishment supply involves cost and time lines that it can ill afford.

Supply Chain Management in the Drug Industry: Delivering Patient Value for Pharmaceuticals and Biologics, By Hedley Rees
Copyright © 2011 John Wiley & Sons, Inc.

Observations, Views, and Experiences of the Author

It has always amazed me what a huge role transport and related activities play in clinical trial supplies. This isn't the amazing part, however—it is the way that drug development companies give scientists and technologists responsibilities in this area without proper knowledge and training. It is then left to third-party logistics providers and other associated contractors to guide, advise, and make good (hopefully, it is not too late).

I remember well a scientist responsible for provision of supplies to a phase II study for a biological approaching me with pain in his eyes. The test material that he and his people had spent three arduous months producing had perished in an airport warehouse for want of a dry ice top-up (dry ice is used to keep temperature-sensitive materials cold). The disappointment was palpable. The lesson he learned was one for all in this area to heed. There is only one entity with overall responsibility and accountability for shipment of materials—the owner.

The mission for the transportation and storage element of SCM should now be clear. It centers on keeping a firm handle on compliance, risk, cost, documentation, and time lines throughout the chain of custody from point A to point B. No easy task in the rapidly developing world of pharmaceuticals. In the text that follows we cover some of the main areas involved but are *not* giving operational or professional advice. The scope of the book precludes an in-depth treatment, so we have placed our emphasis on helping readers in their search for information sources and reference points, which is how I have built up knowledge in this area. Although incomplete, it has served the purpose.

Observations, Views, and Experiences of the Author

While in big pharma, I held managerial accountability for transportation and import–export, although I had not entered the profession through that route. Therefore, on entering the world of biotech where there was no formally trained staff to lean on, I was on a steep learning curve. This meant that I had to acquire the basics by learning from whomever and whatever I could. It led me to contacting HM Customs & Excise, the UK Home Office, environmental agencies, the U.S. Food and Drug Administration, chemical industry associations, the U.S. Drug Enforcement Agency, and many other organizations in furtherance of moving compounds around the world. What I discovered was that the necessary information is always there somewhere; it is a question of following a series of leads until eventually the source is found. This requires first, a determination to reach the source, and second, the patience to refrain from acting before being certain of the ground—falling foul of the competent authorities is not an option.

The sources cited in this section aim to provide as much guidance as possible.

10.2   INTERNATIONAL TRADE AND COMMERCE

As with other areas of the book, here we seek out the meaning and assumptions behind many activities that are often taken for granted. The roots of the discipline of transportation and storage are planted firmly in the world of international trade, that is, transactions between buyers and sellers. In the act of buying and selling, there must be a binding agreement to transfer ownership from one party to another; along with that, in the case of goods, the change of ownership is accompanied by a change of location, often across borders. So transportation and storage are linked inextricably with international trade and commerce. This means that much of this section focuses not only on physical movement, important though that is, but also on the dimensions of trade that underpin that movement. International trade in pharmaceuticals has been subject to global negotiations for many years and is facilitated by the World Trade Organization.

10.3   THE WORLD TRADE ORGANIZATION

The World Trade Organization (WTO)[1] deals with the rules of trade between nations at a global or near-global level. Stated aims define it as:

- An organization for liberalizing trade
- A forum for governments to negotiate trade agreements
- A place for the settlement of trade disputes
- A system of trade rules
- A negotiating forum

There is a tremendous resource of information at the Web site, and we have paraphased below an understanding of the organization's role.

Essentially, the WTO is a place where member governments go to try to sort out the trade problems they face with each other. The first step is to talk. The WTO was born out of negotiations, and everything the WTO does is the result of negotiations. The bulk of the WTO's current work comes from the 1986–94 negotiations, called the Uruguay Round, and earlier negotiations under the General Agreement on Tariffs and Trade. The WTO is currently the host to new negotiations, under the Doha Development Agenda launched in 2001.

Where countries have faced trade barriers and wanted them lowered, the negotiations have helped to liberalize trade. But the WTO is not just about liberalizing trade, and in some circumstances its rules support maintaining trade barriers: for example, to protect consumers or prevent the spread of disease. At its heart are the WTO agreements, negotiated and signed by the bulk of the world's trading nations. These documents provide the legal ground rules for international commerce. They are essentially contracts, binding governments to keep their trade policies within agreed-upon limits. Although negotiated and signed by governments, the goal is to help producers of goods and services, exporters, and importers conduct their business while allowing governments to meet social and environmental objectives.

There is a third important side to the WTO's work. Trade relations often involve conflicting interests. Agreements, including those painstakingly negotiated in the WTO system, often need interpreting. The most harmonious way to settle differences is through some neutral procedure based on an agreed-upon legal foundation. That is the purpose behind the dispute settlement process written into the WTO agreements.

The WTO began life on January 1, 1995, but its trading system is half a century older. Since 1948, the General Agreement on Tariffs and Trade (GATT) had provided the rules for the system. (The second WTO ministerial meeting, held in Geneva in May 1998, included a celebration of the 50th anniversary of the system.) It did not take long for the General Agreement to give birth to an unofficial, de facto international organization, also known informally as GATT. Over the years GATT evolved through several rounds of negotiations.

The last and largest GATT round was the Uruguay Round, which lasted from 1986 to 1994 and led to the WTO's creation. Whereas GATT dealt mainly with trade in goods, the WTO and its agreements now cover trade in services and in traded inventions, creations, and designs (intellectual property). One important outcome from the Uruguay Round is what was termed the *zero-for-zero* duty agreement on pharmaceutical products. This basically involved the pharmaceutical trading counties agreeing reciprocally to lift the duty obligation on companies providing pharmaceutical products in finished form. This was further extended to active ingredients and chemical intermediates through negotiation with the chemical industry associations. If it could be proved that these materials would be used only for pharmaceutical purposes (i.e., would not be sold in competition in the fine chemical markets), they would be eligible for zero-for-zero status. Chapters 29, 30, and 38 and special annexes of the Harmonized Tariff System list the materials that were included.

The next contributor, Matt McGrath of Barnes/Richardson,[2] is an expert and explains in detail.

GUEST CONTRIBUTOR SLOT: MATT MCGRATH

Customs Duty in Pharmaceuticals

Prior to the Uruguay Round, tariffs on pharmaceuticals and their inputs had generally been assessed at the same ad valorem levels as those for chemicals, since finished dosage drugs, bulk active ingredients, and input intermediates are all classifiable for tariff purposes under Chapters 29, 30, and 38 of the Harmonized Tariff System (HTS), which cover single organic chemicals, medicaments, and chemical mixtures, respectively. The zero-for-zero agreement differentiated the pharmaceuticals from the rest of these compounds by, first, designating all medicaments in Chapter 30 as duty free, including both dosage drugs and bulk mixture incorporating excipients ready for dosage processing. Second, the agreement designated all bulk antibiotics, alkaloids, vitamins, and hormones as duty free, without the need to update the list of such compounds. Next, the agreement produced an appendix that contained two primary lists of compounds which would be duty free regardless of where they were classified in the HTS. This includes a list of all active pharmaceutical ingredients (APIs) that have been assigned an INN (international nonproprietary name) by the World Health Organization, and their salt, ester, and hydrate forms, as well as an approved list of sole-pharmaceutical-use intermediates used to manufacture an API. This material must be updated periodically to include any recently approved INN lists as well as new compounds developed by the industry which they would like to have treated as duty-free on a multilateral basis. The agreement appendixes are updated approximately every three years, although the process is essentially a diplomatic negotiation among WTO member states and therefore does not adhere to a rigid schedule.

Industry members may participate in the negotiations and request the addition of new products through an ad hoc global industry group known as Intercept, open to any pharmaceutical manufacturer. The group reviews requests, recommends additions to the negotiators, and vets updated appendixes with national chemical industry associations to avoid opposition based on nonpharmaceutical applications. After international coordinated approval of the updates, each member state follows its own implementation procedures, some of which require legislative endorsement, prior to full duty-free treatment by all participants. It should also be noted that since the WHO applies most favored nation principles in tariff assessment, all the participants must provide the same duty-free treatment to the listed products from any other WTO member country, regardless of whether or not they participate in the zero-for-zero agreement.

Although new bulk APIs and intermediates can only be added to the duty-exempt appendix every three to four years, it is still possible to obtain the benefit of duty suspension or avoidance through local customs procedures which are commonly applied by pharmaceutical traders while awaiting the zero-for-zero update. Among these are (1) national temporary duty suspensions for inputs further manufactured in the importing country (legislative in the United States, administrative in the EU); (2) duty drawback or inward processing procedures (for the recovery of tariffs on imported chemicals used in pharmaceuticals that are to be exported); and (3) the use of foreign trade zones for tariff inversion, which permit dutiable inputs to be entered duty-deferred for processing in the designated zone, then entered from the zone into the custom territory as duty-free dosage drugs classifiable in HTS Chapter 30. It is also common for importers to use bonded entry or special noncommercial classifications for imports of bulk APIs which will be consumed solely in clinical trials in the importing country. This is only necessary to avoid duty prior to a compound's inclusion in the zero-for-zero appendix; after that, it may be entered for consumption without duty, regardless of whether the drug is at the commercial stage or still in clinical trials. All such alternative entry procedures are for customs purposes only; importers must still meet all local food and drug or health ministry requirements for entry, regardless of dutiable status or tax-exempt procedure.

Regardless of the duty status of a compound or the development stage of a drug, customs law requires the declared value to be based on one of five specified alternatives, even if the drug is still at the clinical trial stage or merely in research. Therefore, the shipper and importer must make sure that they have designated an appropriate value for new compounds which have no transaction value but which can be declared on the basis of a computed value or other cost-based equivalent.

10.4   INTERMEDIARY ARRANGEMENTS

A key component of international trade is representation of selling companies where they do not have a presence themselves. This is less of a consideration for multinational companies that have operations all over the world. For smaller companies, however, selling their products in export markets would be impossible without intermediary representation. This is where agents and distributors come in. They will have existing intelligence, contacts, and some level of infrastructure in the market(s) in question. Their role is to work with the selling company to establish markets for a seller's products. There are fundamental differences between agents and distributors. The choice of whether a selling company (the principal) should use an agent or distributor depends on the particular circumstances.

10.4.1   Agents

An *agent* is a person employed by the principal to make sales contracts on its behalf. The agent does not enter into any contractual relationship and it is the principal that takes the risk. Under this arrangement, the principal must maintain separate accounts and deal with all the administration of individual customers, such as raising invoices and credit control. This can result in higher costs than those in a distributor arrangement, but it has the advantage of supporting awareness of the seller's brand in the market and provides more direct access to customers.

10.4.2   Distributors

A *distributor* buys goods from the selling company at an agreed-upon price and resells in the market in question. There is no contractual relationship between the principal and the distributor's customers. This means that the export market may not know anything of the selling company and thereby make it more difficult to raise brand awareness.

It should be clear that the preferred arrangement will be based on the longer-term plans of a selling company. Agents can help get footholds in markets there would be a strategic benefit in penetrating, whereas distributors are more likely to provide an income stream from markets of lesser long-term interest but still good business propositions. Bob Ireland now takes up the tale.

GUEST CONTRIBUTOR SLOT: BOB IRELAND

Selection and Management of Sales Intermediaries

First, to clarify, I am using the term *distributor* to describe any sales intermediary in a market; thus, the organization concerned could be a licensee, distributor, agent, co-promotion partner, co-marketing partner, or other—all independent organizations that utilize sales and marketing skills to sell your product.

I cannot think of any pharmaceutical company that does not use such intermediaries somewhere, somehow, where the manufacturer (the primary supplier) cannot operate economically alone. In pharmaceutical marketing circles the motivation and management of intermediaries gets little air time, and those companies that have established an "alliance management" team have a tendency to focus on the prelaunch (development) stages of alliance; very few managers seem to have direct responsibility for ramping up sales via a distributor network.

Earlier chapters have covered the normally understood marketing drivers: issues of product uniqueness (efficacy, positioning, outcomes, etc.), customers (patients, payers, clinicians, etc.), and the influencers (HTAs, KOLs, patient groups, etc.), but as soon as you appoint a distributor you introduce an additional competitive element, you are now not just in competition with the other compounds in your therapeutic area, you are also in competition with all the other products in the distributor's portfolio. The primary objective is to get an unfair percentage of your distributor's time and attention.

Selection   I shall not dwell on the various market research sources available to establish which companies operate in your therapeutic area with a noncompeting portfolio, a sales team that has credibility with the target clinicians and payers. They are many and varied, so I say only *do your homework*—time spent in reconnaissance is never wasted. However, I would also say that over half of the distributors that I have appointed have materialized serendipitously, so keep your ears and eyes open.

It is better to be in the market in any way rather than have regulatory (and pricing) approval and not be there. Experience beats research every time; it also generates revenue, whereas research expends it. However, the use of market research to fool your distributor into believing that you know as much about his market as he does and that he is quite safe sharing his market data (as you know it all already) is a valuable tool.

Once you have drawn up your short list of intermediaries, having eliminated the line collectors, time sponges, and competitors who wish to bury your product, you begin negotiations. Again there are many sources for the legal issues that have to be addressed, key contract clauses, and commercial terms, so I shall pass over them as well. However do look for a partner who is willing to include a realistic forecast in the contract, one who accepts performance clauses related to marketing investment and sales activity as well as sales generation.

Assess the reasons for the distributor's desire for your product; are they in line with your objectives and strategy? How do their other principals and partners speak of them? How much of your time will they demand? Where will your product sit in their current portfolio and their sales reps' schedules? Does their marketing team understand the therapeutic area? Are the time lines for key performance indicators (KPIs) achievable? And, critically, is the deal balanced? Will the distributor's profit motive be met adequately? Will your return meet the corporate norm? Also, never let them think that this is a one-horse race; have a competitor's literature or annual report visible in your briefcase.

My final three pieces of advice on selection are:

1. Small and hungry is beautiful when entering a market for the first time (the benefits of a large partner are often illusory).
2. Find an independent local expert who has been a soldier in the trenches who can help you.
3. Remember that honesty by the prospective distributor is not likely; he is desperate for your product and will do and say anything to get it.

Management and Motivation   Once a contract is signed and the army of lawyers have retreated back to their burrows, there is the normal desire to sink back in a postcoital glow of an objective achieved. However, now is when the hard work begins. The contract just gives each of you reasons to terminate the relationship, some protection when it does, and some element of theoretical performance—it does not motivate anyone. Get in there, identify your champion inside the distributor who will be the soft underbelly through which you maximize the impact of your product in the marketplace, the person who (unknowingly?) is going to get you an unfair level of time and attention in the distributor's organization.

You must recognize that the reason you are using a distributor is that entering the market directly is not cost-effective and that the distributor is driven by a need to spread the costs of his sales and marketing operation. Thus, as I said above, you will be competing for sales and marketing time and resources against the other products in his portfolio. You must also understand that any distributor recognizes that the more successful he is, the more likely he is to lose your product as it becomes economical for you to take over. Thus, consciously or subconsciously, the distributor will be "economical with the truth" regarding the dynamics of the market, the problems that he has to overcome, and the unique capability of his sales team.

So, what are the key mechanisms that need to be established to optimize the distributor's motivation to generate revenue with your product? First, inside your own organization, ensure that everyone who may be in contact with the distributor [regulatory, pharmacovigilance, medical, marketing, back office (order/invoicing), etc.] is fully briefed on the distributor; his organization, systems, and procedures related to the ordering, shipping, and management of your product; and the key staff: who to talk to when, how they are doing, and what they are doing. Make sure that your company is comfortable communicating with the distributor.

Start the relationship on a high note. This is usually training, so make it of the highest quality and do not make any assumptions regarding the distributor's level of knowledge and competence. Prepare material recognizing the specific market access issues of the distributor's market, show that you understand the challenges that he will face, make it easy for him to integrate your product into his portfolio and (relatively) easy to address the pricing, reimbursement, managed care, and payer hurdles. Much may have been addressed in the earlier negotiations, but revisit, revisit, revisit—market dynamics change rapidly.

While preparing the training material, always remember that quality trumps quantity every time, but ensure that all levels of management in the distributor organization are aware of your product and the benefits that selling your product brings to their company. Think of training as the vehicle to build the relationship. Throughout the alliance management and the building of the relationship—and, of course, the building of revenue—keep as the highest priority incentives for all levels in the distributor firm. The owners and senior managers have profit (and/or cash) as their incentive; lower down (sales, marketing, supply chain, etc.) the staff can be offered a wide range of incentives, from cash to various forms of recognition. Bear in mind that credit and payment terms are an opportunity, not a hurdle. But also remember not to waste your concessions on new products, newness itself is a massive incentive.

Other activities that will keep your product in the forefront of the distributor's mind and product portfolio is a continual, planned stream of communication, both to the ultimate customer and to the distributor's staff. New international promotional campaigns must be communicated to the distributor well before they appear: what they will be and why they are being developed. Getting the distributor to commit to a significant contribution to the promotional budget or activity will also focus his mind on your product (always a good test of your negotiating skills), and a clear and agreed-upon plan for marketing and promotion (including his forecast of profitability) makes the commitment easier and more clearly understood throughout the distributor organization.

Finally, never forget that any distribution deal is destined to terminate either because the distributor becomes so successful that it pays you to enter the market directly, or because he fails to deliver this objective and you move to an alternative. So keep pushing, but always be ready to jump.

Here speaks the voice of experience!

10.5   TERMS OF TRADE: INCOTERMS

Incoterms[3] are a set of rules agreed upon internationally under the auspices of the International Chamber of Commerce. When they are included in a trading agreement, they can be relied upon in any dispute between buyer and seller. They relate to the allocation of risk and cost between the two parties. Recently updated in 2010, they appear in commercial documents as Incoterms 2010. Incoterms do not apply to ownership of title (see Section 10.6). Title is a separate issue and is normally dealt with in another part of a contract for sale or supply agreement. What incoterms do is make it very clear who is responsible for all the costs, activities, and potential losses associated with getting a product from A to B.

The terms are described below. Please note these refer to Incoterms 2000, since they will still be applicable through transition during 2011. In Incoterms 2010, DAF, DES, and DDU are replaced by DAP (delivered at place). DAT (delivered at terminal) replaces DEQ. Incoterms 2010 also create two classes of term: (1) Rules for any mode of transport; (2) Rules for sea and inland waterways.

1. *E-term: Departure.* There is just one E-term, EXW. This term indicates that the seller's obligation is minimal and that the obligation is to make the goods available at the seller's dispatch bay. The seller does not even need to help load the goods onto the transport vehicle unless inclined to do so. Under this term, all risks and costs after pickup from the seller's premises are those of the buyer.

2. *F-terms: Main carriage unpaid*
   - FCA: free carrier (. . . named place). This means that the seller delivers goods, cleared for export, to the carrier nominated by the buyer at the named place.
   - FAS: free alongside ship (. . . named port of shipment). This requires the seller to place the goods alongside the vessel at the named port of shipment, cleared for export. This term applies only to sea or inland waterway.
   - FOB: free on board (. . . named port of shipment). This term requires the seller to deliver the goods over the ship's rail at the named port of shipment. Again, this applies only to sea or inland waterway.

3. *C-terms: Main carriage paid*
   - CFR: cost and freight (. . . named port of destination). The seller must pay the cost and freight necessary to deliver goods over the ship's rail at the named port of destination. This term applies only to sea or inland waterway.
   - CIF: cost insurance and freight (. . . named port of destination). Under this term, the seller must also insure the goods against loss until the handover take place at the port of destination. This will entail the seller taking out marine insurance.
   - CPT: carriage paid to (. . . named port of destination). The seller must deliver the goods to the carrier nominated and is responsible for all costs to bring the goods to the destination nominated. This term may be used irrespective of the mode of transport.
   - CIP: carriage and insurance paid to (. . . named place of destination). In addition to the requirements of CPT, the seller is required to procure insurance against risk of loss during transportation to named destination. Again, this term may be used irrespective of the mode of transport.

4. *D-terms: Arrival*
   - DAF: delivered at frontier (. . . named place). This term requires the seller to deliver the goods to the buyer's frontier but not to clear for import. It is important to name the frontier precisely in the term since the country of export also has a frontier. The buyer's aim in using this term is to have the goods at their disposal in their own country.
   - DES: delivered ex ship (. . . named port of destination). This term requires the seller to deliver the goods on board the ship at port of destination but not

cleared for import. If the seller is to bear the costs and risks of discharging the goods, DEQ (below) should be used.

- DEQ: delivered ex quay (... named port of destination). As DES, but seller has to unload goods on the quay, but still not cleared for import.
- DDU: delivered duty unpaid (... named port of destination). The goods are still not cleared for import, but the seller is responsible for delivery to a named location, normally the buyer's premises. The buyer is responsible for clearance and associated customs duty liability. This term applies to all modes of transport, although for transportation by sea, DES or DEQ may be more appropriate.
- DDP: delivered duty paid (... named port of destination). Under this term the seller is responsible for delivering the goods and paying the customs duty owing. In this term and DDU, the requirement is on the buyer to unload the goods.

With respect to forming trading agreements, the buyer will seek to do business on the most advantageous basis of DDP, whereas a seller will attempt to contract on EXW terms. These terms are important in international trade since they are universally accepted, comprehensive descriptions of the respective obligations on the parties. They therefore make the forming of contracts less subject to ambiguity, thus speeding up the process and reducing the risk of misunderstandings should things go wrong in execution.

10.6   OWNERSHIP OF GOODS: TITLE

An important aspect of international trade relates to ownership of goods. Often termed *holding title* to goods, identification of an owner is vital both to understand who has the trading asset and who is responsible for looking after it in all respects. The obligations we spoke of earlier must fall on the owner of the goods, even if others are performing the actual physical or administrative activities. If a company buys goods and imports them into its home country, that company has the obligation to ensure that the goods meet the regulations of all the relevant competent authorities involved. This means that companies must be very clear on the point of change of title when entering into commercial transactions. Normally, the contract of sale or supply agreement will stipulate the point at which title transfers. If in doubt, the company should seek legal advice. Incoterms do not refer to ownership of goods being limited to the allocation of risk and cost responsibilities.

In the pharmaceutical industry, ownership is very relevant to the concept of a sponsor company or license holder. As mentioned earlier, the term *sponsor* is given to the company making an application to conduct a clinical trial in humans or to market a drug. To supply either the clinic or to market, the sponsor and license holder will need to purchase and add value to materials until the materials become either clinical trial supplies (test material) or part of a finished product for sale. This means that a sponsor owns a significant amount of material and, accordingly, has the responsibilities of ownership. This is not always well appreciated, especially in smaller drug development companies.

The implication is that ultimate responsibility lies with the sponsor company for shipments relating to clinical trials or commercial product supply. Outsourcing to third-party manufacturers or logistics providers does not relieve them of the responsibility for proper governance of materials and activities in the supply chain.

Observations, Views, and Experiences of the Author

This is an area where I often find confusion among clients that I work with. This is part of a broader confusion, I believe, in the world of drug development using outsourced supply chains. There is a perception that the holder and mover of the materials has it all covered while it is in their possession. For example, if a product needs to be shipped, the freight forwarder knows how to do it. Well, yes, he does in most cases, but if it goes wrong, he is not accountable; you are, as the owner of the goods. Similarly, if it needs to be made, the CMO should know how to make it, but they are not the party held accountable by competent authorities. This is an account from the article on virtual pharma reference cited in Chapter 4[4]:

> According to Marla Phillips, PhD, director of the Pharmaceutical Technology Institute at Xavier University (Cincinnati), "The Food and Drug Administration (FDA) is not concerned about the existence of virtual pharma, but rather, their concern lies with how many examples there are of virtual pharma not fulfilling their quality function, which is why they are coming under the spotlight. In the Preamble to the 1978 GMP [good manufacturing practice] Regulations, the commissioner made it clear that *the contracting firm owns the goods and the contractor merely performs a service.* The responsibility for release against the registered information and GxP [good practice] compliance rests with the contracting firm.

10.7 THIRD-PARTY LOGISTICS PROVIDERS

When shipping goods, the owner has a number of options regarding the provision of services to accomplish the physical transportation and associated administration.

1. *Freight forwarders.* A freight forwarder typically deals with larger shipments using a range of transport modes, either self-owned of under contract. They also tend to offer value-added services that lighten the load for those engaged in administration. This could involve raising customs documentation, clearing goods through customs, settling duty and tax deferments and payments, and arranging additional forwarding. Freight forwarders offer a cost-effective solution for large consignments that require less specialist handling.

2. *Express couriers.* Express couriers have established their reputations on moving smaller quantities of goods quickly. Often, they operate with what is termed a hub-and-spoke system, whereby there is a preset network through which all shipments must travel. Hubs are set up at strategic locations around the world, so that any location is accessed by sending to the closest hub and then shipping on to the consignee from the hub. This makes for very cost-effective and predictable service as long as limited specialist handling or treatment is required.

3. *Specialist handlers.* A small cadre of specialist shippers, including World Courier, Marken, Yourway Transport, and Life-Con, has emerged in recent years around the needs of companies engaged in clinical trial supplies. They recognized that material shipments in clinical trials were often time- and/or temperature-sensitive. Sometimes they were even biological hazards governed by stringent regulations.

Both the traditional freight forwarder and express courier had difficulties doing justice to these types of shipments. Pharmaceutical companies were grateful to see a rise in the specialist handlers who could take a much more personalized and knowledgeable approach to their specific needs. These providers were able to monitor the shipment closely and spot any issues. They were able to get into the airport facilities, for example, to re-ice shipments that needed a top-up of dry ice due to an unexpected delay. They could also fill a supportive shipping advisory service to pharma clients, especially biotech and virtual companies. They also charge an associated premium for this level of service, so they must be used wisely.

When selecting and appointing freight forwarders or courier companies, one must be aware that they are only as good as the information with which they are provided; also, vitally important, the responsibility is with the sponsor to orchestrate proceedings. Good companies know their stuff and try very hard, but ultimately, if it doesn't get there, its the sponsor's problem. It is critical to select a provider that meets your needs, to build a strong working relationship, and to remember that a good global forwarder can be significantly more cost-effective for less-specialist shipments.

10.8 CUSTOMS

Worldwide customs information is available from the World Customs Organization.[5] Below is some explanatory information that has been paraphrased from their Web site.

The World Customs Organization (WCO) is the only intergovernmental organization focused exclusively on customs matters. With its worldwide membership, the WCO is now recognized as the voice of the global customs community. It is noted particularly for its work in areas covering the development of global standards, the simplification and harmonization of customs procedures, trade supply chain security, the facilitation of international trade, the enhancement of customs enforcement and compliance activities, anticounterfeiting and antipiracy initiatives, public–private partnerships, integrity promotion, and sustainable global customs capacity building programs. The WCO also maintains the International Harmonized System goods nomenclature and administers the technical aspects of the WTO Agreements on Customs Valuation and Rules of Origin.

Customs Valuation The customs value of imported goods is determined primarily for the purpose of applying ad valorem rates of customs duties. It constitutes the taxable basis for customs duties and is also an essential element for compiling trade statistics, monitoring quantitative restrictions, applying tariff preferences, and collecting national taxes.

How Imported Goods Are Valued Today, almost all customs administrations of the current 153 WTO members value imported goods in terms of the provisions of the WTO Agreement on Customs Valuation (adopted in 1994). This agreement establishes a customs valuation system that bases the customs value primarily on the transaction value of imported goods, which is the price actually paid or payable for the goods when sold for export to the country of importation, plus certain adjustments of costs and charges. Currently, more than 90% of world trade is valued on the basis of the transaction value method, which provides more predictability, uniformity, and transparency for the business community.

WTO Valuation Agreement The WTO Valuation Agreement is formally known as the Agreement on Implementation of Article VII of the General Agreement on Tariffs and Trade (GATT), 1994. It replaced the GATT Valuation Code as a result of the Uruguay Round multilateral trade negotiations, which created the WTO in 1994. The agreement provides a customs valuation system that bases the customs value primarily on the transaction value of the imported goods, which is the price actually paid or payable for goods when sold for export to the country of importation, with certain adjustments.

Where the customs value cannot be determined on the basis of the transaction value, it is determined using one of the following methods:

- The transaction value of identical goods
- The transaction value of similar goods
- The deductive value method
- The computed value method
- The fall-back method

These valuation methods must be used in hierarchical order.

Benefits of the Agreement The agreement is intended to provide a single system that is fair, uniform and neutral for the valuation of imported goods for customs purposes, conforming to commercial realities and outlawing the use of arbitrary or fictitious customs values. By its positive concept of value, the agreement recognizes that customs valuation should, as far as possible, be based on the actual price of the goods to be valued. With the majority of world trade valued on the basis of the transaction value method, the agreement provides more predictability, stability, and transparency for trade, thus facilitating international trade while ensuring compliance with national laws and regulations.

The Harmonized System   The Harmonized Commodity Description and Coding System, generally referred to as the harmonized system or simply HS, is a multipurpose international product nomenclature developed by the WCO. It comprises about 5000 commodity groups, each identified by a six-digit code, arranged in a legal and logical structure, and it is supported by well-defined rules to achieve uniform classification. The system is used by more than 200 countries and economies as a basis for their customs tariffs and for the collection of international trade statistics. Over 98% of the merchandise in international trade is classified in terms of the HS.

The HS contributes to the harmonization of customs and trade procedures and the nondocumentary trade data interchange in connection with such procedures, thus reducing the costs related to international trade. The harmonized system is governed by the International Convention on the Harmonized Commodity Description and Coding System. Further details can be obtained online from the WCO,[6] the International Trade Centre,[7] and the International Customs Tariff Bureau.[8]

10.9   SHIPPING REGULATIONS RELATING TO MATERIALS

10.9.1   Some Important Considerations

Those involved with shipping pharmaceutical products and materials around the world should be cognizant of the importance of compliance with the various national and international laws applied through competent authorities such as the following:

- Registration, Evaluation, Authorisation and Restriction of Chemicals (EU): REACH[9]
- The Toxic Substances Control Act (U.S.): TCSA[10]
- U.S. Department of Agriculture (or EU equivalent): USDA[11]
- U.S. Food and Drug Administration: FDA[12]
- European Medicines Agency: EMA[13]

Recently, this next area has become of increasing importance. Following is material from the UK's Human Tissue Authority to explain.[14]

10.9.2   The European Union Tissue and Cells Directives

The European Union Tissue and Cells Directives (EUTCD) set out to establish a harmonized approach to the regulation of tissues and cells across Europe. The directives set a benchmark for the standards that must be met when carrying out any activity involving tissues and cells for human applications (patient treatment). The directives also require that systems be put in place to ensure that all tissues and cells used in human application are traceable from donor to recipient.

10.9.3   Human Tissue (Quality and Safety for Human Application) Regulations 2007

The directives were fully implemented into UK law on July 5, 2007 via the Human Tissue (Quality and Safety for Human Application) Regulations 2007 (Q&S regulations). The HTA's mission was extended by the Q&S regulations to include the regulation of procurement, testing, processing, storage, distribution, and import–export. The implications for the supply chain are clearly evident.

10.10   A FINISHING NOTE

We finish the chapter with some material from the author's newsletter and Web site.

10.10.1   Biotech PharmaFlow Web Site Case Study

Ineffective logistics outsourcing was causing a UK biotech company costly trial delays, loss of cold chain shipments, excess shipping charges, and much wasted internal activity. Through tendering, using a detailed request for proposal and structured inclusive selection process, it was possible to appoint a preferred provider of third-party logistics services. This significantly reduced internal management activity, provided detailed control information on costs, and increased the reliability and timeliness of service.

This exercise had been prompted by a typical problem: A drug is not available at the site in time for study initiation.

Issues Arising

- Lack of coordination with the contract manufacturer
- Inadequate service from freight forwarders and couriers
- Delays in customs clearance
- Degradation of temperature-sensitive materials
- Damage to material through inadequate transit packaging
- Material expiry
- Good distribution practice compromised on shipment

Some Points to Consider

- Is supply management on the project team agenda?
- Are clear points of contact nominated?

- Is there a simple mechanism to allow for contractor lead times and constraints?
- Are SOPs written and agreed to for distribution logistics?
- Is a preferred specialist logistics provider identified?
- Have transport tests been carried out on the shipping container?
- Is an inventory control system in place?

To provide some background on this, I include a PharmaFlow Newsletter.

10.10.2   Biotech PharmaFlow Newsletter

This month we focus on some aspects of clinical trial supply logistics that are either poorly understood or prone to confusion, often causing delays in delivering drug to investigator sites. Some points to consider are:

- A new active substance (NAS) requires an international nonproprietary name (INN). These are allocated by the World Heath Organization (WHO).
- Goods also need to be classified with a commodity code so that customs can identify them for duty calculation. An internationally agreed harmonized tariff is available, details of which can be obtained from UK HMRC's national advice service, based in Southend-on-Sea.
- Details of the goods to be shipped must be set out on a commercial invoice (or not whether the goods are intended for commercial sale). The value declared must reflect a fair valuation. Declarations such as "research materials, of no commercial value" are incorrect. Often, an end-user letter is included with the shipment to provide customs staff with an easy-to-read summary of materials and study references.
- Storage and shipping conditions must be set and supported by stability data. Temperature data loggers should be included in any shipments where temperature sensitivity exists. The data logger should be calibrated and activated properly by the consignor. The consignee should deactivate the data logger and ensure that the data are returned to the sponsor or other responsible party. Any out-of-specification excursions should be investigated throughly and CAPA-documented.
- Buyers and sellers should be aware of Incoterms 2000. Incoterms define the allocation of cost and risk between buyers and sellers. They have international acceptance and cover a spectrum from Ex Works (EXW), where the buyer accepts all cost and risks outside the seller's premises, to delivered duty paid (DDP), where the seller accepts all costs and risks until the goods are in the buyer's hands. Typically, a buyer will aim to contract on DDP incoterms and a seller on EXW.
- Goods need to be properly insured by the shipment sponsor, as freight forwarders and courier companies provide only meager cover. This cover is often termed

marine insurance and contrary to the suggestion in the name, it covers all modes of transport and designated storage locations. Contact a broker for more information.

The list above should serve as a helpful indicator. None of the points can be regarded as specific advice without knowledge of the particular circumstances. The only sure way is to document your processes with comprehensive standard operating procedures that have been reviewed and approved appropriately.

11 Information Systems and Information Technology

11.1 OVERVIEW

Well-devised information systems (IS) and information technology (IT) can be tremendously enabling when dealing with the complex situations that are prevalent both in pharmaceuticals and in SCM. The converse is also true. Inappropriate deployment of IS and IT can turn a flourishing business into a quagmire of information "quick sand," where it takes increasing amounts of time and effort to keep from being sucked into the abyss that awaits. IS and IT pervade all areas of business, and on the face of it, in this chapter we may seem to cover too wide a scope. The point to remember is that the rigor of compliance and accountability across the entire supply chain leaves almost no area untouched.

The aim is to focus on the enabling potential of IS/IT, while understanding how to steer clear of the quick sand. The first consideration is to understand the distinction between an IS and IT. IS involves the information flows necessary to run an organization or business effectively. Often, paper systems (manual) are all that are needed to satisfy requirements that are simple and straightforward. For example, if all that needs to be achieved is preparation of simple household accounts, then buying and learning to use a computer and software specifically for that purpose may be a waste. However, for a small business owner with a requirement to prepare annual accounts, maintain customer and supplier databases, record inventory, and deal with the many other demands for information that small businesses have, some type of computerized assistance may be a lifesaver. This is where the key enabler of IS, information technology (IT) steps in. IT provides opportunities for electronic (computerized) assistance that can store, process, and transfer information millions of times faster and more predictably than can manual approaches. This is the fundamental distinction between an IS and IT. IS determines the information needs of a business and the associated systems flows and accountabilities (manual or electronic). It must be the responsibility of the business owners, even though stewardship may be invested in a specific functional area. Conversely, those invested with the stewardship of IS must look to the business owners for direction. Information technology is a key enabler and requires technical skills and knowledge for continued delivery of fit-for-purpose and differentiated enablement technology. The combination of these two areas is known

Supply Chain Management in the Drug Industry: Delivering Patient Value for Pharmaceuticals and Biologics, By Hedley Rees
Copyright © 2011 John Wiley & Sons, Inc.

as IS/IT and will be referred to as such from here onward. The starting point is some history on the development of the IS/IT landscape.

11.2   BRIEF LAY HISTORY OF COMPUTER SYSTEMS DEVELOPMENT

When first invented and developed through the twentieth century, computers were a revelation. The speed of processing and the ability to crunch numbers at the apparent speed of light seemed amazing. However, through the 1960s and 1970s, computers became enormous, often needed to be water cooled, and were fundamentally dumb: garbage in, garbage out as the manta went. They were also the domain of computer "experts," who knew all about programming languages, binary logic, central processing units, and a multitude of other technically jargonized snippets of vital information required to operate in the domain. This gave rise to departments [variously called management information services (MIS), IS, IT, computer services, etc.) of computer experts and practitioners who were required to interpret the requirements of people operating in the organization and to deliver computerized business "solutions". These operating people were given the name *users* by the computer fraternity, and something called a *systems analyst* emerged as the translator or interpreter positioned between users and the computer department.

There were, of course, problems with this approach. The giant "mainframe" computers were apparently simple beasts, but they needed to work in very specific ways. This, in combination with the (to be expected) errors in interpretation between users and systems analysts, resulted in enormous requirement specifications having to be written between IS/IT and its users. These had to be "signed in blood," and woe betide any user with a change of heart from there onward. Computers were beginning to seem not what they were originally cracked up to be.

Then came along IBM and others in the 1980s with the personal and desktop PC. For the first time, users had computer power in their own hands, and the novelty was overwhelming. It became possible for users to write simple programs without in-depth knowledge of computer languages. These users were able to deliver worthwhile benefits to themselves in their everyday work without having to go cap in hand to computer experts. The benefits were that of being able to store and retrieve information quickly, carry out calculations rapidly with reliability, and produce reports and graphs to share this information with colleagues in a tailored fashion. As PC hardware became increasingly powerful and software more sophisticated, the growth of desktop PCs became almost exponential, as did the potential for users to run as isolated islands, duplicating data already available in the organization, disconnected from the overall organizational processes. A case of out of the frying pan and into the fire, maybe?

In 1990, along came Michael Hammer with a convincing argument which postulated that irrespective of whether it was a fire or a frying pan, it was deep trouble. Hammer was a professor of computer science at the Massachusetts Institute of Technology who published an article in the *Harvard Business Review* and subsequently went on to write the now famous text with James Champy titled *Reengineering the Corporation*.[1] From this, the acronym BPR (*business process reengineering*) gained recognition and popular usage. One of the prime assertions from the work was that information technology and the use of computer-based automation had become such an obsession that a blind eye had been turned to whether the technology was actually adding value. Existing ways of operating were being computerized without assessments of the value added from these ways of working. In metaphorical terms, organizations were not seeing the forest for the trees. There was a complete disconnection of the needs of an organization from the activities that were being carried out in the name of progress. Hammer advocated radical "tree" surgery.

Indeed, Hammer had identified a phenomenon that had been going on for some time. Computerization had taken on a life of its own and had started to muddy the water of business imperatives. Many shared Hammer's view, as I did, and much was written on the topic. There was little to deny the fact that non-value-added activity and performance failures were associated with misdirected computerization. What was not so clear was how to go about changing it. Whereas radical tree surgery was widespread, results reported were patchy and often retrograde. We have more to say on this topic in Chapter 16 when we explore sustainable change. For our purposes here, suffice it to say that the BPR medicine was potentially more dangerous than the disease itself.

Interestingly, as the work of Hammer and others was being digested by the business world, a new type of technology entered the world of computing in the early to mid-1990s: *client–server technology*. It allowed users to have access to the power of a large-capacity computer (a server) while being able to define and run particular applications located on their own desktop PCs. This began to place the power in the hands of users and helped stimulate a transformation in the relationship between IS/IT and business users. For IS/IT, highly configurable solutions began to emerge from the new technology that paved the way for more integrated, yet flexible ways of working that could be offered to the user. For business users there was significantly more opportunity to specify systems requirements and processes for themselves and be confident that IS/IT had the wherewithal to deliver.

The German software company SAP was quick to capitalize on this new opportunity and developed the next generation of their then existing mainframe system SAP R/2 into a client–server version, SAP R/3. This was probably the genesis of enterprise resource planning (ERP). Up to this point, the computer software solutions tended to focus on a relatively narrow band of processing requirements. Companies would have separate computer systems for such activities as sales order processing, financial accounting, purchasing, and manufacturing. If information needed to be shared between systems, such as inventory details between production planning and accounting, a *batch interface* was required. This meant transferring data between systems at the end of each day. The consequence was that the systems were always at least 24 hours out of synchronization, and more importantly, errors were found retrospectively rather than being identified at point of entry. This resulted in much wasted effort trying to get to the bottom of discrepancies.

SAP R/3 changed all that by developing a fully integrated suite of software across all the business processes, including such areas as financial and cost accounting, sales and distribution, materials management, manufacturing, and warehouse management—even human resources management. The key ingredient was that the interfaces occurred in real time, so that if, for example, fresh items were received into finished goods inventory, the potential was there for sales order takers to view the availability immediately and satisfy demand accordingly. This had clear positive implications for a competitive edge.

There was, however, a sting in the tail with this approach. Whereas with a devolved systems approach, users could work relatively independent of each other, a much greater degree of cross-functional dependence was involved in the ERP environment. For example, the ERP systems contained a multitude of shared tables of base information. Whereas previously, any issue with the accuracy of a table was confined to a narrow group of users, under ERP it could affect the entire company. The whole system could be brought to a standstill as the software demanded a particular field, buried in the complex code, to be filled in by people who had no idea that they were suppose to do something. Implementation of these systems had a very checkered history in the early days, but has matured considerably since.

11.3   IMPORTANT PERSPECTIVES ON INFORMATION SYSTEMS

The area of information systems is huge, so for the aims of this book we focus on some key perspectives, presented through guest contributors. The first is enterprise resource planning (ERP) systems. The author was fortunate enough to gain experience here as part of Bayer UK's implementation of SAP R/3 in the mid 1990s through membership of the initial steering committee and project teams. Next, we listen to real-world experiences of ERP from an expert, Steve Waite.

GUEST CONTRIBUTOR SLOT: STEVE WAITE

11.3.1   ERP at Bayer in the UK

In the mid-1990s Bayer announced the introduction of SAP R/3 as the standard software for their global business. In the UK we found ourselves talking with our many operating divisions and introducing them to SAP, the integrated solution—whatever that meant? We soon realized that each of our divisions believed their business operations were very unique and would demand different system configuration in SAP. We were in danger of accepting this belief and creating multiple processes in SAP. To understand this challenge we decided to map and document our current business processes for all divisions.

We gathered together all stakeholders, who were sitting firmly focused on their functional silos, and reviewed the various supply chain processes. As a result of this activity, we identified and agreed on how our business operated. We soon demonstrated that although selling very different products, the underlying business processes were the same. This was then followed by a period of business process reengineering, challenging the status quo, before committing to a configuration of the new process in SAP.

Implementation of SAP resulted in a clear understanding of end-to-end processes and the ability to see across the process rather than just within each activity. Our business information transformed from being based on 24-hour delayed batch processes to immediate live data. We reported management information much quicker, but at the same time were able to identify any input or processing errors earlier. SAP gave the user a choice in selecting how they viewed reports and information. Sometimes there was too much choice, so we developed and agreed on standards across the business. This also identified the need to establish standard operating procedures which then supported training and identified further business improvement.

With the previous systems the business needed the support services to interpret and extract data for their management control. Now the commercial teams were running their own reports. However, the quality and value of this new information was very dependent on the success of some key activities during implementation. Ensuring correct master data (customer–product–supplier) is core to the accuracy and quality of management information and resulting decision making. Establishing clear business processes and testing these with the main users are an essential part of the implementation before going live. It is often easy to reengineer the processes and forget to focus on retraining the people. Staff then slip back into the old ways of working and create inefficiencies in the new system and reengineered processes.

Managing a new business system through process rather than function requires that the organization develop new ways of working. Staff skills and competencies need to be reviewed to meet these new requirements. An essential part of this is that staff have a clear knowledge and understanding of end-to-end business processes and the ability to manage and monitor these. Establishing these skills should ensure ongoing effectiveness in the supply chain process and enable decisions on process improvements to be made to support continuous business change.

This contribution from Steve Waite can be regarded as evidence of this developing relationship between IS/IT and the business through uptake of ERP systems and focus on business processes rather than functions and also on the potential benefits to be derived. What cannot be expressed in words is the resilience and staying power required to work these implementations through to meaningful conclusions. Even then, a conclusion is never reached because things change, drift, and move on. Readers with direct experience of these implementations will know what is meant here and what lay unspoken behind Steve's words. There is much blood, sweat, and tears along the way. I left Bayer, but Steve remained and moved from project leader in the UK to being the director responsible for the ongoing delivery of business processes for Bayer in the UK. Since these early days, ERP systems have developed and in the main delivered substantial benefits to those companies able to harness the potential. They are now also available as much more compact offerings for smaller companies at lower cost and implementation complexity.

From here on, the language of "systems" started to change to a far more shared and better understood vocabulary between users and IS/IT. Notably, references to "business processes" became far more common and helped create a key connection (this may well have been catalyzed by the work of Hammer et al.). Defining the business process involved understanding what the customer needed, looking at who was doing what, where information was coming from and where it was flowing to. Critically, it relegated any potential constraint of IT to a stage following the essential requirements of the business being identified. If IT could not deliver on the requirement of the business process, that was potentially a damaging compromise for the business. The result has been a growing move toward the activity of business process management charged with defining and maintaining a continual alignment between business users and IS/IT. The key aspect of this is the potential to make IS/IT-based improvements that add to the value proposition (including cost base improvement) and ensure that they are reflected in the practical working methods of the business.

From this, we arrive at the relationship between IS/IT and BPM. Below are some common definitions that can be found online:

> In a broad sense, the term Information Systems (IS) refers to the interaction between processes and technology. This interaction can occur within or across organizational boundaries. An information system is not only the technology an organization uses, but also the way in which the organizations interact with the technology and the way in which the technology works with the organization's business processes. Information systems are distinct from information technology in that an information system has an information technology component that interacts with the processes components.[2]

> Business process management (BPM) is a management approach focused on aligning all aspects of an organization with the wants and needs of clients. It is a holistic management approach that promotes business effectiveness and efficiency while striving for innovation, flexibility, and integration with technology. Business process management attempts to improve processes continuously. It could therefore be described as a "process optimization process." It is argued that BPM enables organizations to be more efficient, more effective and more capable of change than a functionally focused, traditional hierarchical management approach.[3]

Any clearer? Readers could be forgiven for experiencing a certain level of confusion and lack of clarity (as similarly experienced by me). For example, is there a dividing line between BPM and IS/IT? What is the difference between a business process and a system? Does IS involve optimization, or is that reserved for BPM? Drawing on the customary first principles approach taken herein, the following discussion aims to be a helpful clarification.

First, businesses and organizations are complex *systems* made up of people, information, equipment (including computers), physical facilities, and various other interacting components. At this level, systems are not about information in isolation. They include all the multitude of interrelated activities involved in achieving the organizational objective of converting inputs into more valuable outputs. The now famous Toyota production system covered in other chapters is one such system.

For a production or any other complex system to work effectively, information needs to flow between parties interacting with the system to create the desired outputs. In simpler bygone times, information was transferred by word of mouth and other noncomputerized methods, such as pencil and paper. As information flows became increasingly complex and high volume, specific departments (or functions) were set up with responsibility for information, especially in relation to the use of computers. These departments have been given various names over the years and are referred to here as IS/IT.

As IS/IT worked with business users, it became recognized that in the same way that physical "processes" converted goods from one state to another through a series of stages, there was also a requirement for information to be processed in stages to accomplish the needs of a business. Invoices needed to be sent to customers and payment made in return. Purchase orders had to be passed on to suppliers and goods received in exchange. Inventory data needed to be collected to be fed into production plans.

From this, we have firms (or organizations or businesses) as complex systems made up of physical conversion processes and business processes. The former, the physical processes, such as making tablets for pharmaceuticals, should be well defined in readers' minds. The business processes relate to the movement of all the packets of information, forward and return, required to pass through and between businesses in the furtherance of business needs. These needs are fundamental, such as collecting payment from customers, providing regulatory authorities with accurate data, and reporting inventory figures. The key issue is that these processes can be delivered either well or poorly, depending on how effectively they are defined and managed.

To take this discussion forward, Dee Carri will share her considerable experience.

GUEST CONTRIBUTOR SLOT: DEE CARRI

11.3.2   IS/IT and Business Process Management

The wide-scale adoption of technology and modern communications systems [known collectively as information communications technology (ICT)] is powering economic power shifts and enabling the globalization of supply chains. Adopting these technologies, organizations can adapt quickly to new economic conditions, source globally, move activities to new or lower-cost locations, outsource noncore operations, and enter into flexible collaborations quickly and efficiently. Customer management can be serviced from any convenient location through the use of the Web and email, supported by IP (Internet Protocol)–based infrastructure. These technologies are continuing to have a profound and fundamental effect on business cycles, collaboration, and innovation. They accelerate value chain cycles dramatically (e.g., four-day lead time to make, ship, and deliver a PC from time of online order to any location in Europe; nearly instant music downloads, online banking, secure payment systems).

These same technologies are empowering customers. With nearly universal broadband access and Web connectivity, customers now have the power to share information across loosely organized networks, and to conduct their own research and purchase products and services—globally and securely. This growth in Web-based consumerism has spawned the new concept of consumer self-service that is cost-effective and efficient for the consumer (e.g., online purchases, order tracking, music downloads), all of which requires virtual semiautomatic business processes or extensive integration of manual activities, transactional systems, Web-based systems, and virtual processes.

Business process management provides the backbone and integration of all of these manual, automated, and virtual activities across the value chain: from customer self-service through extended supply chains and in the back office. Without strong, integrated business processes, many of the sophisticated systems that we take for granted today would quickly unravel and the companies that are dependent on them would become uncompetitive, and perhaps fail. In today's hyperactive, global economy, BPM is critical to the faster delivery of better, cheaper products.

The Process-Centric Organization   Organizations enjoying success in this era are characterized as *process-centric*. They focus, and organize, around their business value chains, always placing the customer first. Furthermore, their business strategy is aligned with their activities (processes), cutting across the traditional organizational "silos." In addition, stakeholder rewards are linked directly to process outcomes. In process-centric organizations, all stakeholders understand their role in the enterprise and their contribution to its strategic objectives (see Figure 11.1).

In such organizations, value chains and associated business processes are tightly managed. Processes are documented, clearly setting out the way work gets done, for what customer, by whom, to what quality standard(s), in what time frame, for what cost, and according to which business rules. These processes and/or process steps are measured and transparent, enabling rewards to be connected directly to actual

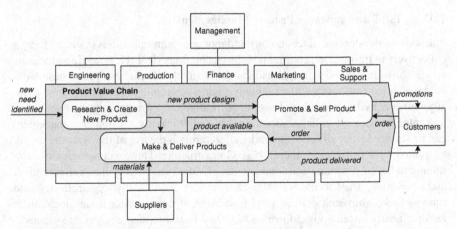

FIGURE 11.1   Example of a value chain. Note that SCM is not yet recognized as a separate discipline. (From Paul Harmon, BPTrends Associates, http://www.bptrends.com.)

process outcomes. This is BPM in the process-centric organization: the connection of strategy, process, and people for the achievement of competitive advantage.

Because existing processes, and therefore the business, are tightly managed, BPM also frees up management to undertake more advanced process analysis and improvement. Process-centric organizations use this time to drive further improvement and to innovate: for example, undertake intercompany and external benchmarks to identify new improvement opportunities; seek out and exploit shared service opportunities across value chains; develop sophisticated process-based responses to external changes; undertake process scenario planning and modeling to gauge the effects of planned or unplanned change; and accelerate time to market for new products and services through the use of process-based techniques and tools (e.g., design for six sigma, quality by design).

Enterprise Process Architecture   Process-centric organizations develop a process architecture that provides a top-down graphical overview of the processes of the organization, by value chain. Taking this top-down approach, it is then possible to decompose the process taxonomy to ever more detailed levels, providing a comprehensive process map for the organization. Process-centric organizations also align their process architecture with the business strategy and the IT architecture.

Conveniently, a number of process frameworks are available to assist an organization wishing to develop its own process architecture (see Figure 11.2). Developed by industry consortia, process frameworks provide a useful starting point and/or a

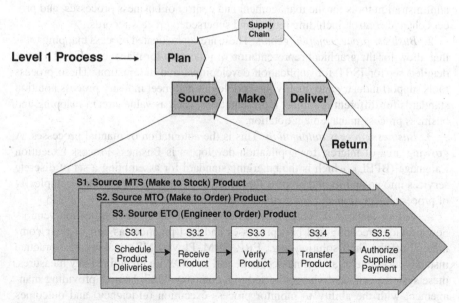

FIGURE 11.2   Example level 1 SCOR process. (From Paul Harmon, BPTrends Associates, http://www.bptrends.com.)

source for best practice review. In addition, most of these organizations also define key metrics for processes and independent benchmarking that enable members to review their process definitions quickly and effectively and benchmark their process performance. Process frameworks range from the specific [e.g., Supply Chain Council's SCOR[4] (Supply Chain Operations Reference)], to the holistic [e.g., AQPC, who provide the Process Classification Framework, covering the generic processes required by most businesses].

The BPM IS/IT Connection   BPM has its origins in quality systems that were traditionally the exclusive preserve of operational excellence and quality functions, with IS/IT involvement being limited to a supporting role through the provision of transactional, content, and information management systems. Recent technology developments, however, are changing this landscape, providing IT leaders and the IT function with many exciting opportunities to contribute actively to the development of the process-based organization and improved business processes. The main developments in BPM technologies are summarized briefly, below.

Service-oriented Architecture (SOA) provides for loose and flexible integration of IT services, allowing for greater agility of IT architecture.

1. *Business process management suite* (BPMS). A BPMS provides tools to manage the process improvement life cycle. The BPMS will contain—at a minimum—a secure process repository, process mapping tools for process documentation and redesign, management tools for process execution (e.g., measures and "dashboards"), administration tools for the management and control of business processes, and process change control, including retired and superseded process records.

2. *Business process mapping tools.* These are sophisticated process mapping tools that allow for the graphical representation of processes for management and a more detailed set for IS/IT for application development and automation. These process tools support industry and quality methodologies and meet industry process notation standards for different graphical representations, such as value stream mapping and business process management notation.

3. *Business process automation.* This is the automation of manual processes. A growing area of interest for application developers is Business Process Execution Language (BPEL), which is the emerging standard for assembling a set of discrete services into an end-to-end process flow, radically reducing the cost and complexity of process integration and automation initiatives.

4. *Vendor-integrated "best processes and practices."* Many application vendors now provide preconfigured best processes and best practices as part of their commercial off-the-shelf solution (e.g., ERP, CRM, PLM, LMS), making best practice instantly available to all businesses, large and small. With predefined key measures, these systems can easily be connected to a company "dash board," providing management with the ability to monitor process execution (efficiency) and outcomes (effectiveness).

5. *Process-based system implementation and delivery.* Using a BPM approach to systems delivery, IT is realizing significant productivity improvements and faster adoption times (e.g., 50% in functional requirements and the design phase, 20% to 25% improvement in the development phase, 30% in quality assurance and testing cycles).

The opportunities offered by BPM technology developments on the IS/IT supply side and increased business expectations are forcing IT to shift from a supporting BPM role to proactively increase its BPM capability and raise its contribution. The focus on BPM by IT management is underscored by research findings from Gartner in its annual CIO survey where BPM is consistently identified as a top priority. This trend is set to continue for the foreseeable future (2012).

BPM Initiatives and the Life Sciences   Until recently, BPM has not been highly visible or prevalent in life sciences organizations. The reasons for this lack of interest are complex but include factors such as the difficulty to achieve consensus across diverse communities and possible overlap with other initiatives (e.g., introduction of new regulations, PAT, six-sigma initiatives, and quality management systems).

Recently, however, some organizations wishing to emulate the success of BPM in other sectors are embracing BPM, evidenced by a growing list of success stories in the sector. Some examples of successful BPM initiatives in the life sciences are the following:

1. *Business process repository:* implementation of a single process repository for the introduction, maintenance, and management of company processes.

    Benefits: A single, global version of the truth; reduction in variation; fast rollout for new operations; improved communication with business partners for interlocking and outsourced processes; local variation visible and linked to global process, enabling global risk assessment and fast changeover to new regulations.

2. *Process-based standard operating procedures* (SOPs): conversion of word-based SOPs to process maps with supporting storyboards to provide additional commentary.

    Benefits: Higher usage of process maps than of traditional SOPs by operational staff; compliance improvements (measured by reduction in CAPA); more effective and efficient SOP training through use of storyboards for SOP training; big reduction in number of SOPs, resulting in faster retrieval and reduction cost of SOP management; process map–based SOPs are particularly useful where many dispersed external parties are involved and/or for seldom-used SOPs (e.g., clinical trial studies, product recall).

3. *PAT implementation:* classic pharma improvement treadmill: linkage of PAT to existing processes, gap analysis, future-state process definition, implementation.

   Benefits: acceleration of implementation and adoption of new processes (up to 40%). Easy collaboration between stakeholders, local and distant (via videoconferencing and process workflow tools).

4. *Direct-to-pharmacy process:* supply chain process transformation, required to control all medicine from point of manufacture to receipt at the dispenser.

   Benefits: drug security; improved governance risk and compliance.

5. *Clinical study process improvement:* mapping of the clinical study process to identify opportunities to improve time to market.

   Benefits: quick identification of critical bottlenecks: data management and clinical decisions; significant improvements (>10 months in discovery life cycle recorded, and achieved in four months).

6. *QMS documentation:* Conversion of word-based QMS to process map–based QMS using the AQPC framework and associated open benchmarking as a basis for best-in-class.

   Benefits: improved use of, and access to, the QMS; reduced cost of QMS management.

7. *Outsource contract management:* contract processes managed and tracked with shared access (on a need-to-know basis) to repository of contract(s), associated process maps, measures, change control improvement suggestions.

   Benefits: improved governance, risk, and compliance; increased innovation in partnership with external partners.

The interesting message that emerges from Dee's words is the increasing focus and benefits to be achieved by following a process-centric path. The follow-on message, though, as seen in other subject areas related to pharma (and life sciences), is that this sector is lagging behind. There are initiatives but they are still being joined up. Readers may wish to consider this in the broader context of some of the industry issues of fragmentation discussed in other parts of the book.

We look next at the specific business processes of SCM.

11.3.3 IS/IT and Supply Chain Management

This will be a brief account of IS/IT in SCM because, in my opinion, far too much emphasis is placed on computer systems in SCM. There is, of course, an absolute and undeniable need for computers to deal with the vast amount of information to be collected, tracked, analyzed, processed, and stored in the name of supply chain operations. The issue is that today's megasolutions arrive with an array of SCM functionality that muddies the waters of necessity. Instead of deciding what a particular situation needs, those buying off-the-shelf packages try to select what they can use from that which is placed in front of them. Normally, that is anything under the sun.

Briefly, before exploring the impact of this, we should follow the development of IS/IT in SCM. Note first that the development of SCM systems support appeared to coincide with the expansion of variety and product complexity in industry. Variety meant many more end items to be planned for expanding customer and supplier bases. Product complexity involved a plethora of components going into subassemblies going into the final product. The net result was hundreds if not thousands if not hundreds of thousands of stock-keeping units (SKUs) to be planned and managed. Details of suppliers needed to be kept on file, purchase orders placed on them, and deliveries booked-in and recorded. It goes on from here until the customer gets what is needed. Enter now materials requirements planning (MRP I), the first attempt to get a handle on things.

Materials Requirements Planning (MRP I)   The pioneers of computers in SCM include Oliver Wight, George Plossl, Hal Mather, and Joseph Orlicky. In their texts, the terminology was not specifically related to SCM in the way in which it has been defined in this book. Most of their work was published under the titles "materials management" or "production and inventory management." Whatever it is called, the work is regarded here as part of the body of knowledge that has been created in relation to the management of complex supply chains.

MRP I is a simple computer algorithm used to determine requirements for the inventory of materials to meet production needs. It uses a bill of material (BOM) to define the quantity relationship between the parent item and component parts (sometimes termed a *parent and child relationship*). It is something like a family tree.

Inventory Code Number   The product can be significantly compromised or even dangerous if a wrong inventory item is included in production; also, each specification must be identified and distinguished from all other, nonidentical items. This involves strict rules on identification to provide unique referencing. A product or item code is typically used to achieve this. The customary rule to decide if a different code should be used is based on fit, form, and function. This means that if two items cannot be used completely interchangeably, they must be regarded as different and have a different number allocated. An example would be a change to an information leaflet in a packet where some additional information is added.

Inventory code numbers are normally categorized within the supply chain into broadly raw materials, work in progress, and finished goods. These are sometimes broken down into more specific categories, such as packaging, chemicals, foil, bulk tablets, and product families. Raw materials are purchased items and work in progress and finished goods manufactured items. Manufactured items will be made from input materials (raw material inventory) and the relative quantities and product structure defined in a bill of materials.

Bills of Material (BOMs)   The components of a finished product and the materials that go to make up the components can be represented as what is known as a bill of materials. Figure 11.3 shows the typical makeup of a simple BOM for a packaged vial of product. The input to the packaged product is a filled, unlabeled vial. The

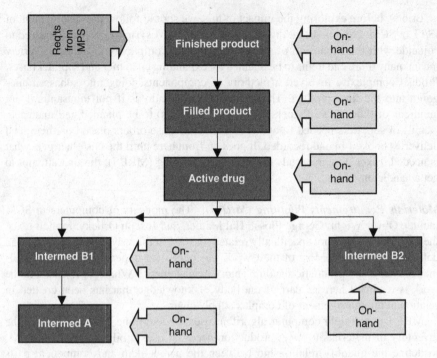

FIGURE 11.3 Simple bill of material structure.

input to that vial is the active ingredient (also with all the other materials) in the solution in the vial. Intermediate stages feed into the solution. Along with the BOM, the algorithm requires information on the available on-hand inventory of all the items concerned and the sourcing lead time of the component parts.

When a customer order (independent demand) arrives, the MRP algorithm checks if there is inventory available to satisfy the order. If there is, it goes no further, other than to reflect the fact that finished inventory has been shipped. If there is no inventory available, it will recommend that more is produced and check the availability of components that are specified in the BOM (dependent demand). For any components that are not in stock, it will suggest a purchase order be placed for a preset amount. The purchase order placement date will be based on the lead time required to source the component. That is all it is!

In theory, it was a wonderful idea. In practice, there were many issues, which are discussed in more detail in the next section. For now, suffice it to say, MRP I was a tool used to determine the procurement needs of the business and did not incorporate manufacturing satisfactorily. A revised approach, MRP II, was developed.

Manufacturing Resource Planning (MRP II)   The acronym was the same, but the words were different. *Manufacturing* replaced *materials*, *resource* replaced *requirements*. Planning stayed the same! Basically, the new approach was devised to address the disconnect observed between what was being procured for use in manufacturing against manufacturing's actual needs. In practice, what was happening was that the raw sales forecasts were being used as the independent demand input. This had two unfortunate effects. First, sales forecasts changed frequently; often well within manufacturing response time. This led to what were termed "nervous" MRP systems, whereby sales orders and forecasts could be entered in to the system that were impossible to satisfy. Since the algorithm was run by a mere dumb machine, it would suggest orders to be raised and delivered in unachievable lead times—very often in the past (past-due messages were generated in volumes that no planner could ever hope to address). When a system starts saying that it needs you to get something in last month, you know there is something amiss somewhere!

The second failing was that the stages of production to meet the forecast had to be planned and completed very much earlier than the finish date in the forecasts. The procurement lead times in MRP I did not take account of this, and therefore dramatic shortages at the start of manufacture were commonplace. MRP II was therefore developed to counter these problems. The developments involved the following:

1. Introduction of orders to instruct production as to when and how much to produce (work orders) as well as the already existing orders to procure (purchase order).
2. The inclusion of product routings. This allowed work centers and labor timings to be established for each product. This meant that there were now two files, one to define product structure and the other to define the operations involved in production.
3. The concept of a master production schedule (MPS).

In one sense, this was a welcome development, as to a certain extent it addressed the issues with MRP I discussed above. In another sense, however, it was a retrograde step because it increased the scale and complexity of these systems to the point where they were (and still are) difficult to control. Keeping the monster fed with up-to-date information, at all the stages, in exactly the form required could potentially be a lifetime's work for an army of people. The benefits needed to outweigh the costs, and for many companies this is not the case. Many have not let that small detail interfere with their plans for IS/IT support for SCM (pharma companies included).

Having said that, there were some prerequisites developed at the time to raise the probability of success. These are summarized from *The Best Investment—Control Not Machinery* by George W Plossl[5]:

1. There must be a complete planning and control system.
2. A valid master production schedule must be developed.
3. The various records used must be accurate.
4. Qualified people and teams must be developed.

Point 2 shows that emerging from MRP II was the important development of a competency set known as master production scheduling (MPS), more recently termed *master planning*. The mission of master planning is to balance the needs of customers for a product with available capacity at the plant. The derived MPS would then be a single agreed-upon set of numbers to drive all activities. Along with the numbers would be rules about how and when changes could be introduced. This started to create the type of stability required to make MRP II more workable.

In addition to MPS, another important development was that of sales and operations planning (S&OP) processes. The aim of this was to engage senior decision makers in managing the interface between the sales teams and the supply chain. This was to counter the tendency of either "side" taking an isolated view of supply to markets. The unavoidable compromises that had to be made when supply issues occurred needed to be made in the light of business impact. Hence, the sponsorship of senior executives with the power to prioritize and spark actions was required.

The final development was ERP, covered in general in Section 11.2. Very simply, it collects all the systems that a company needs to use to run a business into an integrated whole. SCM business processes are included in the whole. The only piece to add here is a word of warning based on the initial comments in Section 11.2. Excessive dependence on computer systems in SCM can divorce practitioners from the nuts and bolts of getting things done. This is definitely the case where MRP II functionality has been used to manage operations on the shop floor. In Chapter 12 we shall see that production systems can be so fast moving that computer technology is inappropriate. That is not because the computer is too slow but because the people using the computers cannot possibly feed them with enough information to reflect what is happening hour by hour, let alone minute by minute. This is where lean thinking needs to take over.

Next we turn to a vitally important area, that of patient safety, a contribution by Adrian Hampshire.

GUEST CONTRIBUTOR SLOT: ADRIAN HAMPSHIRE

11.3.4   IS/IT and Patient Safety

Regulatory authorities around the world are focused increasingly on the risk-based approach to the safety of pharmaceutical products and medical devices when considering their effect on patients. The entire discipline of evaluation of risk is known collectively as *pharmacovigilance*, defined as a "set of methods that aim at identifying and quantitatively assess the risks related to the use of drugs in the entire population, or in specific population subgroups."[6] To gain sufficient data on which to base measurements and predictions of risk, extensive individual data on adverse drug (or device) reactions (ADRs) must be collected from patients rigorously. It is not sufficient to rely on safety data that have been collected during the development of the drug or device, as (1) testing in animals is not analogous to use in humans,

(2) clinical trials are of limited duration and are only indicative of what may occur in real-life usage, and (3) information about rare but serious adverse events may only arise during long-term or extensive public use of a drug or device.

The need for extensive collection of drug safety data has been known for more than 150 years. *The Lancet* started to collect notifications of side effects from anesthetics in 1848. In 1906, the Federal Food and Drug Act required that pharmaceuticals be "pure" and "free of any contamination." In 1937 in the United States, 107 deaths occurred after diethylene glycol was used mistakenly to solubilize sulfanilamides, and in 1952 in France, 100 lethal cases occurred after diethyl tin dioxdide was mistakenly used in a skin preparation. Between 1959 and 1961, multiple reports were made of fetal abnormalities occurring with the use of the new sleep-inducing drug thalidomide. In the United States the law was revised to require drug companies to prove safety and efficacy before the authority would issue a marketing authorization. In 1954, the UK introduced its Yellow Card safety event reporting system. This increasing concern and regulation of the drug production and safety reporting process has continued in a steady and unremitting stream of new legislation and regulations to which companies must adhere. So how do pharmaceutical and medical device companies respond to these ever-increasing demands?

Of course, the ethical industry would never naysay the legitimate demands of regulators who are operating on behalf of the population to whom the companies wish to sell their products. Although the pharmaceutical industry may still find it difficult to shake off the image of snake oil salesmen, their intent is always to ensure that their products are effective and safe. The concern for the pharmaceutical company will be to collect and analyze safety data in the most efficient way possible. And this is why the IT systems come into play.

Given that the total number of individual case safety reports (ICSRs) reported to the regulatory bodies worldwide runs into many hundreds of thousands per year, it would be impossible to generate, process, or analyze these manually. Thus, all companies will use some form of IT system to record and report ICSRs and periodic safety update reports (PSURs) to the regulators, whether these are through the systems that the regulators provide or their own in-house implementation of a drug safety recording and reporting system, such as Oracle AERS or ARGUS, ARISg, Empirica Trace, TrackWise, or any of the other packages available commercially.

In these situations, all the challenges and caveats around validation and properly controlled use of these packages that are explored elsewhere in this book apply in the handling of drug safety cases—but in spades. A pharmaceutical company's drug safety management system is among the most important that the company has and the most critical to keep running in good order. It has been said that there are only four IT systems that are on the critical list in any pharmaceutical company: the system that pays the employees, the system that receives money for products, the system that manages and controls the manufacturing processes, and the drug safety reporting system. If any of these fail, the impact on the company can be huge. If the drug safety system fails and the company is out of compliance with regulations, the regulatory authorities have the power to shut down the company or key elements of the company either permanently or for a period of time. No company wants to risk this, so the highest level of attention needs to be paid to the drug safety system and its proper management and maintenance.

The reason that the regulatory authorities reserve such preeminent power and control is clear. Their concern is focused wholly on the need to ensure the safety of medicines or medical devices that we use. To do this, they must be absolutely sure that all instances of doubt are known about quickly. The "instances of doubt" arise in the form of ADRs, and it is imperative that these are reported in a timely manner. IT systems enable pharmaceutical, medical device, and CRO companies to receive, store, and report ADRs and, without such systems, the speed, extent, and competence of this reporting would not be possible. Beyond this transaction-processing element, IT systems can help illicit information about trends in safety data that is difficult, if not impossible, for a person to derive manually.

In addition to the routine reporting of ADRs, the regulatory bodies are very interested in understanding whether trends within the ADR data might signal some underlying problem with the particular product or class of products. In the broader discipline of IT, we know this as *data mining*. In the world of pharmacovigilance, we mine the data to attempt to generate signals that may indicate a problem, and this is done as part of the approach to managing risks related to therapeutic treatment.

Treatments provide a benefit, but the benefit comes with a risk—a risk of some form of adverse reaction. It is the balance of risk and benefit that the regulators weigh when deciding whether or not to grant a license for the same type of product. Increasingly, though, the regulators are also expecting the producer to take a risk-based approach to the development of a product. Thus, the regulators now look to the producer to be actively monitoring all ADRs and trying to identify any signals that all is not well. Gone are the days when the producer simply reports individual ADRs to the regulator, provides PSURs as required, and that's the end of their responsibility. Now, producers are expected to consider the entire pantheon of risks that their product may generate when used in humans. The body of data that is principally used to try to locate the signals of risk includes the company's own store of data on the product(s) and the data that the regulatory bodies make publically available. Mining this vast reservoir of data cannot be achieved manually. It has to be done by sophisticated programs that operate across vast amounts of data in order to tease out any signals that are implied by the data.

IT systems are therefore critical to the entire process of establishing the safety profile of a product and alerting to any potential change in the level of risk that is involved in use of the product. These systems are essential to the capture, management, and reporting of the basic data that constitute the ADR. The systems also enable the risk-based approach to patient safety that is central to good pharmacovigilance.

If ever there was a case for the utility of IS/IT enablement, the discussion above encapsulates it. Speed and capability to process vast amounts of data securely (when done properly) is enhanced immeasurably by the application of IS/IT. The relevance to protecting patient safety in the supply chain should also not be lost here.

The next section covers areas of IS/IT that were high on the regulatory agenda some years ago, but through the auspices of people such as David Stokes, these risks and opportunities have become much better understood and managed. David explains more in the next section.

GUEST CONTRIBUTOR SLOT: DAVID STOKES

11.3.5   IS/IT and Pharmaceutical Regulations

Computerized systems that are validated are generally understood to be more repeatable and reliable than human beings when executing the same process over and over again. This is not only important from a regulatory perspective in terms of managing risk to product quality and patient safety, but is also a key business consideration in supply chains with significant transactional volumes.

Validation is the process of ensuring that a computerized system meets expectations expressed in terms of the requirements of process owners and that the requirements are clear, complete, and consistent. At a time when supply chains are becoming increasing complex and at a time when regulations in the supply chain area are continuing to develop, it is essential that these requirements include compliance with current good manufacturing practice (GMP) and good distribution practice (GDP).

This is further complicated by new regulations in areas such as labeling in Braille, the inclusion of drug product codes on final packaging (often using two-dimensional bar code labels), and new regulations being introduced to tackle counterfeiting and reimbursement fraud, including pending regulations in the areas of product and package electronic pedigrees and serialization. While GMP regulations have developed relatively slowly over the last decade, this is set to change with the wider introduction of process analytical technology and the adoption of parametric product release, and we are likely to see further regulatory focus on the integrity and safety of highly automated (computerized) product supply chains.

Validation, including revalidation as part of ongoing business process management, plays a vital role in ensuring that our supply chain systems are fit to meet the needs of the business and to ensure product quality and patient safety. This includes compliance with regulatory expectations for the use of electronic records and electronic signatures (ERES). U.S. 21 CFR Part 11 is the most cited regulation in this context, but similar requirements exist in most developed markets, including the European Union and Japan.

When these requirements were introduced, it was extremely complicated to comply technically with such expectations, but it has become technically much easier to use ERES in supply chains, leveraging standard off-the-shelf electronic record solutions and technologies such as encryption. Many of these technology solutions were developed to facilitate growth in online business-to-consumer (B2C) e-commerce rather than business-to-business (B2B) supply chains, but have been incorporated successfully into the majority of mainstream information systems, such as manufacturing execution systems and enterprise resource planning systems.

The challenge remains to identify the scope and content of supply chain electronic records, which may vary from organization to organization, depending on the product profiles involved and which may be linked across complex supply chains. Once identified, the issue of electronic signatures can be further complicated in complex supply chains when electronic records may be signed by personnel from third-party organizations (e.g., a Qualified Person from a contract manufacturer). Generally speaking, the technology exists to solve these issues, but it is important that IS-facilitated supply chains are implemented by teams who really understand the business processes, the applicable regulations, and how to apply the necessary technology in a way that complies with the regulations but that does not make the supply chain inefficient.

The industry "bible" on computer system validation is generally considered to be the GAMP^{TM} Guide, which started in the early 1990s with a focus on process control systems. GAMP now encompasses a broader mission, including IS used in supply chains, and has some specific guidance looking at global information systems. Version 5 of the GAMP Guide also introduced a less proscriptive approach to computer system validation which is applied much more usefully to information systems used in supply chains, and this is now being used to validate supply chain systems in a much more cost-effective and applicable manner.

GAMP 5 focuses much more on the validation of configurable off-the-shelf systems, recognizing that systems such as ERP are used much more widely than custom-built systems (which was the case in the 1980s and early 1990s). It also usefully defines the terms *process owner* and *system owner*, understanding the importance of the business and IS communities working together successfully to implement systems which are now focused on business processes.

Although there are exceptions, in most pharmaceutical companies (and an increasing number of pharmaceutical distributors and logistics companies), the principles of validation and the key concepts of the GAMP Guide are being used to develop and implement supply chain solutions that are "fit for purpose" and meet the requirements of the process owners. However, one of the key issues that is not yet being well addressed is the need to validate complex supply chains across multiple parties, to facilitate product returns and product recalls. Of these, product recall is of specific concern because of the potential impact on patient safety, and there are two underlying issues here.

The first is the understandable focus on optimizing our supply chains for when things work properly and for the 99.9% of the time when we need to manufacture and distribute product as efficiently as possible (reducing costs, minimizing inventories, reducing transportation times, etc.). In many cases we do not think about the minority of cases when things go wrong and we have to accept returns or, even worse, quickly identify the physical location of products in the supply chain and implement a product recall. When everything involved fewer parties and a small number of paper records, this could be done by a small number of people working across a limited number of organizations, consulting their paper records or local information systems and coordinating by phone or fax.

Although our supply chain information systems are being more closely integrated for the 99.9% of cases when things go well, very few companies develop an end-to-end business process for product returns and recalls and ensure that information systems are integrated to support this process, let alone validate the use of these systems to ensure data integrity and reliability. This is one reason why some regulators have expressed a concern that it now takes longer to implement product recalls than in the 1990s, and this is something which the industry needs to address in the future. This can be done by clearly defining business processes for these "exceptions," ensuring that information systems are well integrated to support such processes (increasingly using service-oriented architecture based on standard Web services) and that these processes and systems are validated.

The good news is that all of the knowledge exists within the industry to achieve this – leveraging business process management techniques, newer technologies such as service-oriented architecture to ease the task of integration, and leveraging existing guidance such as the GAMP Guide to validate information systems in a cost-effective manner. In combination, this will extend the benefits of validated information systems to these important (but less frequently used) business processes, will continue to mitigate risks to product quality and patient safety, and thereby ensure the continued efficient operation of highly automated supply chains.

Hopefully, David's presentation has been extremely informative to those wrestling with the complexities of 21 CFR Part 11 and other IS-related regulatory requirements.

11.3.6   IS/IT and SOPs

The earlier contribution from Adrian Hampshire refers to existing processes often being found wanting. Below is an excerpt, contributed by Nicki Haggan, from my company's (Biotech PharmaFlow) newsletter that was prompted by a discussion with Adrian. He said that almost all the IT problems he encountered were actually process issues. He had, because of that, formed an Alliance with Nimbus (Control 2007[8]) to be able to offer a world-class solution to managing business processes. Dee Carri, from whom we heard earlier, is also an advocate and Nimbus partner.

This may seem a trivial question, but increasingly, industry regulators are discovering that SOPs can be found wanting. Often, they are written in isolation without all the relevant stakeholders involved; or changes have been implemented that have unintended impacts on critical areas. Frequently, their adoption across an organization can be patchy, at best. Many organizations take an "impose by edict" approach to the challenge of ensuring that their teams follow the company's SOPs. Although this is a reasonable starting point, greater adoption can be achieved by making the SOP materials, and in particular, information about the process that the SOP defines, much more accessible and useful to the teams.

Replacing lengthy text documents with process maps improves the usability of the existing process documentation and, through this, the level of compliance with the process. The volume of controlled documentation in a quality management system can be reduced significantly by:

- Using flowcharts (or process maps) to capture process information and communicate best practices
- Maintaining a central list of references, roles, abbreviations, and definitions
- Providing clear links between training material, documentation, and support needs for easy maintenance and reduced duplication of information

ICH GxP requires maintenance of extensive controlled documentation. A pending update to the guidance (Q10: A Harmonized Tripartite Guideline on Pharmaceutical Quality Systems) is likely to see an increase in the application of flowcharts, bringing the industry into line with other quality standards, such as ISO 9000. Therefore, proactive application of a business process management–based approach will prepare you for the implementation of this guidance.

Again, Nicki is someone who understands the importance of SOPs translating into sound processes.

12 Improvement

12.1 WHY IMPROVE?

Why improve? may seem an obvious question to some, but little is being taken for granted in this book, so the question is covered here. We start by beating on the same old drum—competitive advantage. In fact, it is the only drum, because much as there seems to be an in-built human need to improve, it seems pretty randomly distributed. In business, random improvement doesn't work; it has to be focused on keeping ahead of the competition in your customer's eyes. That means improving the company's value proposition and cost base. This can only happen through conscious management of the process.

In Sections 1.6.4 and 1.6.5 we touched on industrial progress and attempts to make improvements in the production and supply of products to customers. It is undeniable that significant improvements have been made over the years. New technologies have been introduced, smarter ways of working have been developed, and automation of routine tasks and flows of information has taken place. It has not been a smooth road to travel, however, and there have been spectacular failures along the way. Computers do not always exhibit common sense, robots are ultimately dumb beings, and people often follow the route of least resistance and ignore the smarter option. Nonetheless, progress has been made. The aim of this chapter is to review those improvement efforts, good and not so good, starting at the early stages of industrialization. That should then pave the way for a discussion in later chapters of improvement in relation to SCM. Some readers may be surprised at the scope afforded the treatment here, but let us not forget that the introduction of a new or changed product into a market is a business "improvement" and, as such, holds significant involvement for the supply chain.

Processes for improvement in business have been going for many years, and a plethora of tools and techniques are now available. The genesis of improvement initiatives leads back to the Industrial Revolution and efforts of the early entrepreneurs to maximize productivity of their resources: people, land, and capital. Since supply chains are heavy consumers of all three, much of the early attention was paid here, and many of the gains made were accrued in the supply chain. Readers wondering why this is the case should remind themselves of how the supply chain is made up. It is the sum total of all the production, delivery, and waiting stages required to take products to market. In the case of pharmaceuticals, it is the resources tied up in producing raw materials, intermediates, active ingredients, drug product, and finished

Supply Chain Management in the Drug Industry: Delivering Patient Value for Pharmaceuticals and Biologics, By Hedley Rees
Copyright © 2011 John Wiley & Sons, Inc.

packaged product, followed by the route to market via the wholesalers, pharmacies, and clinics involved. This is not an insignificant amount of people, land, and capital that are tied up.

To be clear also as to terminology, the supply chain as considered here is synonymous with a production system. So when we talk of improvement in the supply chain, we are speaking about improvements to the production system. This is another drum that I am beating throughout the book, and this is as good a place as any to give it another few thumps. The supply chain (or production system) starts at the design of a product. It does not (and should not) start some time after the designers have had their say and produced the final design drawings. Thus, improvement in supply chains begins at the earliest stage and continues through the life cycle of the product.

Before moving into a treatment of the subject area, it should be mentioned that I have purposely avoided the term *continuous improvement*, which has become popular in recent years in loose translation of the Japanese term *Kaizen* (*kai* = change, *zen* = for the better). Once a proponent of the concept, my views have changed in the light of more recent personal experiences.

Observations, Views, and Experiences of the Author

Kaizen will appear in the text to follow, but before that I wanted to emphasize what I believe now to be something of a crisis in the world of business improvement. We hear the term continuous improvement *used so often, as if just the mention of the word is a badge of honour. Whole armies of people chase every minute opportunity to claim a gain here or a win there. Just because it is a continuous search, however, does not guarantee that it is an improvement. As we shall see later, improvements can only be judged by their impact on the entire production system or subsystem. Teams running kaizen events can easily convince themselves that there has been genuine improvement without having the entire picture to allow them to tell. At the Lean Enterprise Research Centre Annual Conference in 2009[1] (held at Celtic Manor Resort, the venue for the 2010 Ryder Cup), several speakers referred to the unrealistic scale of cost savings often claimed by six-sigma and lean initiatives. One speaker reported annual savings claims in excess of the company's total turnover for the year! Something is wrong there somewhere, don't you think?!*

The reason is clear after some thought. In calculating savings, if cash is not actually prevented from leaving the business, it is not a real saving. It is not unusual for improvement teams to take time saved on a particular set of activities and convert that into money saved. Potentially it is, but if that time saving is not converted into a reduced wage bill, no money is saved (and hence there is no improvement in the competitive cost base). Similarly, teams may identify improved working methods that save the cycle time on a particular machine or process and claim major benefits to the business. However, if there is no impact on customer measures of value to them (such as getting the product more quickly), it is not a genuine improvement.

This is not to argue for reduced improvement efforts—in fact, the reverse. My argument is that improvement effort should be focused on activities that make a difference. We seem to have become obsessed with the word continuous *at the expense of the important word* improvement. *The fact is that improvement is important whether continuous or discontinuous, and sometimes the only solution is discontinuous improvement (i.e., radical change). The vital consideration should always be: What is the impact on the total system and the related subsystems that are employed in delivering sustainable competitive advantage?*

Our comments above should set the tone for the chapter, which will decouple improvement from any particular methodology that has gained favor in recent years. We trace through history and explore developments that have been proposed and have taken place in the name of improvement. We do not dwell any longer than is necessary to gain the fundamentals of the approach, so the reader does not have to wade through reams of text. Hopefully, we allow the reader to make objective judgments based on common sense.

12.2 IMPROVEMENT AND PRODUCTION SYSTEMS

The target for improvement should be made crystal clear before moving on to specific approaches. To that end, this section is about improving production systems. It should be well understood now from earlier chapters that SCM operates on systems of production, made up of production stages, delivery stages, and waiting stages that (eventually) deliver goods to customers. These are termed *production Systems*, and many readers will be familiar with TPS, the Toyota production system. Toyota, along with other Japanese companies, such as Nissan, Honda, and Matsushita, have all demonstrated that they can create highly effective production systems. Toyota, particularly, has received a massive amount of attention in pursuit of finding their "secret of success." Much has been written on TPS and on lean thinking that emerged from the analysis. Sadly in my opinion, the world has misinterpreted the findings and been extremely selective in the lessons learned. In fact, as reported in the introductory chapter, as this book was being written, as if by mysterious coincidence, Toyota suffered a massive blow to its mighty reputation for quality and speed of response. Defective breaking systems and accelerator pedals were detected in cars that had reached the market and were in use by customers. When the investigation is finally complete and the causes assessed, no doubt it will involve lessons learned in relation to some of the basic principles of production systems. That is the spirit in which to read this chapter on improvement. No company walks on water. It is basic good working principles that must be followed, not the path of those who know them.

Observations, Views, and Experiences of the Author

Anyone keeping abreast of discussion groups on business improvements on the various networking sites will be aware of the huge battles of divergent opinion that take place in the name of finding the "right path." Questions are raised such as to what is best, lean or six sigma? Is agile better than lean? Is the theory of constraints the best way to go? We might just as well ask: Is the Bible better than the Koran? The ensuing discussion would be equally long and as pointless as those cited above from the networking sites. The real question is, of course: By what principles should we run our lives (production systems)?

With that assertion, I confidently propose the following. There is no such thing as an agile supply chain when taken end to end. Parts of a supply chain, particularly downstream in conjunction with a postponement strategy, can be quick to respond. However, in my opinion, the term creates false expectations. Dan Jones quoted the Coca-Cola supply chain as being 300+ days end to end. How can that be agile when upstream suppliers are starting to produce 300 days ahead of final customer consumption?

There can also be no such thing as a lean supply chain as it has been commonly interpreted under the predecessor concept of just-in-time (JIT). This is not, in my opinion, as a result of Womack and Jones's presentation of their facts and findings. It seems to me to be due to a kind of selective adoption of the principles by those wishing to learn from them. The problems began with JIT as people hit on the possibility, if things were done correctly, of timing in-bound deliveries in close synchronization with the production process. Companies went to JIT deliveries without doing the underpinning work required, such as reducing system variability and defect levels. The ensuing requirement for small and frequent deliveries drove suppliers wild and led to more shortages that they saved. Lean has been similarly misinterpreted—and I do wish that it had been given a different name. People associate lean *with* mean. *The belief is that making savings in waste really means cutting jobs. Then, when we hear talk from the lean world of single-piece flow, batch sizes of one, single-minute exchange of dies, and inventory-less systems, people give up the ghost.*

My plea is, therefore, that we get away from these various pseudo-supply chain and production system "religions" and focus on the best way to run production systems. Toyota has one that is world class, but ultimately it is theirs alone—and we now know that it has been fallible. In the rest of the chapter we cover improvement in this light, the only meaningful measure being how it affects products and customer service.

12.3 THE IMPROVEMENT JOURNEY

12.3.1 Early Attempts at Improvement

Adam Smith, in his work *The Wealth of Nations*,[2] introduced the notion of division of labor. This is a fundamental that still pervades our attitude to work. His aim was to improve the people's productivity by making them concentrate on very specific elements of work so that they became increasingly efficient at the task in hand. The basis of this was the fact that the learning-curve effect of simplicity and repetition made operators increasingly productive. This set the idea that it was a good thing to break tasks down into smaller and smaller bites. It may be worth noting, though (and the reader may well have picked up on this), that in Smith's day, the stimulation and motivation of the operator was not high on the list of priorities for business owners. The rationale for improvement was purely to increase productivity (defined, in simple terms, as getting out more with the same resources or using fewer resources to get out the same amount).

Following on from Smith, F. W. Taylor appeared on the scene to further the "science" of work and productivity improvement. As mentioned in Chapter 1, Taylor was dubbed the Father of Scientific Management and took the early notions of Smith to an entirely new level. That level included the application of something termed *work study*, which was made up of work measurement and method study. Work measurement involved taking a stopwatch to time operators doing the work and also assessing the pace at which the operator worked (termed *rating*). From this it was possible to calculate a standard time for the job, and this was often used to judge financial rewards under schemes known as *piece work*.

It was obviously in the interest of the operator to have the allowed standard time set as high as possible, and this often could lead to "fun and games" on the shop floor. It was not unusual for impediments to speed (such as the wearing of gloves) to be introduced temporarily by the operator during the period of study. More on that later, for now the point to be made is that there were more than a few problems in getting improvement to stick in practice.

Along with Taylor, others developed novel approaches to the measurement of work, notably the Gilbreths. Frank and Lillian Gilbreth reduced all motions of the hand to combinations of 18 basic motions. These included grasp, transport loaded, and hold. They named the motions *therbligs* ("Gilbreth" spelled backward with the 'th' transposed). He was a strong advocate of the "one best way" and accordingly, studied work in immense detail. This led to what were called "synthetic" time standards, whereby time could be worked out from a database of times taken for smaller elements of work. Hence a work study engineer could record a job and then go back to the office and compile a time based on theoretical standards. None of this was, of course, very popular with the workers!

The other branch of work study, that of *method study*, was less controversial but almost equally difficult to work in practice. Whoever enjoyed someone else telling them how to do their job! Method study basically involved recording all the activities connected with undertaking a piece of work, be it making a batch of product, producing a component, or carrying out office work. The method study practitioner would observe the work and break down into specific activities. These activities were then recorded under one of five headings: operation, inspection, temp hold, store, transport. The job was then analyzed with a view to eliminating, combining, and simplifying the steps. From that the work study engineer would define how the work should be carried out.

From small beginnings, Taylor was able to build an entire approach to industrial improvement, which eventually led to formation of the discipline known as *industrial engineering*. Although Taylor was not the exclusive creator, his work does form a major component of the discipline, and certainly his thinking pattern was an important inspiration to many in the field. One final point to note is that Taylor's work did lead to significant improvements to the working methods and productive capability of industry at that time. Many of his approaches and those from industrial engineering to follow are incorporated into the lean and six sigma methodologies of today. Process flowcharts, statistical process control, and waste elimination, for example, are all products of the F. W. Taylor School. That is a major reason to maintain an objective view toward all improvement methodologies that have emerged over the years—they don't need to belong to any particular club, they just need to suit the job at hand.

12.3.2   Industrial Engineering

Industrial engineering grew into a well-known staff activity through the work of others in addition to Taylor, building a common knowledge base. It began to gain widespread interest through the auspices of members of the American Society of Mechanical Engineers (ASME). One of the pioneer mechanical engineers was Henry R. Towne, who wrote an article entitled "The Engineer as Economist," suggesting that the development of management techniques was important for the progression of the engineering profession. From this work, industrial engineering built an impressive armory of tools and techniques with the potential to raise productivity levels significantly.

In 1948, the American Institute for Industrial Engineers (AIIE) was opened and began to provide professional authenticity for practicing engineers. Up to this time industrial engineers really had no specific place in the hierarchy of a company. The ASME was the only other society that required its members to have an engineering degree prior to the development of the AIIE.

A textbook definition[3] defines IE as follows: "Industrial engineering is concerned with the design, improvement and installation of integrated systems of people, materials, information, equipment and energy. It draws upon specialized knowledge and skill in the mathematical, physical, and social sciences together with the principles and methods of engineering analysis and design, to specify, predict, and evaluate the results to be obtained from such systems." That is something of a mouthful, to say the least! But the words do emphasize that the study of the effective use of resources in integrated systems has been around for some time. In a nutshell, the discipline is about making complex systems of people, processes, and equipment operate together more effectively. This includes such things as identifying and removing non-value-adding activities, improving production yields, reducing machine change over times, and simplifying process and product flows.

These days, a typical syllabus of a university degree in IE would include such elements as inventory and resource management, risk analysis, logistics, ergonomics (*ergo* = work, *nomos* = study of), production planning, operational research, quality and process control, value analysis and value engineering, time and method study, design of experiments, and expert systems. Most, if not all, of these topics have rolled forward into further iterations of improvement activities over subsequent years.

There was, however, one powerfully undermining aspect to IE— it was the tool devised by owners and management to fulfill management ends. Historically, productivity improvements invariably meant more work and were almost exclusively converted into additional profits for the bosses. The industrial engineer, especially when wielding a clipboard and stopwatch, became an object of suspicion and was often regarded as a management stooge. The work of Taylor et al. was beginning to become counterproductive as resistance to close supervision and control started to mount.

At the same time, cracks were beginning to appear in the whole concept of mass production. The focus on volume and narrow bands of work, to drive down cost per unit of production, was having a dehumanizing effect. People were beginning to lose connection with their jobs and employers. Increases in product and component variety, spurred on by competitive activity, also prompted a spiral in "systems" complexity. This all resulted in less predictable demand patterns, more convoluted flows through the "process village,"[4] and poorly motivated workers—the impact being a significantly greater propensity for things to go wrong.

The improvement potential contained within Taylor's scientific approach to management appeared to be found wanting. The knowledge of the tools was invested in those without the power to act and there was a distinct waning of interest in industrial engineering. Sadly, this was something of a case of throwing the baby out with the bathwater. The discipline itself was a well-rounded approach to improvement in systems of people, machines, and materials working together to produce products for customers. The issue was around motivation of those doing the work to join in (see Chapter 16 for more on this topic). There had, as well, been some interesting experimentation carried out in the name of productivity improvement (à la Taylor's way) that had delivered some startling results.

12.3.3 Hawthorne Experiments

These studies resulted in what is now commonly termed the *Hawthorne effect*. They were carried out in the 1920s and 1930s at the Hawthorne Works[5] (a Western Electric factory outside Chicago). The intention of the studies was to explore, in good old scientific fashion, the effect on worker productivity of varying lighting in the production environment. The surprising finding was that worker productivity improved irrespective of how the lighting was changed: higher or lower intensity. Other workplace changes were also introduced, and the result was the same. When the studies were concluded, productivity returned to the previous levels.

The conclusion drawn by the investigators was that the attention being paid to the workers was the driving force behind improvements. This was powerful evidence that treating workers as factors of production was a limiting industry's potential to improve. From then on there was increased awareness of the human dimension of working in an industrial setting. Questions were being asked about the wisdom of focusing exclusively on the study of work without consideration of the workers themselves.

12.3.4 Douglas McGregor

Douglas McGregor, a management professor at the MIT Sloan School of Management, fueled the fire further after the publication in 1960 of his now well-known text *The Human Side of Enterprise*.[6] In the book, McGregor defined two very different sets of assumptions about people and work. Theory X assumptions regarded workers as being in need of cajoling and coercing to get them to work: a version of what we now call today *management through command and control*. The deep assumption about human nature was that workers were not naturally motivated to give of their best. Close supervision and direction were essential to get the best results for the company. Theory Y assumptions took the opposite view. Under the right circumstances, employees will direct their own efforts through an innate desire to deliver good-quality work. Theory Y assumptions had clearly not been a component of the scientific movement of Taylor et al.

The interesting fact was, and this seems to be a frustrating aspect of the world's response to improvement initiatives, that McGregor was instantly associated with being a proponent of Theory Y. Others around him, such as the mighty Ed Schein, observed that McGregor was disappointed with the fervor and unbending allegiance to Theory Y assumptions that emerged. It seems he had identified two extremes but was not suggesting exclusive use of either. He saw his work as a starting point for others to experiment with and build on. Instead, the message for many was that scientific management was dead and there was no further role for structure and control. This was not the intended result. Further study of McGregor's work also reveals that he was a strong advocate of the use of these assumptions by people to constructively challenge their own particular assumptions in the world of management at work. Assumptions drive behavior, and behavior drives managerial actions. It was a means of improving personal and managerial performance.

As an aside, readers should consider McGregor's experience in relation to the current view of lean thinking. Many have pounced on aspects of lean methodology that were not intended to be the main focus.

12.3.5 W. Edwards Deming and the Total Quality Movement

Concurrent with McGregor's work on industrial improvement, W. Edwards Deming was equally questioning of the way that mass production was failing to deliver. In the early 1950s he was invited by the Union of Japanese Scientists and Engineers to help Japan employ methods that he had applied successfully in the United States during the war effort. His work in the United States was only partially successful because management appeared reluctant to fully embrace the concepts and associated necessary changes. In contrast, Japanese management and workers quickly absorbed the teachings in their totality. His early work in Japan was around statistical methods to control defects by reducing variability and opportunities for error. It is believed that Deming's major contribution was no so much the techniques (SPC had been known and used in Japan for many years) as his ability to communicate the mathematical concepts to workers so that they used them in the work environment. He gave simple, understandable tools to those actually responsible for performing the primary value-adding activities. The Japanese workers used the tools willingly to improve their working methods—on a continuous basis, later to be termed *kaizen*, so popular in lean parlance. Readers should note here that this is possibly the greatest power within the success of Japanese industry—the ownership of those doing the work for the quality of their own output.

Deming made a significant contribution to Japan's later reputation for innovative high-quality products and its economic power. He is regarded as having had more impact on Japanese manufacturing and business than any other person not of Japanese heritage. Despite being considered something of a hero in Japan, he was only just beginning to win widespread recognition in the United States at the time of his death. From Deming's success in Japan emerged a set of principles that grew from his own experiences of mass production methods, which he believed were flawed. In one of his books, *The New Economics for Industry, Government, Education*,[7] he had this to say: "The prevailing style of management must undergo transformation. A system cannot understand itself. The transformation requires a view from outside. The aim of this chapter [from his book] is to provide an outside view—a lens—that I call a system of profound knowledge. It provides a map of theory by which to understand the organizations that we work in." At last, this was recognition that industrial enterprises were complex, interrelated systems. His major assertion from this was that much of what happened, especially when things went wrong, was down to the system, not the people working within it.

Deming identified four elements of his system of profound knowledge:

1. *Appreciation of a system:* understanding the overall processes, involving suppliers, producers, and customers (or recipients) of goods and services
2. *Knowledge of variation:* the range and causes of variation in quality and the use of statistical sampling in measurements
3. *Theory of knowledge:* concepts explaining knowledge and the limits of what can be known
4. *Knowledge of psychology:* concepts of human nature

Deming described the system:

"The various segments of the system of profound knowledge proposed here cannot be separated. *They interact with each other*. Thus, knowledge of psychology is incomplete without knowledge of variation.

A manager of people needs to understand that *all people are different*. This is not ranking people. He needs to understand that the performance of anyone is governed largely by the system that he works in, the responsibility of management.

The appreciation of a system involves understanding how interactions (i.e. feedback) between the elements of a system can result in internal restrictions that force the system to behave as a single organism that automatically seeks a steady state. It is this steady state that determines the output of the system rather than the individual elements. Thus it is the *structure of the organization* rather than the employees, alone, which holds the key to improving the quality of output.

The knowledge of variation involves understanding that everything measured consists of both "normal" variation due to the flexibility of the system and of "special causes" that create defects. Quality involves recognizing the difference in order to eliminate "special causes" while controlling normal variation. [Deming taught that making changes in response to "normal" variation would only make the system perform worse]. Understanding variation includes the mathematical certainty that variation will normally occur within six standard deviations of the mean.

As we will cover exemplar thinking in Chapter 15, the links between Deming's system of profound knowledge and all subsequent approaches to improvement should begin to emerge. For example, consider the following four questions:

- *Point 1:* What is this in essence if not the principles behind value streams?
- *Point 2:* What is this if not six sigma?
- *Point 3:* What is this if not the concept of continuous improvement through systematic problem solving?
- *Point 4:* What is this if not respect for people?

My underlying assertion is that Deming was the master pointing the way, and the world studied one of his star pupils while the master remained on the sidelines.

Deming offered 14 key principles for management for transforming business effectiveness. The points were first presented in *Out of the Crisis*.[8] The 14 points are listed below in a very truncated fashion that aims, based on key phrases that Deming uses, to emphasize the critical essence of the messages:

1. Create constancy of purpose.
2. Take on leadership.
3. Cease dependence on inspection.
4. Minimize total cost.
5. Improve constantly.
6. Institute training on the job.
7. Institute leadership.
8. Drive out fear.
9. Break down barriers between departments.
10. Eliminate slogans, exhortations, and targets.
11. Eliminate work standards (quotas) on the factory floor; eliminate management by numbers and numerical goals.
12. Assume pride of workmanship.
13. Emphasize education and self-improvement.
14. Transformation is everybody's job.

These 14 points could only have grown out of Deming's disenchantment with mass production practices and principles. They refer massively to the role of the individual within the production system, whether as worker or manager. The historical reliance of mass production on numbers, targets, productivity, and technology is stark by its absence. He puts the onus on the systems of work and organizational working rather than on those within it.

In my opinion, these teachings of Deming pointed to solutions for problems we are still wrestling with today. Anyone currently working in our industrial society would find it difficult to challenge those principles in a way that would be anything other than nitpicking. The difficulty seems to be that while nodding agreement to the principles, it is not clear how a person can go about improving matters. Perversely, the message is that people cannot, unless and until they set about understanding systems; and that is not enough. They then need to know what to do to change matters; and that is not enough; they need to be able to work on ways to implement change for the better; and that is not enough; they need to see those changes implemented and then move on to the next systemic issue.

We now continue the journey through the various improvement initiatives. In doing so, keep in mind the impact on systems parameters, as defined by Deming, that these initiatives may have. Some readers with a pressing interest in getting to the nub of systems thinking in relation to improvement efforts may wish to move on to Chapter 15.

12.3.6   Value Engineering and Value Analysis

Value engineering and value analysis were covered in Section 8.7 and are raised here again to illustrate the link with systems. As we have learned, variety and variation are the sworn enemies of systems, since they seek a steady state to operate effectively. Having defined these two activities as basically the removal of all but the essential elements in a product structure, it should be clear how they contribute. The necessary standardization and simplification required to implement VE and VA provide a supporting undercarriage for the associated production system.

12.3.7   Master Production Scheduling Emerges from MRP II

The notion that production systems work best with stable schedules and standard routines started to take hold as MRP II failed to deliver the expected results. Not only were forecasts always wrong, but very often, the Forrester effect made them positively wild. For those who are not familiar with this concept, it relates to the amplification of demand that takes place through the tiers of a supply chain as small changes of demand in the market result in massive increases in orders.

The first evidence of this realization was the emergence of master production scheduling as a functional discipline in P&IC. This role was identified as the interface between the market and the plant to ensure that schedules were realistic while also remaining cognizant of market requirements. Previously, MRP I systems had used sales forecasts to generate plant requirements and made the process very "nervous." This meant that they were prone to frequent and significant change. The aim was to redress the balance so that plant constraints could be accommodated while still meeting customer demand. This was the forerunner to the lean concept of *heijunka*[9]—level loading, to be discussed later.

12.3.8   Theory of Constraints

Readers familiar with supply chain management may well have read *The Goal*[10] by Goldratt and Cox. This was a seminal text at the time because it exploded some of the myths of mass production related to the blind focus on people–machine utilization and production volume. It also called into question (correctly in my opinion) the accountants' view of production economies. Goldratt originally helped develop and sell a software product called Optimized Production Technology (OPT). OPT was billed as the first software to provide finite-capacity scheduling for production environments. During his activities, Goldratt realized that the habits and assumptions (paradigms) of employees and managers prior to using the software were still prominent and influenced results negatively after implementation.

The Goal was a great success. The systems link was the assertion that the supply chain is only ever as good as the weakest link, or the limiting constraint. Goldratt included a metaphor of a troop of scouts walking in line, all having to walk to the pace of the slowest member. This made the point that running machinery and equipment to full-capacity potential was a fruitless exercise if it were not a constraint in the supply chain. All that was doing was producing material that the system did not have capacity to consume. It was destined to sit around waiting until the constraint eventually caught up.

12.3.9   World-Class Manufacturing

Richard J. Schonberger was a student of Japanese manufacturing techniques. He wrote the book *World Class Manufacturing*,[11] which was his own personal take on best practice ways of operating based primarily on Japanese ways of working. Schonberger identified the four prime pursuits of world-class manufacturing (WCM) as total quality control, just-in-time (JIT, later to morph into *lean*), total preventive maintenance (TPM), and employee involvement.

He also defined his principles of *good management of manufacturing*, which he declared as his own action agenda for manufacturing excellence. This involves 17 points:

1. Get to know the customer.
2. Cut work-in-process.
3. Cut flow times.
4. Cut setup and changeover times.

5. Cut the flow distance and space.

6. Increase the make or deliver frequency for each item required.

7. Reduce the number of suppliers to a few good ones.

8. Cut the number of part numbers.

9. Make it easy to manufacture the product without error.

10. Arrange the workplace to eliminate search time.

11. Cross-train for mastery of more than one job.

12. Record and retain production, quality, and problem data at the workplace.

13. Assure that line people get first crack at problem solving (before staff experts).

14. Maintain and improve existing equipment and human work before thinking about new equipment.

15. Look for simple, cheap, movable equipment.

16. Seek to have plural rather than singular workstations, machines, cells, and lines for each product.

17. Automate incrementally when process variability cannot otherwise be reduced.

These points are reproduced here for readers to be able to compare Schonberger's ideas with Deming's 14 key-principles. These also appear to be recommending actions that operate on the overall production system to create stability, repeatability, and responsiveness to external change (discussed further in Chapter 15).

12.3.10   Business Process Reengineering

A number of organizations, having recognized that they had grown fat through the 1970s and early 1980s on a diet of captive markets and a stable business environment, acted clearly and decisively in slimming down to become fit for the competitive rigors of global business. Notably, General Electric, under the leadership of Jack Welch, introduced sweeping changes in the mid-1980s, which included de-layering as a key component. Senior managers at GE Appliances at the time were quoted as describing the eliminated levels as "loaded with high-priced, high-quality staff who massaged data, briefed one another, passed thing up the line . . . and back down again." There is no doubt, that organizational structures can become top-heavy, which can impede a company's cost base and ability to innovate.

Business process reengineering (BPR) became a classic solution and in cases where it has been applied appropriately to the need, it has resulted in dramatic improvements. Much of BPR was founded on changes to organizational structures: that is, taking managerial layers out of an organization. *De-layering*, as it became known, was regarded as a key element in a cocktail of organizational change initiatives including BPM. The aim was to reduce bureaucracy and thus improve business indicators. It also, by the way, cleared the channel for the organizational "system" to operate in an atmosphere of significantly reduced "noise." This is another "helpful" systems effect and is discussed further in Chapter 15.

12.3.11   Just-in-Time

JIT came along packaged for consumption by Western industrial society. It majored on the success achieved by Japanese companies in working with much lower levels of inventory in the supply chain. It seemed miraculous, almost too good to be true; and that's what it was. Companies found themselves sailing close to the wind in the name of JIT; quite a few found themselves capsized. The way it was interpreted in the West led to companies putting the cart before the horse. Realization started to emerge that some important things needed to happen before JIT could work. Lean thinking came along to provide some answers.

12.3.12   Lean Thinking and Enterprise

Lean (along with six sigma, to be covered below) is probably the most current example of proposed exemplar thinking. Particularly in pharmaceuticals at this time, many companies are adopting lean approaches to solve some of their problems. It is appropriate, therefore, to start building an understanding of lean thinking and its application to the entire enterprise. There is no shortage of excellent material on lean and the toyota production system on which lean was founded. Lean is based on the work of Womack, Jones, and Roos and is documented in the now famous text *The Machine That Changed the World*.[12] It describes a landmark study of the automobile industry based on the largest and most thorough study ever undertaken in any industry. Sponsored by the International Motor Vehicle Programs (IMVP) of the Massachusetts Institute of Technology, this was a $5 million five-year 14-country study of the worldwide auto industry. Termed the NUMMI study, it made a thorough investigation of Japanese methods of manufacture and supply and demonstrated that they could be transferred successfully into a Western-based organization (General Motors in Fremont, California).

The title of this section purposely includes the term *enterprise* to reflect the applicability of lean thinking throughout an entire organization. To date, the uptake of lean thinking has been confined broadly to production and operational areas. It does, however, have utility in any part of a business where people work to achieve productive ends, be it designing a new product, creating a service offering, or even running, say, an advertising campaign. The reason for this misconception is not totally clear, but it is undeniable that the mainstream business schools have not picked up on lean as a core approach to business management (see also Owen Berkeley-Hill's commentary in Section 15.3). That is what it is, however, surprising as that may be to some readers. The Toyota production system, on which lean is based, along with similar approaches from Japan, is a complete approach to designing, making, marketing, and selling products.

The strategic marketing method of customer segmentation, explained so expertly by Malcolm McDonald in Section 6.6 (and widely used in business schools) is reflected in the principles of lean. The first principle is: "Specify value from the standpoint of the end customer by product family."[13] What is that about if not market segmentation? The issue, possibly, is that as with all of lean, there has been selective hearing of the principles. The first principle is taken as a one-size-fits-all customer, and it is often skipped over. The last phrase, "by product family," drops off many versions of the principles as they are reported out. In fact, it is a critical phrase.

The point is that as seen in the ICI example in Chapter 6, customers for similar products can be very, very different. The design of their products and supporting production processes may need to accommodate these differences. The Japanese manufacturers proved themselves to be accomplished in their level of understanding of their customer segments, but where is that reflected in lean principles? It is in that little phrase "by product family." What it doesn't do is explain how product families should be set, that is, how to move from a one-size-fits-all approach to a segment-based approach.

Hopefully, this has given a flavor of this book's treatment of lean enterprise. We see it as a massive contribution to the body of knowledge on the challenges of becoming increasingly effective in supplying products and services to customer markets. We also recognize, though, that there have been errors in translation of the principles and details that have led to widespread confusion. Lean is regarded as "mean," "cost-cutting," "random removal of waste," and "fast-track," for example. Let us stop at fast-track, because I have personal experience of this.

Observations, Views, and Experiences of the Author

I was asked to spend time at a UK manufacturing site that was part of a Swiss-based big pharma firm. The assignment was to examine their processes in preparation for their implementation of SAP advanced planning and optimization (APO). They were already experienced users with SAP R/3 ERP. I had worked for the site director previously while in permanent employment and had a lot of respect for the incisiveness of his thinking. It was under his sponsorship that the consultancy exercise was carried out.

I won't go into the details of findings, other than to say that one of the ailments they were suffering from, which seems common in big pharma organizatioons, was running too many variants on long-changeover, high-speed machinery. Their overall equipment effectiveness (OEE) was typically in the low to mid 20%. Production planning was based on the capacity they thought they should achieve rather than what they achieved regularly in practice. This led to huge capacity overloads and firefighting based on that well-known "priority of the loudest voice."

The feedback I gave reflected these findings and provided details and suggestions. The point of interest here is that some of the products manufactured at this site had been designated as lean brands. This was part of the headquarters initiative to drive lean into the organization. When I heard the term lean brand I was mildly suspicious. Value streams (see later) become lean rather than brands. Brands typically have more than one product family under the umbrella. For example, in pharmaceuticals they may contain injectables, different types of solid-dose, topical creams and lotions, inhalers, and so on. The production flows (value streams) for these would need to be totally different. Lean can only be applied at this level.

My suspicions were confirmed a week or so into the assignment. There was a two-tier system in operation whereby the lean brands had shorter conversion lead times allocated. So a lean brand item received into stores would need to pass through receiving inspection in two days; nonlean brands could take five days. Lean brands were treated in a similar fashion when loaded onto production equipment. Miraculously, however, if products required the same processing, say blister packaging, they went through the same set of equipment. Which do you think received priority? What sort of service levels do you think customers for nonlean brands were getting?

They had, of course, completely missed the point of lean. It is not about doing things quicker or cheaper or slicker. We go into this in much more detail in Chapter 15. For now, some of the thinking processes of lean are explained and reviewed so that readers here are not subject to similar misconceptions. This will be brief because the references provide ample opportunity to dig deeper. The main aim here is to create an appetite for understanding the capabilities contained within lean, not the tools.

Five Principles of Lean[14]

1. Specify value from the standpoint of the end customer by product family.
2. Identify all the steps in the value stream for each product family, eliminating whenever possible those steps that do not create value.
3. Make the value-creating steps occur in tight sequence so that the product will flow smoothly toward the customer.
4. As flow is introduced, let customers pull value from the next upstream activity.
5. As value is specified, value streams are identified, wasted steps are removed, and flow and pull are introduced. Continue until a state of perfection is reached in which value is created with no waste.

Figure 12.1 shows a schematic representation of the benefits of a lean approach (value streams segmented by product family approach, compared with the mass production approach of a process village)

Policy Deployment The way these principles are developed into concrete implementations of lean ways is through policy deployment or management (*hoshin kanri*). It is described by Womack and Jones in their book *Lean Thinking*.[15] It involves the interaction of objectives, projects, cash targets and improvement targets, to deliver plans, typically on an annual basis. One of the important outcomes is often identification of the need to break down organization of the production system along *product*, rather than production process lines (functional, as in the process village). This is to support principles of engagement with the market above. Value stream analysis is normally used to develop the approach.

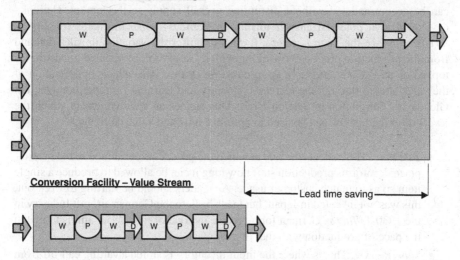

Short run times and queues; quick change-overs; short transfer distances; low in-process inventory

FIGURE 12.1   Comparison of a lean product family arrangement versus a process village.

Value Stream Analysis   This leads to the mapping of value streams, which is an activity that defines how value is (or is not) delivered in the current-state arrangement. Following is the stage of defining one or more future states that act as a basis for improvement efforts. The mapping specifies the physical flow of material and the information flows. There is an established methodology to carry out the mapping, supported by material and information icons. There are important points to note about mapping that are raised by lean experts such as Womack and Jones. First, data and information collection should be based on actual observations, not third-party accounts of what is happening. Second, the current-state mapping should not become the work of a lifetime. The purpose of mapping the current state is to be able to indentify and implement future-state improvements. Third and vitally, authority should be delegated to one person (the value stream manager) with a complete focus on the value stream (end-to-end supply chain). That person is required to possess a range of competencies so as to manage the value stream in support of customer need.

Heijunka   In today's complex demand environment, products have inherent uncertainty that cannot be predicted accurately. For example, a product manager dealing with minor markets with complex dynamics will find it hugely difficult to forecast accurately on a month-by-month basis. In senior management review meetings, the manager can be castigated for causing her own supply problem through lack of forecast accuracy. This can turn into a mutual "blame allocation" event between supply planners and the product manager!

The solution is to design the supply system is such a way that forecast inaccuracies can be accommodated without disrupting overall supply to the market. Heijunka developed as a potential answer to this problem. *Heijunka* translates roughly as *levelization* (see the *Lean Lexicon*). It aims to buffer the variation in sales demand from the production process by working with a "reservoir" of finished goods that is topped up at a steady rate from the production facility. This allows optimization of the value stream through the increased stability and learning for repetition (see Ian Glenday's contribution in Section 15.3). This creates an environment in which the levers described below can be used to optimize flow and value delivery.

- *Takt time*. This reflects the rate at which the product is consumed in the marketplace. It informs production staff how long it can be allowed to produce a single item so as to match customer usage. As readers should be starting to work out, this was not invented in Japan, but leads back to the German aircraft Industry in the 1930s! (*Takt* is German for a precise interval of time.) The aim is to match the pace of production with that time allowance.
- *Supermarket*. This is where the input inventory is stored awaiting call-off from the downstream process. The idea is that the producer can see what is being consumed and make the necessary arrangement for replenishment based on standard rules.
- *Kanban*. This is a signal to the upstream operation, from the supermarket, to produce a specified quantity and then stop.

This is the basis of what is termed *pull scheduling*, called for in lean principle 4. We can now see that this is very different from the MRP II logic supporting batch and queue operation.

Five S's   This is basically the concept of "a place for everything and everything in its place." It is used in the workplace to underpin effective working methods. The English translation of the Japanese terms (both quoted in the *lean lexicon*) is *sort*, *straighten*, *shine*, *standardize*, and *sustain*. What that means in practice is to clear away all that is not needed to do the work on a daily basis. Then arrange items so that they are easy to locate and use. Finally, always clean up and maintain the discipline of working to the standards.

Single-Minute Exchange of Die   This technique was made famous by Shigeo Shingo, after whom the Shingo Prize was named. He was a consultant to Toyota who became a specialist in setup reduction and error proofing, both so necessary for lean to become truly effective. The driver in mass production was always to maximize batch sizes between each changeover, and this had been recognized as a barrier to modern manufacturing methods. Shingo responded to the needs of lean for short, easier changeover procedures. Dies were in common use in car manufacture to form components. Each die would be specific to the component being produced. Machines running a range of components therefore had to be changed over as the component range changed.

Shingo was successful by distinguishing between work that could be completed while a machine was still running (external operations) and that which required that the machine be stopped before the work could be carried out. By identifying and completing all the work that could be completed externally (such as acquiring and preparing the new die "machine-side" for rapid insertion), impressive setup time reductions were achieved. (Think of the example of changing tires on racing cars.)

One final thought on SMED. The principle can also be applied to product development by converting work carried out in series into concurrent work streams.

Every Product Every Interval   This is a fundamental concept of lean that is so often missed. It is the ultimate determinant of production lead times, which is so important in supply chains. This is covered in detail by Ian Glenday in Section 15.3. For now, a metaphor may help.

A Helpful Metaphor

We see examples of this commonsense way to run production systems around us every day. McDonald's, for example, operates a "supermarket" out of which the associates draw the product as customers arrive and place their orders. The "feeders" behind can see how the inventory is moving and can replenish accordingly. How would it work, do you think, if customers had to forecast their orders a few days before so that batches could be made up in anticipation?

Take another example, the London Tube (or New York Metro). I love the certainty of knowing that the production system (moving me from A to B) works such that if I miss one train, the next is only minutes away; and in missing this train, my ability to get a connection is not affected, because when I arrive, the next train is only minutes away. Could anyone imagine having to forecast their journey and connecting trains to ensure a place on the train? This seems ridiculous, but this is the equivalent of the way we work in supply chain management where batch and queue predominates (that includes pharmaceuticals). We ask customers to forecast their requirement ahead of time to allow for the extended lead times to manufacture. Most often the lead time taken for granted and is unchallenged. If product is not forecast, sometimes three or six months ahead, requirements will not be fulfilled. Once submitted, there is normally no option to cancel if circumstances change.

So what did the people who run the Tube do? They divided the production system into subsystems that process similar products, that is, products with similar routings. For example, the Central Line carries passengers (products) who have a routing to central London destinations. When a product joins a queue, it is limited to similar products, so there is no jostling for position with competing product families; also, only those turning up for travel on that day are in the queue. There are no reserved slots in anticipation of phantom passengers turning up.

On the London Underground there are 11 different lines covering a discrete set of locations, with a degree of overlap. I select the line I need to process me according to my needs as a product. That line then runs on a fixed cycle. They vary the frequency of trains at different times of the day. At rush hour, a train may run every two minutes, so if you miss one, there will be another one through in two minutes. This is especially important if there are connections and the train you are on is delayed. In less busy times, the frequency reduces, but the passenger still knows roughly how long to wait for the next train without forecasting beforehand! This is not quite a full pull system whereby the system operates only when demand arrives, but it does give a flavor of how repeating cycles can work.

In fact, by way of crude comparison, the UK mainline rail network (in contrast to the Underground) has actually instituted a system of prebooking seats for a defined leg of the journey, putting labels at the back of each seat reserved. If it were not so inconvenient, it would be funny. Train passengers (or "customers" are we are now called) often arrive at their train with only minutes to spare, so do not have time to search for their seat. If the train is busy, it's impossible to walk the corridors to search anyway. So the net result is that people ignore the seating system and work on the first-come first-served principle—except that there is the occasional amount of calm or heated debate over who occupies a seat for the journey.

12.3.13   Six Sigma

The formation of the six-sigma approach is normally attributed to Motorola in the early 1980s and gained rapid usage by early adopters such as GE. It is made up of a problem-solving methodology and a set of improvement tools. The methodology is termed DMAIIC (define, measure, analyze, improve innovatively, and control). The tools draw heavily on statistical approaches (many of those employed by Deming in the early 1950s) and improvement processes such as flow process charts. One of the distinguishing features of six sigma as it has developed is the levels of associated competency. Thus, there are yellow belts, green belts, black belts, and master black belts. (equating with belts in the martial arts).

The aim of six sigma is to attack the variation that so often interferes with process performance. It spread awareness in Western companies (it was already there in Japan) of the need to aspire beyond historical quality targets. These had previously been to contain the number of defects produced by a process to three-sigma levels (approximately 70,000 defects per million repeats). Six-sigma levels moved that target up to 3.4 defects per million repeats. This particular way of packaging an improvement methodology was used by many to derive significant benefits.

Surprisingly (to some), there is very little new in six sigma compared to what Deming and others taught in the 1950s and 1960s. As a trained industrial engineer, I can remember studying statistical process control and many of the other tools and techniques as part of my undergraduate coursework.

12.3.14   Process and Operational Excellence

The final approach to consider is more an extension to lean and six sigma. Process and operational excellence combines lean, six sigma, and design excellence into a complete set with which to run an organization. Organizations such as Johnson &

Johnson pride themselves in taking process excellence seriously and run company-wide programs maintained by in-house staff.

It should not have escaped the readers' attention that the word *process* appears again, and that should not be a surprise. We finish the chapter by reinforcing that point. *Improvement* activities act on *processes* within *production systems*. The only measure of the worth of improvement activity is in relation to its impact on the production system. All those involved in improvement activities in organizations should keep that reality at the forefront of their thinking at all times.

13 Bringing the Holistic Together

13.1 SETTING THE SCENE

Having stepped through the discrete but interlinking processes of supply chain management, it is now time to look at how they must all work together in practice. This is best achieved by considering the case of a company responsible for the entire end-to-end supply chain. There are two reasons for this. First, it is the most challenging case for supply chain management as it involves cognizance of both the management of in-plant resources and the interrelationship between third parties involved in the flow to market. Second, outsourcing of the supply chain is so prevalent in the pharmaceutical industry these days that this is a very common arrangement to encounter. I will set the scene.

Observations, Views, and Experiences of the Author

A fair portion of my career has been spent working with emerging pharma companies operating fully outsourced supply chains. By emerging, I mean biotech firms with aspirations to commercialize their precious compound (or, occasionally, compounds) by retaining rights to supply to a licensing partner(s). They may possibly also wish to co-promote the product in conjunction with their larger partner(s). This means that they will be responsible for running a commercial supply chain and managing expectant (even demanding) customers.

Once the licensing agreement has been struck, their thoughts turn to delivering on their commitment to supply. This is normally the stage at which I or someone like me is invited to join. In my own case, initially it was as a permanent employee, but in more recent years it has been as either for short-term consultancy or as an interim contractor. The process I adopt is the same in every case, and the following is an account of the stages that it typically involves: first to define what is needed and then to satisfy those needs in time for launch. It involves using all that has gone before, from the most strategic level down to the minute detail of individual inventory records. Every piece is vital to success.

Supply Chain Management in the Drug Industry: Delivering Patient Value for Pharmaceuticals and Biologics, By Hedley Rees
Copyright © 2011 John Wiley & Sons, Inc.

13.2   THE PROCESS EXPLAINED

13.2.1   Collecting All Relevant Information

Figure 13.1 shows the breadth of information that must be collected in order to get a clear picture. Data collection is not always an easy process in sponsor companies because of the distributed functional responsibilities. It typically involves talking with members of the project team, such as pharmaceutical technologists, process development staff, and marketing and regulatory staff, and piecing together the picture.

13.2.2   Mapping Current-State Physical Supply Chain

When all the information is collected, the next stage is to produce a current-state map of the physical supply chain. Figure 13.2 shows a typical schematic of an overview which generally reflects the emphasis on development from start to finish. The farther along the supply chain, the less work has been completed. The map stages in the analysis are shown in Figure 13.3. This reflects a clinical trial supply chain in place that is being extended to package and supply a commercial product.

This may all seem very simple until the typical information flows around the supply chain are identified, as shown in Figure 13.4 (this is a simplified version!). This shows the volume of complex interactions and document flows that take place during the operation of such a supply chain. Although this is not information typically associated with supply chain management (e.g., orders, forecasts, schedules), it must all take place properly for the supply chain to succeed. A hiccup anywhere along the way can have dramatic consequences. This makes it incumbent upon those overseeing the supply chain to make sure that all necessary arrangements are in place. It makes the following a very important assessment process. Some might call it a risk assessment; others, a maturity path assessment. Whatever it is called, it is important.

Figure 13.5 shows the initial target-state supply chain when both clinical and commercial requirements are taken account of. Note the information flow that is needed to support the scheduling process. This moves us on to understanding the profile of independent demand.

13.2.3   Developing Demand Profiles

Forecasting uncertainty is always greatest prior to the product being launched. Marketing has the responsibility to position the offering for maximum impact and then predict sales for business planning purposes. Typically, the forecasts will consider such things as the following:

- The epidemiology of the indication (the study of factors affecting the health and illness of populations)

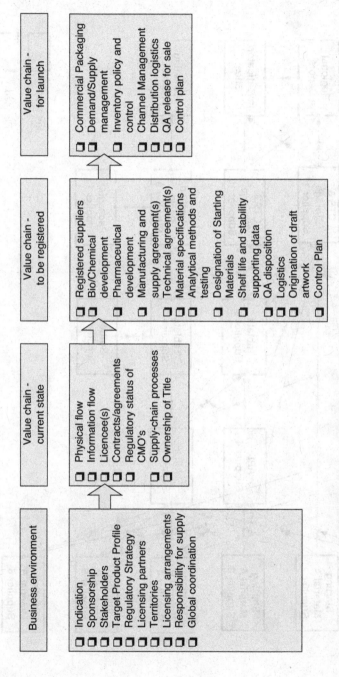

FIGURE 13.1 Information needing to be collected for supply chain assessment.

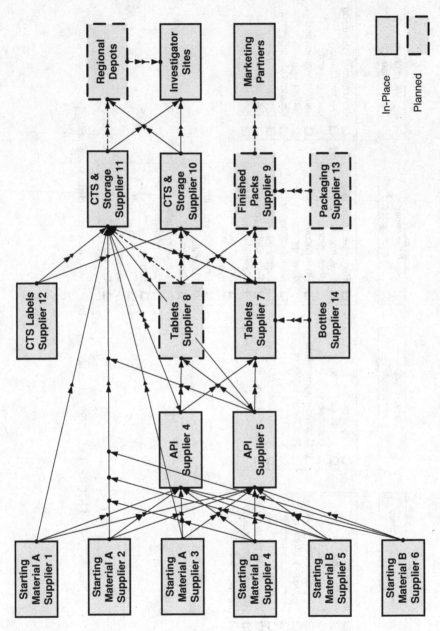

FIGURE 13.2 Generic supply chain: material flow.

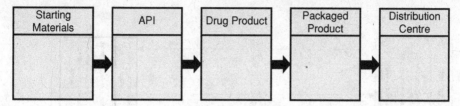

FIGURE 13.3 Material flow stages in setting up for commercial launch.

- Levels of diagnosis
- The label claim likely to be achieved to differentiate the product
- The potential market share
- The treatment regimen
- Seasonal factors
- Pricing levels

These factors go together to arrive at an initial estimate of the amount of a product that will be sold in the market. (More on this is beyond the scope of this book. One company specializing in this area with which I work closely is Apex Healthcare Consulting.[1]) As far as possible, all the assumptions used to derive the forecast should be identified. This is only the starting point, however. The chances of that forecast being absolutely correct are next to nil, given the range of variables. Some bounds now need to be placed on the probable spread of possible sales outcomes. This is what can be termed the *envelope of uncertainty*. The two basic variables for planning purposes are the volume (the forecasts above) and the launch date (based on projected regulatory approval dates).

The most likely case (base case) should be the set of assumptions on which the initial forecasts are based. There are two further sets of assumptions developed, one set based on everything going positive and the other based on the converse. This gives boundaries to the envelope, resulting in three scenarios:

1. *Base case:* most likely launch date, most likely volume
2. *Optimistic case:* earliest launch date, highest volume
3. *Pessimistic case:* latest launch date, lowest volume

The next step is to test each demand load on the supply chain.

13.2.4   Pressure Testing the Current-State Supply Chain

Armed with these figures from marketing, it is possible to test out the capability of the end-to-end supply chain. This is done by using a very simple master production schedule (MPS) and materials requirements planning (MRP I) system, as described

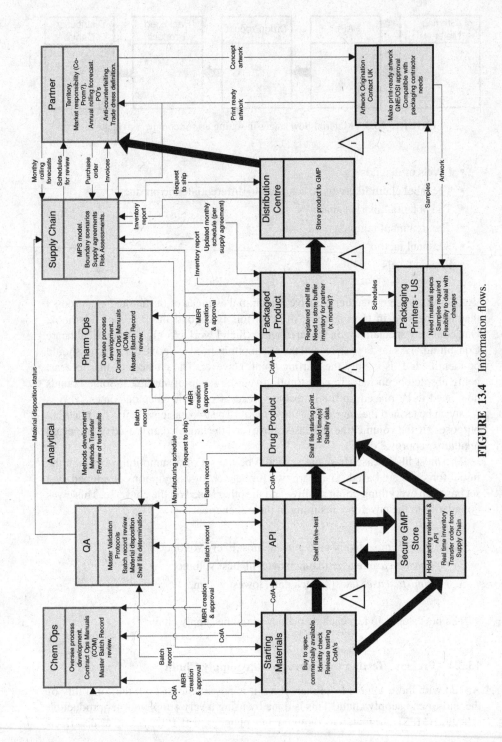

FIGURE 13.4 Information flows.

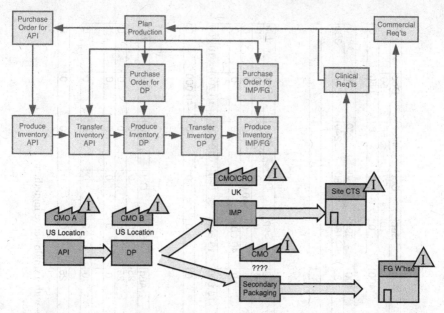

FIGURE 13.5 Demand/supply information flows for clinic and commercial purposes.

in Chapter 11. A simple spreadsheet is enough for this. Figure 13.6 shows the inputs, outputs, and information needed to process an MPS; Figure 13.7 shows an example of the layout and calculations involved. The supply chain is explored under the various demand profiles above. The boundary conditions are:

1. Early launch/high volume
2. Late launch/low volume

The vital point to appreciate is that there can only be one schedule for the amount of stock to be manufactured for launch and planned for postlaunch supply. The material

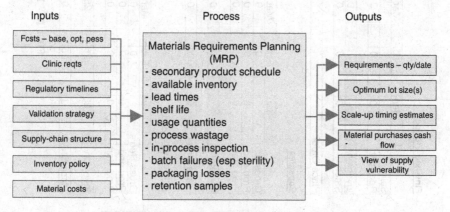

FIGURE 13.6 MPS/MRP information processing.

Finished Product

	Jan	Feb	Mar	Apr	May	June	Jul	Aug	Sep	Oct	Nov	Dec	Jan
Sales	0	0	0	0	0	0	0		10	60	60	60	60
Receipts	0	0	0	0	0	0	0	400	0	0	0	650	0
Inventory	0	0	0	0	0	0	0	400	390	330	270	860	800
Safety	0	0	0	0	0	10	70	130	180	180	240	300	360
Place Order													

Capsules

	Jan	Feb	Mar	Apr	May	June	Jul	Aug	Sep	Oct	Nov	Dec	Jan
Gross Req's	0	0	0	0	0	0	26,400	0	0	0	42,900	0	0
Prod end	0	0	0	0	0	40,000	0	0	0	40,000	0	0	0
Prod start	0	0	0	0	40,000	0	0	0	40,000	0	0	0	0
Inventory		0	0	0	0	40,000	13,600	13,600	13,600	53,600	10,700	10,700	10,700
Place Order	0	40,000	0	0	0	40,000	0	0	0	0	0	40,000	0

Active ingredient

	Jan	Feb	Mar	Apr	May	June	Jul	Aug	Sep	Oct	Nov	Dec	Jan
Gross Req's	0	0	0	25	0	0	0	25	0	0	0	0	0
Prod end	0	0	0	0	0	0	0	25	0	0	0	0	0
Prod start	0	0	0	0	0	0	25	0	0	0	0	0	25
Inventory	25	25	25	0	0	0	0	25	0	0	0	0	0
Place Order	0	25	0	0	0	0	0	0	0	0	0	0	0

FIGURE 13.7 Base MPS/MRP for soft gel capsules with a single active ingredient.

planned for validation is already defined. With the spreadsheet model we can use the three conditions to determine the necessary support schedule. The MPS is initially calculated using the base-case forecasts and an inventory policy that allows what is regarded as an acceptable starting point. Given the immaturity of the supply chain, the finished inventory holding may be much higher than preferred at later stages of maturity. At this stage there are no prizes for cutting things fine. When the analysis is completed, based on validation quantities, the resulting MPS will be set.

That MPS is then tested under the boundary conditions. In the optimistic case, inventory will deplete far more quickly than planned. The test demonstrates how long the inventory will last before a stock-out. If that period was sailing too close to the wind, a revised schedule can be calculated to meet more cautious assumptions. For the pessimistic case, exposure to obsolescence is the risk, and the amount and cost of product involved can be determined. This may not alter a decision to err on a higher schedule for launch, but it will sensitize all to a potential outcome if volumes do not meet expectations.

13.3   DEVELOPING AN ACTION AGENDA

Above we have described how the production planning and scheduling for launch can be determined for optimum effect. Concurrent with this work, further preparation and possible remedial work are required. (See Figure 13.8 for possible outcomes if this

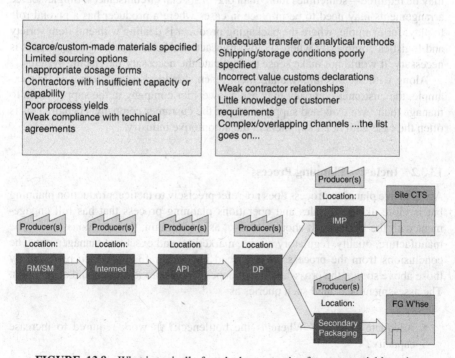

FIGURE 13.8   What is typically found when preparing for commercial launch.

is not done.) I have developed a series of prerequisites that must exist, or be installed in the supply chain, to underpin success. These have not been devised theoretically through research and scientific rigor; therefore, readers should not treat them as such. They are more akin to a checklist and a to-do list combined. They are described below.

13.3.1   Well-Defined Robust Supply Base

The supply base should be made up of producers that are competent to deliver both compliant processes and systems and satisfy the needs of the market. This means more than quality assurance audit as is required by the regulators. It should involve a complete assessment of the producers as to their maturity to enter into commercial supply arrangements. This will look at the way they procure materials and manage their supplying producers, their competencies in supply chain and operational disciplines referred to in this book, and a range of other factors.

A key consideration that is often missed is the architecture of the end-to-end supply chain. Supply chain architecture relates to the structuring of producers in the chain. It is similar to building a house. An architect will design it so that it is fit for the purpose intended. Houses may have different needs, depending on where they are built, who will occupy them, how long they are to last, and what use they will fulfill, for example. Supply chains must similarly be built to deal with the challenges of the product, its market, and the supply base strengths and weaknesses. Backup sources may be required—sometimes more than one in special circumstances. Single-source arrangements may need to be in place in cases where a producer has a pivotal role to play: for example, where the packaging producer is dealing with end-item variety and logistics complexity where a close transactional relationship with customers is necessary. It would not make sense to duplicate the necessary interfacing systems.

Along with architecture, management reach should also be determined. For example, the customer company may ask a lower-tier company in the supply chain to manage their own extended supply chain on the customer company's behalf. This is often the case with tier 1 suppliers in the automotive industry.

13.3.2   Inclusive Planning Process

An inclusive planning process does not refer precisely to tactical production planning but is more akin to a sales and operations planning process that has full engagement with the business. It should involve, as a minimum, those responsible for the manufacture, quality, regulatory affairs, marketing, and executive management. The conclusions from the process, as described in Section 13.2, are then reviewed by those above so that the cross-functional dependencies are identified and acted upon. The assessment is around such queries as:

- Adequate capacity? Where is the bottleneck? Is work required to increase capacity?
- Appropriate scale of manufacture? When do we need to scale up? What time scale is involved?

- Outputs of risk assessments? What are the mitigations? Who will instigate action?
- Sourcing and Inventory policy? Do new sources need to be qualified? Is inventory buildup required?

This is all documented and becomes the basis for a control plan. This plan is then used for management of the supply chain on an ongoing basis through the cross-functional meeting.

13.3.3 Accurate Records Management

Accurate records management refers, first, to clear identification of inventory items throughout the supply chain, so there is appropriate segregation of items and materials that are different. Having achieved that, every piece of information relating to the individual items should be recorded accurately. This includes lot numbers, quality status, location, and expiry dating, for example. This information then provides the basis for material control and traceability or pedigree.

Computer systems are often used to deal with the shear volume of records, and care must be taken that 21 CFR Part 11 is understood thoroughly and incorporated (see Chapter 11). The vitally important aspect is that SOPs reflect practices that enhance accuracy levels and actually convert into a process where responsibilities are allocated unambiguously so there is no confusion as to who is recording what.

A final point to remember is that change control and material disposition practices can be problematic aspects in maintaining record accuracy. Practitioners should be vigilant whenever a process or product change is proposed.

13.3.4 Sound Agreements

Agreements abound in commercial supply chains. This is particularly the case at present with the complex networks in place between third parties. This makes this an important area for attention. The contribution by James Ryan in Section 9.6 provides excellent reference. Also bear in mind the following points:

- Contracts can be formed by performance, so the fact that nothing has been signed with a particular contractor does not mean that certain obligations do not exist. If a contractor is doing work on a company's behalf in full cooperation with employees of that company, care should be exercised to make the necessary contractual reviews.
- Watch out for letters of intent and a memorandum of understanding. These must be regarded as contracts in themselves and should never be signed as a commitment to enter into a further "unspecified" contract, as a way of expediting work to begin.
- Leave lawyers out of the discussions until there is agreement on the main "heads of terms." These include factors such as price, exclusivity, revenue splits, and royalty rates, for example. Lawyers cannot determine the essence of an intended

business relationship; their role is to crystallize that intention into a document that will stand up to legal scrutiny.

- Consider using a "cause or convenience" termination clause so that the relationship is deemed to continue unless there is good cause or it is convenient for one or both parties to terminate. The agreement then specifies how costs will be borne in the event of a split. This is particularly beneficial in relationships that involve a mutual dependence, such as is often the case with contract manufacturing organizations.
- Watch compliance to agreements closely. It can be invaluable to make a one- or two-page summary of the obligations on both sides. In this way the contractual obligation to meet submission dates for orders, forecasts, sales figures, and so on, can be tracked and met.

13.3.5   Appropriate Relationship Building

Contractors and Suppliers

- Use portfolio analysis to determine category segmentation.
- Secure a "continuity of supply" relationship with critical suppliers. This does not necessarily mean investing effort in getting to know each other. As a company you would probably rather not be here. The main thing is to prevent supply failure by opening a dialogue and exploring contingencies.
- Aim to build longer-term working relationships with contractors in the strategic box. This means forming an agreement on how to work together for mutual benefit. That may or may not be underpinned by a formal agreement. The important aspect is a shared view of the future.
- With strategic suppliers, invest time and sometimes money in face-to-face contact and functional interchange. Engage in two-way development activities, learning from each other's specific competency areas. Work out gray areas that exist in between any formal agreements, and most important of all, deliver on commitments.

Route to Market or Clinical Trial Sites

- Understand the stages and players in getting a product to market or investigator sites to carry out clinical trials.
- Start at the end destination and track back to the point where the product is under a chain of command.
- Ensure that a completed supply chain is in place, both physically and in terms of the information flows required to manage supply.

13.3.6   Measurement

- Remember to keep to the "vital few"; also, that leading indicators of performance are far more powerful than lagging indicators. For example, monitoring OEE on a pacemaker or rate-limiting constraint is likely to identify future problems for OTIF (on time, in full) delivery. That is because reduced OEE leads to reduced output, which leads to reduced stock availability for shipments. If this is picked up at the time of OEE issues, short-term corrective measures to increase capacity can be put in place.

- Consider these as your key metrics (reader may also wish to explore the SCOR[2] metrics):
  - Service level (OTIF)
  - Working capital investment (days of inventory on hand)
  - Productivity (output per direct employee; output per indirect employee)
  - Responsiveness (lead time from receipt of customer order to shipment)
- Seek feedback from stakeholders.

13.3.7 Improvement

- Develop an end-to-end perspective for improvement activities in the supply chain.
- Carefully establish product families so as to optimize the value stream (refer to Chapter 11).
- Organize around the value stream with a value stream manger given full authority. Make sure that any upstream and downstream connections are secured.
- Engage stakeholder involvement, especially functional support for the value stream.
- Develop current-state:
  - Material flow
  - Information flow
- Analyze the current state according to the principles described in Chapters 7 to 12.
- Define a future state that aims to maximize throughput efficiency (percent of value-adding time vs. total time).
- Define a feasible future state that improves throughput time in an achievable way. Aim to reduce cycle time by employing the every product every interval scheme (EPE) (see Ian Glenday's explanation in Section 15.3).
- Repeat, focusing on maintaining improvement and further reducing EPE, no matter how marginally. This is the notion of *continuous improvement.*

13.4 CASE STUDY

Some years ago I was asked to join a U.S.-based emerging pharma company to help launch their drug, which was in phase III development. They had rights to supply their marketing partner with finished product. The partner was a large U.S.

biologicals company success story, experienced and demanding. They questioned the minor partner's ability to manufacture and supply to meet their requirements, given that the company had never done it before. In response, the company had undertaken a systems software assessment to decide which production and inventory management package they should implement. They were gearing up for an implementation to go forward from their decision on the software vendor. This is not what they needed at a time when they were faced with a major product launch on which the company's credibility and future depended.

Observations, Views, and Experiences of the Author

Luckily, the vice president for regulatory and manufacturing issues, was an experienced executive and was open to taking my recommendation, which was to put the system implementation on ice until the launch was in the bag. The complexity associated with a single-product, three-presentation launch did not warrant an all-singing, all-dancing software package. It was completely doable, in an outsourced supply chain, with a simple but robust spreadsheet.

I requested that a team be formed so that we could install the supply chain competencies and processes required to bring raw and starting materials through to intermediates, APIs, drug products, and eventually, a finished, packaged product. It showed the typical picture, similar to that in Figure 13.2, whereby much work had gone into the upstream supply chain to develop sources, but relatively little had been done closer to the market. I have mentioned previously the tendency in drug development to start at the beginning and work forward. Time lines drift out and are not corrected because there is little or no connection with time lines to market. (In this case it left the drug product producer in a very powerful position once there was no time to qualify an alternative source.)

The team comprised representatives from clinical trial manufacturing, quality, compliance, regulatory affairs, and finance. My role was that of project leader and supply chain expert. The first task was to get everyone onto a base level of knowledge in supply chain management. This involved running three two-day workshops in two U.S. locations, one near Denver, Colorado and the other on Long Island, New York. To help with this, Mike Dale[3] and Theo Gray, then of S. A. Partners, provided facilitation for the workshops. We ran through current-state mapping of the end-to-end supply chain, supported with education on lean thinking using, for example, a game well known to lean practitioners: the children's block game. This resulted in the team being able to sign up for a future-state arrangement that they felt confident could be placed in front of senior management as a proposed way forward for launch. This was given executive approval and formed the basis of preparations for launch.

Concurrent with this, we produced a simple master production scheduling model for use by the team. Armed accordingly, we were able to model various loads on the supply chain along with the possible outcomes predicted. This was then shared with our "demanding" partner, along with our groundwork. Their confidence level soared and we were able to keep them up to date with our plans as things progressed through our manufacturing launch meetings in their West Coast offices. That compound was launched successfully in the United States in 2004. The two companies had worked hand-in-glove to build a working supply chain through to patients in need.

One other turn of events should be mentioned as a footnote. The product was in a class where there was a competing product, with a lesser label claim, already on the market. The competitor was in the process of running its own clinical trials to improve the label claim. Forecasts from our partner company had factored in a successful outcome for the competitor. As it turned out, the trial failed to meet its end-point, which converted the majority of demand from the competitor's product to ours. Actual sales were four and a half times forecast!

In the modeling we had explored a top boundary condition of six times forecast and therefore knew that we could supply immediate needs and invoke replenishment supplies on an acceptable time line, which of course we did. That work allowed us to move straight into a selection and implementation process for ERP-based production and inventory management. Mike Dale, who I have immense respect for as a strategist and process expert, again provided valuable consultancy inputs to the team. It enabled the specification of supply chain requirements to become an extension of the work already done. The net result was a fully validated, supply chain enabling, supporting system infrastructure.

PART III
Planning and Executing Supply Chain Change

14 Improvement in Pharmaceuticals

14.1 WHERE ARE WE NOW?

In Chapter 1, the topic of twenty-first-century modernization was raised and welcomed. These initiatives form the basis of the main regulatory structure for meaningful improvement in development science as applied in the industry. Along with this, there has been a dramatic influx into the sector of people with lean and six-sigma competencies and also training in these areas made available to those already in the sector. As with twenty-first-century modernization, the objective is to make similar step changes in performance demonstrated in other sectors.

Consistent with the approach throughout the book, the emphasis is on translating the topic into relevance for the supply chain and overall business performance. As mentioned, blind focus on tools and techniques can often disguise the ultimate objective of a job at hand. Similar to regulations and guidelines, it must be clear what they are attempting to achieve as an output and then applied in that context. There will therefore be a minimum of technical exploration of the guidelines from me, although some guest contributors qualified to do so will take on that task.

We begin with some personal experience of mine.

Observations, Views, and Experiences of the Author

I presented a workshop at the Marcus Evans Summit conference in 2005, referred to in Chapter 1. The title of the workshop was "Building, Managing and Perfecting Supply Chains in Biotech." Prior to that, I had listened to Jon Clark's keynote presentation and it was the first time I had been exposed to the FDA's plans for modernization. It was fascinating to hear such terms as lean, six sigma, process capability, and critical to quality attributes (see Table 14.1) being used by a senior FDA official. Up until this point, although my knowledge of other sectors was that these were terms associated with dramatic improvements in supply chain performance, in pharmaceuticals they were frowned upon (for reasons discussed in later chapters). When I checked the FDA Web site, I found information on the critical path initiative and the commentary

TABLE 14.1   Definition of Terms

Term	Explanation	Source[a]
Acceptance criteria	Numerical limits, ranges, or other suitable measures for acceptance which the drug substance or drug product or materials at other stages of their manufacture should meet to conform with the specification of the results of analytical procedures.	Q6a, Q6b
Control strategy	A planned set of controls, derived from current product and process understanding, that assures process performance and product quality. The controls can include parameters and attributes related to drug substance and drug product materials and components, facility and equipment operating conditions, in-process controls, finished product specifications, and the associated methods and frequency of monitoring and control.	Q10
Critical process parameter	A process parameter whose variability has an impact on a critical quality attribute and therefore should be monitored or controlled to ensure the process produces the desired quality.	Q8(R2)
Critical quality attribute (CQA)	A physical, chemical, biological or microbiological property or characteristic that should be within an appropriate limit, range, or distribution to ensure the desired product quality.	Q8(R2)
Design space	The multidimensional combination and interaction of input variables (eg, material attributes) and process parameters that have been demonstrated to provide assurance of quality. Working within the design space is not considered as a change. Movement out of the design space is considered to be a change and would normally initiate a regulatory post approval change process. Design space is proposed by the applicant and is subject to regulatory assessment and approval.	Q8(R2)
Drug product	The drug substance is the material which is active and subsequently formulated with excipients to produce the drug product.	Q6a, Q6b
Drug product	A pharmaceutical product type that contains a drug substance, generally in association with excipients. Drug substance (Bulk material): The drug substance is the material which is subsequently formulated with excipients to produce the drug product. It can be composed of the desired product, product-related substances, and product- and process-related impurities. It may also contain excipients and other components, such as buffers.	Q6b

TABLE 14.1   Definition of Terms (*Continued*)

Term	Explanation	Source[a]
In-process control	Checks performed during production in order to monitor and if necessary to adjust the process and/or to ensure that the intermediate or API conforms to its specifications.	Q7
In-process tests	Tests which may be performed during the manufacture of either the drug substance or drug product, rather than as part of the formal battery of tests which are conducted prior to release.	Q6a
Life cycle or product life cycle	All phases in the life of a product from the initial development through marketing until the product's discontinuation.	Q8(R2), Q9
Process analytical technology (PAT)	A system for designing, analyzing, and controlling manufacturing through timely measurements (ie, during processing) of critical quality and performance attributes of raw and in-process materials and processes with the goal of ensuring final product quality.	Q8(R2)
Process robustness	Ability of a process to tolerate variability of materials and changes of the process and equipment without negative impact on quality.	Q8(R2)
Product knowledge	The accumulated laboratory, nonclinical, and clinical experience for a specific product quality attribute. This knowledge may also include relevant data from other similar molecules or from the scientific literature.	
Proven acceptable range (PAR)	A characterized range of a process parameter for which operation within this range, while keeping other parameters constant, will result in producing a material meeting relevant quality criteria.	Q8(R2)
Quality	The degree to which a set of inherent properties of a product, system or process fulfils requirements.	Q9
Quality attribute	A molecular or product characteristic that is selected for its ability to help indicate the quality of the product. Collectively, the quality attributes define the adventitious agent safety, purity, potency, identity, and stability of the product. Specifications measure a selected subset of the quality attributes.	Q5e
Quality by design (QbD)	A systematic approach to development that begins with predefined objectives and emphasizes product and process understanding and process control, based on sound science and quality risk management.	Q8(R2)
Quality risk management	A systematic process for the assessment, control, communication, and review of risks to the quality of the drug product across the product lifecycle.	Q9
Raw material	Raw material is a collective name for substances or components used in the manufacture of the drug substance or drug product.	Q6b

(*Continued*)

TABLE 14.1   Definition of Terms (*Continued*)

Term	Explanation	Source[a]
Real-time release	The ability to evaluate and ensure the acceptable quality of in-process and/or final product based on process data, which typically include a valid combination of assessed material attributes and process controls.	Q8(R2)
Risk	The combination of the probability of occurrence of harm and the severity of that harm	Q9
Risk analysis	The estimation of the risk associated with the identified hazards.	Q9
Risk assessment	A systematic process of organizing information to support a risk decision to be made within a risk management process. It consists of the identification of hazards and the analysis and evaluation of risks associated with exposure to those hazards.	Q9
Specification	A specification is a list of tests, references to analytical procedures, and appropriate acceptance criteria with numerical limits, ranges, or other criteria for the tests described, which establishes the set of criteria to which a drug substance or drug product or materials at other stages of their manufacture should conform to be considered acceptable for its intended use.	Q6a, Q6b
Specification-release	The combination of physical, chemical, biological and microbiological tests and acceptance criteria that determine the suitability of a drug product at the time of its release.	Q1a(R2)

[a]International Conference of Harmonization Studies.

from Janet Woodcock, then director of the Center for Drug Evaluation and Research (CDER). These are some extracts taken from the FDA Web site.[1]

Three years ago, when we launched the Critical Path Initiative, it was conceived as a way to bridge the gap between basic scientific research and the medical product development process. The public and private sectors have made massive investments in basic biomedical research over the past three decades. At the same time, investment in development science, or what we call "regulatory science," needed to predict and evaluate product performance, has lagged significantly. FDA researchers and reviewers tried to bridge this gap, but resources were lacking, and we were never fully successful in explaining the crucial importance of independent research into product characterization and manufacturing, analytical and other test methods, animal models, toxicology, biostatistics, clinical trial design, and other subjects that are crucial to developing safe and effective products. And with the emerging application of genomics, proteomics and other molecular technologies, advanced imaging techniques, nanotechnology, robotics, etc. to medical uses, the gap was growing wider.

The first Critical Path paper, published in March 2004, was intended as a wake-up call to all stakeholders: that without significant investment in development science, our ability to evaluate and predict product performance would continue to be quite limited, and the path to market and beyond, fraught with problems. We called for a collaborative cross-sector effort to modernize development by performing the research needed to incorporate new genomic, imaging, statistical, methodologic, analytical and informatics tools into the development and review processes and standards.

The basic idea is to reduce uncertainty about product performance throughout the product life cycle through scientific research. We have set up a large number of collaborations with partners to get this research done, in areas as disparate as drug manufacturing and clinical trial design.

The full piece can be found on the FDA Web site. It is abridged here for the sake of brevity, but still the message is extremely powerful. Basically, it says that the industry must get significantly better at developing new drugs. This is supported by the U.S. GAO report, where one of the key conclusions was: "There are limitations on the scientific understanding of how to translate chemical and biological discoveries into safe and effective medicine." The attrition rates quoted in the report and repeated in Chapter 1 bear witness. Of 250 compounds that enter preclinical development, only five survive the journey to clinic. Of those five, only a single one will make it to market. What other conclusions could be draw from those figures?

We all know the issue, but what is the solution? In my opinion, the key lies in making the connection between the supply chain and drug development. A commercial supply chain is the result of a successful development program. In fact, as we have said many times throughout the book, it is the only reason for the existence of development; similarly for discovery research. Without sales a business cannot survive. This means that all eyes should be on the end result. At the moment, this is far from the case. Eyes are presently on the next endpoint, whether that be proof of safety, proof of concept, or definitive proof. This makes quality by design and the other initiatives founded on sound development practices just empty promises.

To explore further, in this chapter we summarize the main areas that affect the pharmaceutical supply chain and then discuss some of the issues, challenges, and opportunities that exist. Throughout the chapter, regulatory modernization will be regarded as the total of the work conducted and recommendations made by the ICH (United States, EU, and Japan) and the U.S. FDA. In addition, industry-sponsored modernization, in response to the initiatives, is considered. It is highlighted here and the theme continues throughout: that the message from regulators to the industry is to become *less* dependent on *them* for specific guidance. The message is explicit in the words of Janet Woodcock in launching the FDA initiative in 2002. Dr. Woodcock clearly laid down the gauntlet by asking for "a maximally efficient, agile, flexible manufacturing sector that reliably produces high-quality drug products *without* extensive regulatory oversight." To do this, the implication was that pharmaceuticals would emulate other sectors—with moves toward strong quality systems, emphasis on process understanding and capability, inclusive "design for manufacture" processes, and rigorous risk management and mitigation approaches.

In my opinion, the emphasis therefore has to be on embedding safe and effective ways of operating into the fabric of our processes for producing modern medicines.

Less regulatory oversight must, by definition, mean more industry engagement in modern methods of increasingly effective drug manufacture. This means instantly that guidelines (and this is all they are) are only part of the solution. Guidelines are a starting point, but as with any attempt of one body to guide an alternative way of working of another, it is the subject of the guidance that must convert them into demonstrated reality. Those framing the guidelines cannot do that on their behalf. Asking for further guidance when problems and issues occur is not a solution. There are questions of organization, leadership, and customer orientation, for example, that are also important elements of any sustainable solution.

This is not to suggest that the big pharma players in the industry are holding back on resources in tackling the modernization challenge. Nor are they sitting back simply waiting for further regulatory guidance. It should, however, be emphasized that there is more to it than resources and technology alone. Other sectors had to reconsider in depth their ways of working to respond successfully to a changing world. This is, surely, the chalenge for twenty-first-century modernization.

There is also evidence that the changes are not happening quickly and that in many instances, they are not happening at all. In discussions with a good and knowledgeable industry contact of mine over a period of several years, this aspect has been explored in some detail. Below are answers to some questions put in a recent telephone conversation between the two of us.

GUEST CONTRIBUTOR SLOT: MARTIN LUSH

Modernization and Regulation

Hedley Rees: Martin, you spend your professional life working with and training quality control personnel in pharmaceutical production best practices. How would you describe the current status of understanding with respect to modernization?

Martin Lush: This is not the first time we have discussed this, Hedley, is it! Nothing seems to have changed since we last spoke. There seems to be a small percentage (2 to 5%) of what I would call visionaries (even mavericks!) who have embraced the opportunity with open arms. Otherwise, the level of awareness and interest appears dismal. For example, at a recent workshop that I ran for quality control professionals, when we discussed risk-based decision making, only three people in a class of 15 had heard of quality management systems (Q10), let alone read it! I had a similar response on another workshop on Q10—and these were aspiring qualified persons!

H.R.:   That really is shocking given the time these guidelines have been in development and use. Any ideas what could be behind this apparent apathy?

M.L.:   Well, I can only speak for those I work with who tend to be at the "coal face" of commercial production. First, their minds are more focused on job security, which tends to keep them focused on doing more of the same. There has been so much change in the industry; just keeping a job has become a major preoccupation. Second, initiatives like Q9 are regarded as projects that will eventually go away, rather than fundamental changes to ways of working. Many companies write their risk management policy, run a few courses on failure mode and effects analysis (FMEA), and then check the box: Q9 implemented—job done. In reality, the old ways of working and thinking remain and nothing really changes. It's incredibly frustrating to see Q9 only being used reactively, rather than proactively, where risk-based thinking really adds value. The other factor I notice is that very few actual leaders seek our help and advice. Site heads and vice presidents of quality control tend to send delegates to collect intelligence on what the next regulatory initiative is. For them, if it is not going to add to their pain of compliance, they would rather not get involved. Unless initiatives such as Q9 and Q10 are pushed by well-informed leadership, they fail. This is not rocket science.

H.R.:   Doesn't modernization, though, have full sponsorship of regulatory bodies worldwide? Surely the guidelines wouldn't have been written if they were there to be ignored?

M.L.:   Good question and I would tend to agree. At the highest level there appears to be a real drive for change, particularly from the U.S. FDA. The trouble is we are not seeing it permeate down to field investigators or inspectors. For example, Q10 (QMS), being in place only relatively recently, is off the radar screen for the time being. Q9 has been out longer, but the interpretation has been restricted to the need to carry out FMEAs. So we now have companies believing they have adopted Q9 principles by having FMEAs documented and on file. As you know, the aim and utility of Q9 is much more encompassing than that. Interestingly, those companies that are taking up Q9 and seeing benefit are generics companies. I would say that only about 10% of those I deal with are pushing forward with Q9 in any meaningful sense.

H.R.:   What in your opinion would be helpful to further the cause of modernization in the industry? I know you have researched lean and six-sigma adoption for yourself and found a mixed bag of opinion.

M.L.:   Well, I think people are wondering if it is all going to take off or just roll along gently. We should remember that 15 years ago, the FDA signaled that systems-based audits were the way to go, and here we are, even to this day, with 70% of U.S. companies not performing systems-based audits. It seems that companies do these things only if it is a nonnegotiable regulatory requirement. Old habits die hard! The trouble is the world has changed and this old style of thinking—maintain the status quo—is no longer good enough. Eventually, pure economics will drive modernization and new ways of thinking. My only concern is that some companies will have left it too late. When I say the word *modernization* I find my self smiling. For other industries the Q8, Q9, and Q10 approaches have been in use for the last 40 years! If Deming was listening in, he would be screaming "I told you all this 60 years ago!"

If Martin is correct, and he is well positioned to know, there is something of a road block on the way to modernization. The author finds equivalent levels of disinterest, scepticism, and confusion in his everyday contacts in drug development.

Let's look next at another account from one who should know, Emil Ciurczak.

GUEST CONTRIBUTOR SLOT: EMIL W. CIURCZAK

(Reprinted with kind permission of Putman Media.)

Rationales Behind QbD and PAT

If there is a failing with Q8, it's that it has been so hard for the industry to decipher and implement. As with many documents, many workers in the field have only read parts or synopses of parts of Q8 and not the document itself. Some of the key concepts are worth reiterating here, so I will do so. Perhaps the largest leap of faith for devout GMP-ers is the concept of continuous process verification in lieu of the time-worn approach of three strikes (er, batches) and you're finished.

The original GMP document (the new cGMP document was issued in November 2008) suggests a minimum of three production-level batches to set process conditions. [*Minimum* is often read as "that's all we need."] The problem here is that the process cannot be considered static and unchanging: raw materials, APIs, ambient conditions, operators, and equipment all change over time and must be taken into consideration. This flies in the face of the traditional cGMP interpretation by compliance and quality assurance staff of setting everything in stone in the MMF (master manufacturing formula), or *Quieta non movere*.[2]

What is needed is simply called *continuous process verification* in the guidance. This is an alternative approach to process validation in which manufacturing process performance is monitored and evaluated continuously. It takes into consideration that all aspects change over time and that each batch is unique. It seems that change comes slowly to the pharmaceutical industry and for a number of legitimate reasons: It is very heavily regulated and simultaneously, highly competitive. However, *Quinon proficit deficit*.[3]

Years ago, the phone company was highly regulated but was also a monopoly, so the regulations were mere inconveniences. When pharmaceuticals only had to worry about generic competition, the strict guidelines had, in fact, full-employment benefits. It was often remarked that the majority of jobs in the industry were to fulfill some FDA-mandated purpose. Thus, we owed our jobs to the regulations. At a time when a patent-protected product meant seven to ten years of undiluted income, the "regs" didn't bother many people. However, today, with mergers, cutbacks, and fewer blockbusters, anything that can save waste and expense needs to be considered. The idea of never settling on a "final process" is old hat to nearly every chemical and engineering industry in the world but, for some reason, seems alien to the pharmaceutical industry. Now the FDA, EMEA, and ICH all say that it's OK to enter the twenty-first century.

A major concept introduced in the guidance is called *design space*. Briefly, this is the multidimensional combination and interaction of input variables (e.g., material attributes) and process parameters that have been demonstrated to provide assurance of quality. In simple terms, since a fixed set of conditions does not allow the production staff to react to changing materials and conditions, ranges of settings are needed. This combination of ranges needs to be shown to give a quality product. The region of (imaginary) space bounded by these allowable variations is known as design space. By *quality* the Guidance means the suitability of either a drug substance or a drug product for its intended use. This term includes such attributes as the identity, strength, and purity from ICH Q6A.[4]

Working within the submitted design space is not considered as a change; thus, making a change within, for instance, hardness parameters or weight limits is certainly allowed. Movement out of the design space is considered to be a change and would normally initiate a regulatory postapproval change process. Design space is proposed by the applicant (producer) and is subject to regulatory assessment and approval. The design space is determined by experimentation.

The results of a *formal experimental design* will, using multivariate math (e.g., partial least squares) point to the major effects on product quality and limits of "acceptable" values for them. It is defined as "a structured, organized method for determining the relationship between factors affecting a process and the output of that process." This is also known as *design of experiments*. A number of software programs are commercially available for the design of experiments; most are quite easy to use. The work comes in when the actual runs need to be done.

One key to the design space is known as *process robustness*. In short, this is the ability of a process to tolerate variability of materials and changes of the process and equipment without a negative impact on quality. The more robust the process, the greater range of incoming raw material variation will still give an acceptable product. (One example might be for a solution; if the material in question is simply to be dissolved, particle size limits might be redundant. It would be smarter to state merely "stir until dissolved" rather than specifying a set mixing time.)

Another important term introduced in Q8 is the *life cycle* of a product. This refers to all phases in the life of a product from the initial development through marketing until the product's discontinuation. It implies that we can and should control the facets of the product from development until it is no longer made by the company. This requires much more integrated discussions from the synthesis steps through production to stability testing and, eventually, the decision to discontinue production.

The ability to control all the steps is the basis of *process analytical technology* (PAT). In a nutshell, PAT is a system for designing, analyzing, and controlling manufacturing through timely measurements (i.e., during processing) of critical quality and performance attributes of raw and in-process materials and processes with the goal of ensuring final product quality. It is based on each step of a pharmaceutical process "passing muster" before being allowed to proceed to the next step. For example, a dry blend is measured for maximum uniformity before it is wet granulated. Then, when being dried, it must meet certain criteria (percent solvent, particle uniformity) before being allowed to proceed to lubrication, and so on. PAT generates documentation for product improvement as well as controlling each batch to obviate failure.

You might ask, "Why the Latin quotes?" Well, quite simply, *Quidquid latine dictum sit, altum videtur*.[5]

Throughout this section by Emil, the regulatory intension 'behind' the regulations begins to emerge. As with all the modernization guidelines, they aim to empower pharmaceutical drug developers and manufacturers to act. To act in what way? To encourage them to act as masters of their own destiny. The technology or particular sentence in the guidelines is in many respects irrelevant. The question is about making changes for the better through the life of a product based on sound science, understanding, and management of risk. As Emil quite rightly points out, this is something embedded in almost every chemical- and engineering-based company in the world. Why not pharmaceuticals?

Observations, Views, and Experiences of the Author

As a practitioner in the industry, I encounter much scepticism about the future of modernization. Many agree with the principles but fail to see how the implementation is going to work. This appears to be founded on the fact that the regulators do not have instant answers to questions; but how can they? They have grown up in the same industry, with the same assumptions and issues as everyone else. If they had the answers they could only have come from another planet. The point is that answers can only be found through those doing the work finding out for themselves, by doing things differently, albeit safely.

To do that, there must be a clear picture of what the end game means in real-world terms. Let me try and explain. The world of chemistry manufacturing and controls (CMC) has since its inception been a scientific and technical undertaking. What has always been missing is the realization among those involved in specific stages of the process that they are actually part of building a supply chain to patients. I can make that assertion with confidence because I often mention it to colleagues in CMC and get a wry smile of "that's what you think!" in return. The penny has been slow to drop, even with the advent of modernization. Until the penny drops, no amount of guideline direction is likely to be enough. In the same way that we can't inspect quality into a product, we cannot police quality into the development process—there will never be enough policemen.

The penny dropping would have CMC specialists view themselves as any other participant in manufacture from other industries: that is, upstream developers with downstream customers. This finishes off with yet another beat on an important drum; those customers are not the regulators.

With those sentiments, we move forward to give a brief rationale and account of the modernization guidelines from regulators. This will then be followed by an expansion of the principles by an experienced guest contributor (Ed Narke) and then my own critique of industry attempts to respond. This will conclude by looking at the issues that still need to be addressed, with suggestions for further work and improvement based on learning throughout the book. The review incorporates ICH Q8, Q9, and Q10 and twenty-first-century modernization.

14.1.1 Pharmaceutical cGMPs for the Twenty-First Century: A Risk-Based Approach

The first report was issued on February 20, 2003 and can be found on the FDA Web site.[6] The stated objectives were as follows:

- To encourage the early adoption of new technological advances by the pharmaceutical industry
- To facilitate industry application of modern quality management techniques, including implementation of quality systems approaches, to all aspects of pharmaceutical production and quality assurance
- To encourage implementation of risk-based approaches that focus both industry and agency attention on critical areas
- To ensure that regulatory review and inspection policies are based on state-of-the-art pharmaceutical science
- To enhance the consistency and coordination of FDA's drug quality regulatory programs, in part by integrating enhanced quality systems approaches into the agency's business processes and regulatory policies concerning review and inspection activities

14.1.2 International Conference on Harmonization Q8, Q9, and Q10

Following is part of the text of a press release dealing with step 4 for the ICH6 program, dated July 17–18, 2003:

The Steering Committee was pleased to hear the positive outcome of a brainstorming workshop on initiatives related to a risk-based approach to Drug Product Quality. This session was attended by more than 60 designated experts from the six ICH parties, observers and non-ICH parties. The workshop discussion led to a general agreement on a high level vision: *a harmonized pharmaceutical quality system applicable across the lifecycle of the product emphasizing an integrated approach to risk management.*

The Steering Committee agreed that the experts from the six parties will work further on two areas:

- On Pharmaceutical Development incorporating elements of Risk and Quality by Design, and covering the product lifecycle.

- On a better definition of the principles by which Risk Management is integrated into decisions regarding Quality including GMP compliance both by the regulators and industry.

Industry will, in addition, produce a Quality Systems Scoping Document including GMP as a subset, which should address areas of perceived differences in the three regions.

The work of ICH resulted in three guidance documents being produced: Q8, Q9, and Q10. An important point to bear in mind is that although these are separate guidances, they form a holistic set, much in the way of supply chain processes. The unifying theme is that they describe principles of working that minimize the scope for error in the making of products for patient needs.

ICH Q8 Pharmaceutical Development   This guideline describes the contents suggested for the 3.2.P.2 (pharmaceutical development) section of a regulatory submission in the ICH M4 common technical document format (see Chapter 3).

The pharmaceutical development section is intended to provide a comprehensive understanding of the product and manufacturing process for reviewers and inspectors. The guideline also indicates areas where the demonstration of greater understanding of pharmaceutical and manufacturing sciences can create a basis for flexible regulatory approaches. The degree of regulatory flexibility is predicated on the level of relevant scientific knowledge provided.

The guideline does not apply to contents of submissions for drug products during the clinical research stages of drug development. However, the principles in this guideline are important to consider during those stages as well. In fact, in my opinion, regulatory emphasis should become increasingly demanding at this stage. This is where the spirit of healthy supply chains lives and needs to be considered seriously. If pharma companies are to be expected to know more about their processes and materials at the design stage, this is the obvious point to seek evidence of attempts being made to do that.

The guideline goes on to say that changes in formulation and manufacturing processes during development and life-cycle management should be looked upon as opportunities to gain additional knowledge and further support establishment of the design space. This concept of design space is a critical aspect for manufacturing improvement. It means that a company should not just define and validate output from equipment or a process operating within a specific or constraining range of parameter settings. It should identify and vary the critical parameters to prove that the output product is acceptable within a range: the design space. A simple example would be to vary mixing speed for a blending operation across a range and document the range over which product quality is unaffected. In this way the company would have the latitude to make changes without having to revert to the regulator. Design space is proposed by the applicant and is subject to regulatory assessment and approval. Working within the design space is not considered a change. Movement out of the design space is considered to be a change and would normally initiate a regulatory postapproval change process.

At a minimum, those aspects of drug substances, excipients, container closure systems, and manufacturing processes that are critical to product quality should be determined and control strategies justified. Critical formulation attributes and process parameters are generally identified through an assessment of the extent to which their variation can have an impact on the quality of the drug product.

In these situations, opportunities exist to develop more flexible regulatory approaches: for example, to facilitate:

* Risk-based regulatory decisions (reviews and inspections)
* Manufacturing process improvements, within the approved design space described in the dossier, without further regulatory review
* Reduction of postapproval submissions
* Real-time quality control, leading to a reduction of end-product release testing

To realize this flexibility, the applicant should demonstrate an enhanced knowledge of product performance over a range of material attributes, manufacturing process options, and process parameters. This understanding can be gained by application of, for example, formal experimental designs, process analytical technology, and/or prior knowledge. Appropriate use of quality risk management principles can be helpful in prioritizing the additional pharmaceutical development studies to collect such knowledge.

The design and conduct of pharmaceutical development studies should be consistent with their intended scientific purpose. It should be recognized that the level of knowledge gained, not the volume of data, provides the basis for science-based submissions and their regulatory evaluation.

Process Analytical Technology (PAT)   PAT aims to facilitate the implementation of quality by design through the use of analytical tools to aid process monitoring, understanding, and control. The results can them be used in making risk-based decisions in relation to product quality. A wide array of technology enablement has been developed and is in the process of development. The FDA has this to say on PAT[7]:

The scientific, risk-based framework outlined in this guidance, Process Analytical Technology or PAT, should help pharmaceutical manufacturers design, develop, and implement new efficient tools for use during product manufacture and quality assurance while maintaining or improving the current level of product quality assurance. The framework we have developed has two general components:

1. A set of scientific principles and tools supporting innovation
2. A new regulatory strategy for accommodating innovation

Focus placed on the science of manufacturing. The Manufacturing Science working group, which was established at the launch of the Pharmaceutical cGMPs for the 21st Century initiative, is involved in identifying efficient approaches for characterizing and controlling critical manufacturing process parameters and quality assurance. The primary focus of its activities is to find new ways to use the knowledge acquired during pharmaceutical development, scale-up, optimization, and production during regulatory risk-based decisions. The Manufacturing Science working group will work with the PAT team in a number of efforts. First, efforts are underway to develop a broad regulatory strategy that ensures that existing application review and cGMP programs are based on sound state-of-the-art scientific and engineering knowledge. We hope the new regulatory strategy will encourage manufacturers to develop and implement the latest technologies in pharmaceutical manufacturing processes.

Continuing international cooperation. The plan will emphasize an integrated approach to risk management and science. Several actions were outlined to implement this vision. An expert working group (EWG) will be established on pharmaceutical development, which will incorporate elements of risk and *quality by design* throughout the life cycle of the product. A second EWG was established to better define the principles by which risk management will be integrated into decisions regarding quality, including cGMP compliance both by the regulators and industry. This group will develop a risk management framework intended to lead to more consistent science-based decision-making across the life cycle of a product. These two expert working groups will work in parallel and exchange information on a regular basis.

ICH Q9   It is important to understand that product quality should be maintained throughout the product life cycle such that the attributes that are important to the quality of the drug (medicinal) product remain consistent with those used in the clinical studies. An effective quality risk management approach can further ensure the high quality of a drug (medicinal) product to patients by providing a proactive means to identify and control potential quality issues during development and manufacturing. Additionally, use of quality risk management can improve the decision making if a quality problem arises. Effective quality risk management can facilitate better and more informed decisions, can provide regulators with greater assurance of a company's ability to deal with potential risks, and can beneficially affect the extent and level of direct regulatory oversight.

These aspects include development, manufacturing, distribution, and the inspection, submission, and review processes throughout the life cycle of drug substances, drug (medicinal) products, biological and biotechnological products [including the use of raw materials, solvents, excipients, and packaging and labeling materials in drug (medicinal), biological, and biotechnological products]. Two primary principles of quality risk management are:

1. The evaluation of the risk to quality should be based on scientific knowledge and ultimately link to the protection of the patient.
2. The level of effort, formality, and documentation of the quality risk management process should be commensurate with the level of risk.

Quality risk management is a systematic process for the assessment, control, communication, and review of risks to the quality of the drug (medicinal) product across the product life cycle. Quality risk management activities are usually, but not always, undertaken by interdisciplinary teams. When teams are formed, they should include experts from the appropriate areas (e.g., quality unit, business development, engineering, regulatory affairs, production operations, sales and marketing, legal, statistics, and clinical) in addition to people who are knowledgeable about the quality risk management process. Decision makers should take responsibility for coordinating quality risk management across various functions and departments of their organization; and assure that a quality risk management process is defined, deployed, and reviewed and that adequate resources are available.

ICH Q10 Pharmaceutical Quality System   ICH Q10 describes a comprehensive model for an effective pharmaceutical quality system that is based on International Standards Organization quality concepts. Implementation of ICH Q10 throughout the product life cycle should facilitate innovation and continual improvement and strengthen the link between pharmaceutical development and manufacturing activities. The guideline considers the product life cycle and includes the following technical activities for new and existing products.

- Pharmaceutical development
  - Drug substance development
  - Formulation development (including the container and closure system)
  - Manufacture of investigational products
  - Delivery system development (where relevant)
  - Manufacturing process development and scale-up
  - Analytical method development
- Technology transfer
  - New product transfers during development through manufacturing
  - Transfers within or between manufacturing and testing sites for marketed products
- Commercial manufacturing
  - Acquisition and control of materials
  - Provision of facilities, utilities, and equipment
  - Production (including packaging and labeling)
  - Quality control and assurance
  - Release
  - Storage
  - Distribution (excluding wholesaler activities)
- Product discontinuation
  - Retention of documentation
  - Sample retention
  - Continued product assessment and reporting

There are three main objectives:

1. *To achieve product realization:* to establish, implement, and maintain a system that allows the delivery of products with the quality attributes appropriate to meet the needs of patients, health care professionals, regulatory authorities (including compliance with approved regulatory filings), and other internal and external customers.

2. *To establish and maintain a state of control:* to develop and use effective monitoring and control systems for process performance and product quality, thereby providing assurance of continued suitability and capability of processes. Quality risk management can be useful in identifying the monitoring and control systems.

3. *To facilitate continual improvement:* to identify and implement appropriate product quality improvements, process improvements, variability reduction, innovations, and pharmaceutical quality system enhancements, thereby increasing the ability to fulfill quality needs consistently. Quality risk management can be useful for identifying and prioritizing areas for continual improvement.

These were the objectives of this modernization initiative—but there have been some concerns, as described below.

14.2 SUBSEQUENT DEVELOPMENTS SINCE INCEPTION

The dissemination and implementation of the guidelines has not been without problems. See the extract below from the Final Concept Paper[8] from the ICH Implementation Working Group (IWG) on ICH Q8, Q9, and Q10, *dated and endorsed by the Steering Committee on November 1, 2007.*

Type of harmonisation action proposed: Implementation Working Group

Statement of the perceived problem: In Brussels 2003 a new quality vision was agreed on. This emphasised a risk and science-based approach to pharmaceuticals in an adequately implemented quality system. As a consequence, the guidelines on Pharmaceutical Development (Q8), Quality Risk management (Q9) and Pharmaceutical Quality System (Q10) were drafted. As these concepts and principles are rather new in the pharmaceutical area, it is important that, due primarily to departure from the traditional approaches to quality guidance, proper implementation of these concepts is provided by bringing clarity, further explanation and removing ambiguities and uncertainties.

Background to the proposal: It has become apparent, based on public workshops or other symposia, that deviating views have been observed, setting up non harmonised interpretation and new expectations beyond the intention of these ICH guidelines. Concerns have been raised in the two ICH-Q strategy sessions identifying the need for an ICH Q IWG. An ICH sponsored implementation is considered necessary to ensure the globally consistent implementation of Q8, Q9 and Q10 and to ensure that maximum benefit is achieved from the interaction between these guidelines.

Issues to be resolved: The following issues have so far been identified and will need to be addressed:

- Technical issues and related documentation: common understanding of terminology; address inter-relationship between Q8, Q9 and Q10; applicability to both review and inspection; final status after partial implementation is established (e.g. level of details in the dossier)
- Additional implementation issues: influence on existing ICH guidelines
- Communication and training: e.g., Q&A, briefing packs from ICH; external collaborations; workshops.

Having taken a high-level walk through the regulations and discussed some of the emerging problems, we now hear from Ed Narke, an expert with in-depth experience of CMC, regulatory and quality issues, and QbD.

GUEST CONTRIBUTOR SLOT: EDWARD NARKE

14.3   A BLUEPRINT FOR QUALITY BY DESIGN

If the regulators at the U.S. Food and Drug Administration (FDA) and the European Medicines Agency (EMEA) truly change the way they regulate, could the future "desired state" of manufacturing science and the related regulatory processes[9] actually be realized? Well, the agencies may have changed already. This concept of quality by design (QbD) was introduced into the chemistry manufacturing and controls (CMC) development process as a result of the pharmaceutical current good manufacturing practice (cGMP) for the 21st Century Initiative with the objective of achieving a desired state for pharmaceutical manufacturing.

Expectations were formally sketched out in 2004 with the announcement of the process analytical technology (PAT) guidance entitled "A Framework for Innovative Pharmaceutical Development, Manufacturing and Quality Assurance,[10] and more recently (2006–2008) through the International Conference on Harmonization (ICH) guidelines Q8(R1), Pharmaceutical Development,[11] Q9, Quality Risk Management,[12] and Q10, Pharmaceutical Quality Systems.[13] This emphasis on a risk-based "QbD approach" encourages sponsors and manufacturers to make larger investments earlier in the product life cycle during process development in advance of approved commercial operations. The objective is to identify and develop a design space (discussed further in Section 14.3.3) which accommodates a range of defined variability in the process materials and operations and still produces the correct product quality outcomes. In 2005[14] the FDA launched its initial pilot program, and in 2008[15] a second program was begun for biotechnology products to obtain more information on, and to facilitate agency review of, risk-based QbD approaches. These pilot programs were initiated to assist regulators in developing further guidance for industry on QbD and risk management. With the publication of the ICH's "Note for Guidance on Pharmaceutical Development, Q8(R2) in 2009,[16] the opportunity now also exists for sponsors to develop a "process understanding that takes into account the need for different design spaces to accommodate future changes in the scale, economics, or other aspects of the manufacturing process in the later stages of the product life cycle."

For the pharmaceutical industry, QbD has ushered in a new approach to regulatory filings, and perhaps even more important, the way in which drugs are developed. The regulators at both the FDA and EMEA, along with a number of other world health agencies, have challenged the industry to achieve a consistent level of understanding through controlling variability and assuring product quality. The concepts described in the PAT guidance and the Q8, Q9, and Q10 guidelines lay the foundation for the shifting regulatory review process. As the paradigm shifts to the perception that doing more comprehensive up-front work is vital for understanding the product and process, and as more QbD submissions are submitted, companies are going to have to start paying more attention to the investigation phase and the consequential shift of review attention at this phase as the QbD approach takes hold.

How does quality compliance change across the entire manufacturing network? How much does the new environment raise the bar? And just as important, does it raise it out of reach for small companies? The intention of this discussion is to lay out the regulatory considerations relating to the implementation of QbD. From a regulatory perspective there are no "right" or "wrong" choices in this regard. The difference comes in the regulatory authorities' expectations of the amount of data needed to support any proposed approach and the consequent regulatory agreement desired. Essentially, what regulators are concerned about primarily as they review the CMC sections of future clinical trial and marketing applications can probably be summed up in a single question: How well do you know your product? The questions that flow from that are related to the product's target product profile, including its quality attributes and control of the manufacturing process, effecting critical attributes and stability over time. Industry will eventually reach a point where a discussion of QbD with regulatory authorities will be necessary. The timing of the discussion should ensure that any proposals or strategy changes allow sufficient time before submission to fully develop analytical and process data to support the proposal or regulatory expectations. Will the industry change as a direct result of the evolving guidance? Maybe it already has.

14.3.1 A Regulatory Perspective

To QbD or Not to QbD   It is expected that sponsors who adopt a QbD approach, together with a quality system as described in the Q10 document, Pharmaceutical Quality Systems, will achieve this "desired state." Ideally, despite variations in materials and processing that in the past would have resulted in unacceptable product batches, the ability to achieve the appropriate quality outcome consistently must be designed into the process itself. Alignment with the QbD principle recommendations in the ICH guidance documents can help facilitate fundamental implementation, including identification of the overall target profile and critical quality attributes (CQAs) that are of significant importance to product safety and/or efficacy; a design of the product and processes to deliver these attributes; a robust control strategy to ensure consistent process performance; confirmation and filing of the process, demonstrating the effectiveness of the control strategy; and finally, ongoing monitoring to ensure robust process performance over the life cycle of the product. As we will discuss, risk assessment and management and the use of statistical approaches and process analytical technology provide a foundation for these activities. This effort increases product and process understanding, reduces process variability, and can move manufacturing toward real-time quality assurance.

Why Apply QbD Principals, and When?   Taken as a whole, QbD promotes an understanding of product design space in the forefront of development efforts, providing the coherence and continuity that trial-and-error approaches lack. Eventually, this will save time together with money and work. By introducing the QbD principles with regular risk assessment sessions early in the drug project, many potential future problems can be avoided. Sponsors should expect a significant payback in the cost of scale-up and postapproval changes made to the process later in the product life cycle. The regulatory authority's new dedication to science-based regulation and risk-based enforcement would result in significantly reduced risks of costly deviation investigations or rejects, consequent enforcement actions, reducing risks to customers and therefore to the business itself. Although more explicit guidance on process science is still awaited from both European and U.S. regulatory authorities, many of the elements have already been established as a result of the ICH guidance documents.

With the full implementation of QbD, the traditional end-product testing soon may no longer be compulsory to define ultimate product quality. Rather, through regulatory agreements (or contracts) and predefined protocols using current or new technologies in conjunction with the full establishment of a quality system, consistency and predictability of product quality could be demonstrated using formal experimental design and/or prior knowledge to establish understanding and knowledge of the process most affecting the quality attributes of the product. In summary, the resulting regulatory benefits are significant:

- Increased use of QbD in product development not only increases product and process understanding, but also demonstrates how to produce a product with a predictable and consistent quality.
- This science-driven risk-based approach to development and eventual regulatory filing relies on communicating greater scientific understanding of the product to the probability of producing a high-quality drug, reducing the risk of inconsistent quality.
- A QbD approach should lead to smoother transitions from investigation applications (e.g., INDs, CTAs) through post-licensure.

The application of QbD and quality risk management may initially mean more experimental activity and paperwork. However, it is well documented that the QbD approach can provide many advantages. First, and most important, it offers an effective tool for faster and more focused process development. Second, as a consequence of the risk analysis performed, any nonrobust process steps can then be identified and possibly eliminated. This new regulatory environment has also highlighted new ideas regarding process development in manufacturing. Additionally, it has focused renewed attention on two very important areas of process science that until recently may have been somewhat neglected in the pharmaceutical industry: Design space development and design for manufacturing. Ultimately, QbD implementation may yet yield improved regulatory flexibility, with less postapproval evaluation, as it becomes more of the archetypal way of doing business.

Product knowledge may allow regulatory authorities to use a science risk-based assessment to perhaps shorten or reduce the CMC review process. More significant for industry, QbD provides a chance to develop new ideas and opportunities to explore new options to meet regulatory requirements and operational flexibility.

The Business Case   Industry and the agencies already may agree on the mutual regulatory or scientific benefits that can be realized by QbD implementation, as this approach is in alignment with the existing regulatory guidance documents. However, industry, academia, and the regulatory agencies need to work together to pursue these opportunities to overcome the challenges and realize the significant benefits that QbD has to offer. These benefits can translate into significant reductions in working capital requirements, resource costs, and time to value. The bottom-line gains, in turn, pave the way for additional top-line growth. When fully implemented, QbD means that all critical sources of process variability have been identified, measured, and understood so that they can be controlled by the process itself. The potential business benefits are noteworthy:

- Reduced batch failure rates, reduced final product testing, and lower batch release costs
- Lower operating costs from fewer failures and deviation investigations
- Increased predictability of manufacturing output and quality
- Reduced raw material and finished product inventory costs
- Faster tech transfer between development and manufacturing
- Faster regulatory approval of new product applications and process changes
- Fewer and shorter regulatory inspections of manufacturing sites

As an added benefit, this collaboration has the potential to drive the adoption of better practices and sustain the business benefits of higher levels of process predictability and quality compliance across the entire manufacturing network.

14.3.2   Design Through Product Understanding

Pre-IND to Phase I/II Regulatory Opportunities   Phase I is the initial introduction of an investigational new drug (IND) into humans through clinical studies designed to determine the product's metabolic and pharmacological actions in humans and side effects associated with increasing doses. Identification of the quality target product profile and critical quality attributes (CQAs) lay the foundation for the design and control of the process. An effective QbD "regulatory strategy" is critical to ensure that neither the manufacturing process nor the control strategy of the product imposes any potentially unacceptable human safety risk. In phase I it is too premature to think about:

- Manufacturing "consistency"? (think manufacturing "control")
- Test method "validation"? (instead, think "suitable for use, robust and scientifically sound")
- Maximum product "shelf life"? (rather, think "stable for the length of the proposed study")

The most essential goal is to ensure that an effective compliance strategy is in place for the drug product. To help understand the type of manufacturing compliance controls that follow good scientific and QbD principles that are applicable at phase I, sponsors can use FDA's specific considerations for INDs[17,18]: for example, in combination with ICH Guidelines, so the pathway for QbD regulatory compliance risk control is fairly well defined.

Sponsors can incorporate QbD principles during the early planning stages for the preparation of an investigational application. You need to address:

- What the company intends to submit
- The overall submission strategy
- A proposal for change reporting

Determine how information on quality attributes and the process design space and control strategy will be integrated. A sponsor's effort to implement a QbD approach early provides a potentially valuable model for discussion, focused in particular on any challenges in defining CQAs. It is suggested that a separate pathway be developed on CQAs, leaving room for the other development efforts to focus on process-related issues where the approaches are more universal in nature and less product-specific.

Identifying the Quality Target Product Profile (QTPP)   The QTPP should be established as soon as a product has been identified as a feasible candidate for investigation and should be revisited at each of the key stages of development, with any changes approved and documented by the appropriate governance. However, it's never too late to start. The initial design of the product will set limits for what the product and the process is capable of delivering (e.g., small molecules if you eliminate the capability to degrade, or large molecules if you eliminate the ability to aggregate, or if you eliminate the deamidation sites). You can really limit the inherent variability of the product. The QTPP is defined as a "prospective summary of the quality characteristics of a product that ideally will be achieved to ensure the desired quality, taking into account safety and efficacy of the drug product." This includes the dosage form and route of administration; dosage form strength(s); therapeutic moiety release or delivery; and pharmacokinetic characteristics [e.g., dissolution and performance (bioavailability)] appropriate to the dosage form being developed as well as quality criteria (e.g., sterility and purity) appropriate for the intended marketed product.

Identifying Critical Quality Attributes That Define the Product Product quality attributes, principally those deemed a critical quality attribute (CQA) play a key role in the QbD model from early process development through validation to specification setting and ensuing manufacturing changes. Without having a real, well-defined approach to CQAs, it is difficult to move forward with the rest of QbD. Therefore, once the QTPP has been defined, the next step is to identify the relevant CQAs, defined as "a physical, chemical, biological or microbiological property or characteristic that should be within an appropriate limit, range, or distribution to ensure the desired product quality."[19] Identifying CQAs requires a certain amount of product knowledge: possible mechanism of action; key attributes of the drug substance and raw materials; impurities and their impact on quality, safety, and how the drug product excipients; and overall product formulation product performance.

Pharmaceutical products, especially biologics, can have numerous quality attributes that can potentially affect safety and efficacy; therefore, CQA identification is best accomplished by using risk assessment in accordance with the Q9 guidance. The product quality attributes can be laid out on a criticality scale, with attributes known to affect safety and efficacy ranking high in criticality and those known to have no impact on safety and efficacy ranking low. This risk assessment should account for the design of the molecule. Define "potential" or "presumptive" CQAs "very early on in development" or pre-IND, and refine the CQA designations as more structural–function understanding is gained based on product knowledge and clinical experience. Classify quality attributes into two categories:

1. *Critical quality attributes:* those required for the intended function of the molecule or for safety reasons. Establish release specifications behind critical quality attributes.
2. *Noncritical quality attributes:* intermediate or final product quality attributes not likely to be critical for the intended function. Continue to monitor these as a measure of process performance and consistency.

Risk is considered lower if product-specific clinical data are available and clearly demonstrate no adverse impact on safety or efficacy. By contrast, risk is high if clinical data indicate otherwise. In cases for which product-specific clinical data are not available and estimation of criticality relies on product-specific, nonclinical data or data from another platform product, criticality may fall between these two extremes. Initial assessment followed by experimentation with multivariate studies using appropriate scale models provides an understanding of the relationship between the process parameters, material attributes, and product quality attributes and their criticality. This helps identify robust process conditions and acceptable limits. Prior knowledge coupled with investigational data helps establish product quality attribute specifications. In addition, a final overall risk assessment might serve as the basis for the development of the control strategy for the manufacturing process. Risk assessment should involve independent evaluation of each CQA. Various CQA classes exist, and each class can have more than one associated quality attribute. Some commonly observed classes (process and product related) and their attributes are as follows:

1. Large-molecule product variant attributes
   - Process modifications (aggregation, oxidation, glycosylation, fragmentation)
   - Purity (cell culture media components, viral purity, host cell proteins, DNA, and endotoxins)
   - Protein A (for MAbs)
   - Cell related–materials (methotrexate, antifoam, insulin, etc.)
2. Small-molecule process-related impurity attributes
   - Process modifications (polymorphs, solvents, genotoxic impurities)
3. Drug product attributes
   - Particles, clarity, color, osmolality, pH, concentration, potency, volume
   - Endotoxin, bioburden, sterility
   - Novel excipients
   - Host cell modifications (glycosylation, phosphorylation, truncation, glycation, methylation and isomerization)
   - Leachables

Under QbD, release and stability specifications would be set to CQAs based on the knowledge of the relationship between that attribute and product performance. We are not empirically deriving these quality attributes exclusively from either the lots that were used or from process capability. Instead it is defined by real knowledge of what impact that attribute has on clinical performance. Setting specifications should be a data-based exercise that uses statistical tools and allows for incorporation of data as they become available throughout the product life cycle. If your process is well controlled and you never get to step very far outside that control point within the clinical experience, you are always going to be "critical." Explore ways to get out of the box. Purposely varying the attribute and testing it in nonclinical studies early on is one way to get out of the box. Once all CQAs have been identified, the concept of quality can be extended to define a product design space. This should be documented in the regulatory filing in the form of in-process and drug substance or release specifications that define the acceptable variability in the CQAs.[20] Design space can depend on a multitude of factors, including process robustness or capability; the capability of the analytical methods; stability of the drug substance and drug product; and the level of understanding of the impact of a CQA on the safety and efficacy of the product, including the clinical and nonclinical data for the product. In the regulatory application, CQAs are included in defining and justifying specifications. It is generally becoming a regulatory expectation that you have a justification of specification section in which you discuss whether an attribute is critical or noncritical.

Dealing with the Risk   Risk analysis forces one to employ structured thinking. Identify what could go wrong, how it can go wrong, and the impact on product quality and patient safety. Once risk analysis is well understood and done properly, it's really not difficult. ICH Q9 lists several structured risk analysis methods, and the guidance spells out clearly what to work on and why, to focus attention on the more important issues. As the saying goes, "anything is possible, but not everything is equally probable." Risk analysis allows a product sponsor to spend resources on the most likely problems. The best preparation is to study simple risk assessment methods such as preliminary hazard analysis and failure mode effects analysis. Both are commonly used to assess the severity of a failure, the probability of CQA going out of the acceptable range based on process capability, and the ability to detect it based on proposed in-process and lot release testing.

14.3.3 Design Through Process Understanding

QbD introduces the concept of a design space: that is, the multidimensional combination and interaction of input variables (e.g., material) and process parameters that have been demonstrated to provide assurance of quality. Identifying and verifying the design space is a principal task of QbD. Three approaches can be used alone or in combination:

1. A first-principles approach that combines experimental data and mechanistic knowledge, physics, and engineering to model and predict performance
2. A statistical design of experiments approach that employs efficient methods to determine the impact of multiple parameters and their interactions
3. A scale-up correlations approach that employs a semiempirical approach to translating operating conditions between different scales or pieces of equipment

When moving toward a QbD approach, critical process parameters driving variability in the CQAs will need to be identified and understood during process development. This is what the ICH means by *process understanding*. The traditional approach to product development and manufacturing often involved the use of empirical methodologies, in particular to relate the process to the product and the product to the clinic. In contrast, QbD is defined in the ICH Q8 guideline as "a systematic approach to development that begins with predefined objectives and emphasizes product and process understanding and process control, based on sound science and quality risk management." It requires a culture of continuous improvement, and close collaboration between the process development and manufacturing teams, along with deployment of appropriate enabling technologies. You'll want to identify in the filings your thought process about how you got from where you were with this process to what is truly critical, and how you arrived at those conclusions.

As noted, QbD is a systematic approach to development that begins with predefined objectives and emphasizes product and process understanding and process control, based on sound science and quality risk management. Sponsors are well advised to invest in process science and process characterization and really get to know the manufacturing process and its outcome and effects on the critical product attributes. Process scientists will get excited about design of experiments and process analytical technologies. Quality assurance staff will get excited about failure mode effects analysis and consensus quality risk assessments, and regulatory personnel will get excited about change control with reduced reporting requirements. But this investment should be made wisely. Understanding the science does not come cheap. Facing today's tight financial environment and the reality that only slightly over half of drug products that transition from phase II into phase III actually make it into the marketplace, sponsors have to be selective in how limited time, resources, and money are invested. The goal is to increase the level of product and process knowledge and understanding, not just to generate volumes of scientific data. QbD can be a challenge, and it becomes more demanding for complex manufacturing processes or processes that produce biological products. Quality by chance (QbC) had previously been the norm for manufacturing. This was due to the fact that pharmaceuticals are manufactured using batch processes. QbC is a very risky option moving forward.

Phase II to Early Phase III Regulatory Opportunities   The transition from phase II clinical trials (studies to evaluate the effectiveness of the drug for a particular indication in patients) to phase III clinical trials (expanded studies intended to gather the additional information about effectiveness and safety needed to evaluate the overall risk–benefit relationship of the drug) is a major milestone for a sponsor. By the end of phase II a company has devoted considerable time, expertise, and expense to understanding the science of how the drug product works in humans and how to administer the drug product clinically to maximize its medical benefit and minimize its medical risks. But have similar resources been expended to understand the science of how the drug product can be manufactured consistently to yield the desired quality? Gone are the days when a manufacturing process that was successful in preparing clinical product for phases I and II was also considered good enough to go forward into later-stage clinical trials and even commercial manufacturing. Today, under QbD, basing manufacturing decisions scientifically on enhanced product knowledge and product performance data over a wider range of material attributes, processing options, and process parameters is fast becoming the norm. Full QbD implementation is critical at this stage to ensure that all activities necessary for eventual marketing approval are being planned for, and any identified CMC development impediment is under discussion with the regulatory agencies. This is the revolutionary expectation by the regulatory authorities in the twenty-first century as stated in ICH Q8: The aim of pharmaceutical development is to design a good-quality product and manufacturing process to deliver the intended performance of the product consistently. The information and knowledge gained from pharmaceutical development studies and manufacturing experience provide scientific understanding to support the establishment of the design space, specification, and manufacturing controls.

An investment in process science will pay off in improved manufacturing process control for later clinical stages and commercial production. Sponsors need to encourage communication and teamwork with the regulatory authorities. Meetings between the company and the regulatory authorities can help provide assurance to sponsors that there will be no major CMC strategic surprises that could significantly delay the marketing application review and approval. Somehow industry will have to take a leap of faith based on our scientific prowess and education to move from "chance" to "design." If we can take this jump, we will be a step closer to a well-defined process.

Want to avoid regulatory delays? Seek out regulatory authority advice. This sounds easy, but for some sponsors it also sounds intimidating. What if the regulatory authority wants much more to be done than is currently scheduled? What impact would that have on the corporate-determined marketing approval date? Sponsors must understand that it is not about a company believing that it knows more about its process and product than the regulatory authority; it is about involving the regulatory authority as a team player. Since the regulatory authority ultimately controls the drug product's fate, it can only be an advantage for a company to ensure that the reviewer clearly understands the science behind the manufacturing process and product. Sponsors need a reality check for their QbD regulatory and compliance strategy at this transition from phase II to phase III, and the regulatory authorities can provide it. Both FDA and EMEA see the value of CMC-focused end-of-phase II (EOP2)/scientific advice meetings with drug sponsors. They consider these meetings a critical interaction and particularly important. Regulatory stringency is lowest at the start of the process development effort and increases as the clinical trials process into later stages, reaching its highest level during commercial manufacturing operations. The best opportunities to explore the edges of the required envelope of the control space and develop the scientific support and experience necessary to maximize the predictability and quality of the manufacturing process are therefore available during process development. Once commercial operations begin, these opportunities are much more limited.

Defining the Process Design Space   Process parameters such as time, temperature, pH, and concentration can also have an observable impact on the quality attributes of the product. Design space foundation is based on CQAs and really is related to assessing the criticality of CPPs using the assessment of the interaction of the process and the quality of the product. Design space does not affect a CQA by itself, because you will need to disconnect criticality from process capability. However, the design space itself can affect how you control the CQAs (e.g., a unit operation where you can vary the parameters widely and it really doesn't affect a particular CQA). Do you need to have control over that CQA or a measure of that CQA at that unit operation—say, an in-process control—regardless of how critical it is?

The concept of a process design space is well understood in the manufacture of MAbs, therapeutic proteins, and peptides. The "mantra" of biologicals, unlike with small molecules, has traditionally been that the process is the product, which of course does not mean that you are really doing QbD solely because you focus so much on process. However, once process variability has been established in the form of the product design space, process characterization studies can be used to define the acceptable variability data from comparability and product characterization studies, from clinical and nonclinical studies, and from the capability of the process and analytical methods. The acceptable normal ranges operating (NORs) and proven acceptable ranges (PARs) for a process can then be documented in the regulatory filing. Traditionally, processes are operated with fixed controls, transferring variability in inputs and materials to variability in product quality. In the QbD paradigm, a "dynamic control strategy" is used to operate the process in a different way, and thus manage the variability in inputs and materials (e.g., variability in raw materials, solvents, or media components procured from different vendors) to achieve consistent product quality. The QbD model preaches "dynamic manufacturing" as well, in that the process can be changed to fit the material inputs, and the product attributes can be assured in real time. It should be emphasized that a combination of acceptable ranges based on univariate experimentation does not constitute a design space. The acceptable ranges must be based on multivariate experimentation to develop a proper design space.

The sponsor can choose to establish independent design spaces for one or more unit operations, or to establish a single design space that spans multiple operations. While a separate design space for each unit operation is often simpler to develop, a design space that spans the entire process can provide more operational flexibility. For example, in the case of a drug product that undergoes degradation in solution before lyophilization, the design space to control the extent of degradation (e.g., concentration, time, temperature) could be expressed for each unit operation or as a sum over all unit operations.

Key steps in defining a process design space defined in literature include performing risk analysis to identify parameters for process characterization, designing studies using design of experiments and using qualified scaled-down models, and then executing these studies.

The Role of Design Space Development   The concept of design space has gained in popularity as a tool for process development scientist. A control space within the design space is proposed by the applicant and is subject to regulatory assessment and approval. As the product matures in its life cycle, factors such as scale-up, economics, and others can require changes in the control scheme for the process. The scientific basis for moving or expanding the control space is usually developed out of necessity to cope with process shortcomings long after the original process development work was done. Working within a design space would not be considered as a change; however, movement out of a rigidly defined design space would be considered to be a change and would normally initiate a regulatory change control process. That could be a costly and inefficient process because it could possibly trigger the need for new clinical studies.

With the publication of ICH Q8, the opportunity now exists to develop an approvable design space in advance of commercial launch that anticipates and accommodates continuous improvement. This allows manufacturers to make changes that move the process from one control space to another within a design space, as necessary, without the need for regulatory approval, provided that both control spaces remain within the approved design space.

To realize the benefits of such a design space approach, the process development and manufacturing team must develop and document the scientific basis for the justification and approval of the design space in the CMC Module 3. The information used for this work comes in part from appropriately designed experiments that define and test the outer limits or edge of failure of the intended design space to understand the effects on the CQAs. At the time of process scale-up or tech transfer, data and information about the control spaces, as well as the CPPs within which the control spaces operate, must be readily available before transferring or scaling the manufacturing operation.

DOE and Statistical Approaches for Data Analysis Use of statistical approaches for designing experimental studies and performing data analysis has emerged as a fundamental activity for implementing QbD. A large number of raw materials and process parameters typically affect any given unit operation in a process. Understanding the impact of each raw material and input parameter on each output parameter is not practical. A combination of risk assessments and design of experiment has emerged as the approach of choice to facilitate this task and can be found throughout the literature.

Similarly, use of multivariate data analysis (from a Bayesian approach or through Monte Carlo methods) to support some of the key activities required for successful manufacture of products, including scale-up, process comparability, and process characterization, has gained significant momentum of late. Such techniques can be used successfully as a diagnostic tool to identify root causes by collating process knowledge and increasing process understanding.

14.3.4 Design Through Robust Analytics

Defining a Control Strategy: Connecting the Dots QbD control strategy has been defined as a "planned set of controls, derived from current product and process understanding that assure process performance and product quality."[21] Reliable analytical methods suited for their intent and purpose is the foundation for any control strategy. The methodology described for design space can also be applied in the control strategy and, more specifically, to the analytical methods (the wheel does not need to be reinvented). For example, chromatography is a laboratory method but also a unit operation. By the same token, technology transfer ideas can also be applied in method transfer procedures, and method transfer and site transfer could be treated using similar principles.[22] In a traditional control strategy, any variability in process inputs (such as quality of the starting material or raw materials) results in variability in the quality of the product because the manufacturing controls are fixed.

As defined in a dynamic control strategy, the manufacturing controls can be altered (within the design space) to remove or reduce the variability caused by process inputs, thus resulting in more constant product quality. Process capability may be the best control strategy. This should be established in small-scale studies, followed by a confirmation during process validation runs. An approach for defining the control strategy can include in-process control testing, raw material controls, process monitoring, specifications, product characterization, and comparability studies along with the process validation testing. For attributes that are known to be critical in terms of their impact on safety and efficacy, several or all of the above-listed elements might be required to define a vigorous control strategy. Using the same assumption, for attributes defined to be noncritical, not as many controls may be required. The control strategy might include material controls (i.e., qualification and specifications of raw materials, excipients, the active, packaging material, etc.), procedural controls (equipment, facility, quality system, etc.), process monitoring and controls (critical and key process parameters), and testing (in-process and lot release testing). The overall control strategy is then refined to ensure that the CQAs remain within the acceptable ranges.

QbD for Analytical Methods   One of the most complicating factors in the change management process is the uncertainty around the power and reliability of the analytical methods on which the process rests. QbD dialogue should always encompass analytical methods. There has been a tremendous amount of work by both industry as well as regulatory agencies around the world to develop the concepts of QbD for the product and process, and these are becoming quite well accepted. Regulators and industry should be, and are, turning their attention to how the new QbD approaches can be applied to analytical methods and their development to help strengthen this link in the control chain. These concepts all seem to apply to methods just like they do for product and process, and can have similarly significant benefits. For example, thousands of regulatory changes every year occur around the world, and about one half of those are due to analytical method changes. Imagine the reduction in workload that implementing an approach like this would bring.

The traditional approach is: "Don't look for things you don't want to know. You already have the specification, the method is approved." The QbD effort here involves changing the analytical paradigm. Carry out a much more expanded version of robustness at the beginning of method development and carry that detailed information all the way through as you finalize and validate the method - so that you have in effect created the method design space. Over the long-term, identify the critical method attributes and the critical method parameters during the QbD development process, and illustrate the supporting experimental data in the application.

The principles and processes involved may include:

- Relating the analytical method target performance profile, defined as the targets for each analytical method that must be met so that the data it produces are fit for the purpose
- Making very clear what you want with the method before truly developing the method, by providing a clear description of the performance profile

This essentially defines the method's design space. Analytical methods are an essential piece of QbD, so QbD does not necessarily mean less analytical testing. It is the right analysis at the right time, based on science and risk. Some benefits from applying QbD to analytical methods are:

- Facilitation of continuous improvement and technological innovation
- Enhanced method robustness
- More flexible regulatory approaches based on data provided and acceptable quality systems at the sponsor's or third party's analytical testing Lab
- More effective utilization of industry and health authority resources

14.3.5   Validation or Conformance

Phase III to Commercial Regulatory Opportunities   Completion of phase III clinical trials, along with completing the definition of the manufacturing process and control strategy, is a major milestone for a company. Activities now focus on preparing the appropriate marketing application for the FDA (the new drug application and the biologics license application) and/or for the EMEA (the marketing authorization application). The goal of this submission from a CMC perspective is to provide enough information in the CTD Module 3 to permit the respective regulatory authority to determine whether the designed approach used in manufacturing the drug and the controls used to maintain its quality are appropriate and adequate to ensure the drug's identity, strength, quality, purity, and safety.

Manufacturing process changes are inevitable, and even desired, during the course of clinical development, whether for scale-up to increase capacity; to improve process consistency, quality, or safety; or for reduction in cost of goods. However, demonstrating product comparability following such manufacturing process changes can be very challenging. This is especially true for biotech products. The ICH guideline, Comparability of Biotechnological/Biological Products Subject to Changes in Their Manufacturing Process, Q5E, provides invaluable guidance on how to accomplish this.[23] The good news for many biotech products is that they are no longer bound to the old adage "the process defines the product." The bad news is that as with small molecules, there is no guarantee of product comparability after a change in the manufacturing process. The urge to quickly fix everything at this late stage (make the process more robust and commercial) is frequently the result of discovering holes in the scientific understanding of the manufacturing process during preparation of the CTD Module 3. Additional process improvements may be desired at this late stage, but they must be entered into cautiously. On the other hand, process changes will be easier to address if you are within the desired state of manufacturing.

QbD Impact on Process Validation   After the control strategy has been defined and the product and process design spaces are established, process validation might be performed to demonstrate that the process will indeed deliver a product of acceptable quality if operated within the design space. This can also confirm whether the small and/or pilot-scale systems used to establish the design space can accurately model the performance of the manufacturing-scale process. The regulatory filing compiled to date is updated and should include the acceptable ranges for all key and critical operating parameters that define the process design space, in addition to a more restricted operating space (control space), typically as described in the more traditional application for pharmaceutical products. The traditional approach of three consecutive confirmation batches should not be necessary in these types of applications. Continuous process verification at full scale is what is required. What that translates to for formal validation is something that you are going to have to learn both through the experience with your product and agreement with the regulatory authorities.

If you have a design space defined and are looking for approval to report certain process changes in the annual report, you may need to implement acceptance criteria that are tighter than your specifications, in line with ICH Q5(E) on comparability studies, as observations of out-of-trend events may suggest product differences that warrant additional analysis. The filing documents would include the product design space, a description of the control strategy, the outcome of the validation exercise, and a plan for process monitoring (you'll need to verify your conclusion continuously). In the QbD paradigm, and with regulatory agency agreement, the filing could also include comparability protocols (or expanded change control protocols) that would allow for future flexibility in process changes with respect to preapproved criteria. As noted, QbD specific regulatory guidance has yet to be provided by the many local regulatory authorities, and when this occurs it is likely to affect the filings made to those jurisdictions.

How to Validate Based on Knowledge Gained from Design Space   The more work that can be done up front in development, the bigger the impact on overall required design of experiment (DOE) studies, design space, and validation work. If something isn't there, you don't have to control it, you don't have to do DOE studies around it, and you don't have to validate it. The amount of work that research can do for you in those very early stages can save you a huge amount of time, effort, and money farther down the line. The development of the design space creates an understanding of what is critical and noncritical for your performance parameters and therefore allows you to focus on what is important when you execute validation. There is little point in spending a lot of time validating performance parameters that really don't affect the quality of your product. A hypothesis is that development of design space would allow for wider validation acceptance criteria. If you don't do QbD or DOE studies, you have to validate a process within the ranges of the experience you have during development. If you have made only three lots and you only varied between X and Y, there is not much choice for the regulatory authorities to give you much wider acceptance criteria since there are simply no data to use to understand what is going to happen to the process if you go outside those experience limits. FDA has recently revised its process validation guidance[24] stating: "Data gathered (during the Continued Process Verification stage) might suggest ways to improve and/or optimize the process by altering operating ranges and set-points, process controls, components, or in-process materials." So the FDA is stating clearly that it expects manufacturers to study, learn, and improve their processes.

Classical process validation where you run straight down the middle at a set point does not validate anything regarding the acceptance criteria for the operating process parameters that have been set. Running confirmation runs at set point does not validate parameter limits. Confirmation runs are really more an experience of what it is like to run at full scale with your trained personnel following the SOPs and pushing the right buttons. With QbD in mind, you have to rethink the term *validation* and what it means; and specifically what design space does for what you are doing now. The validation of design space is essentially assuring that the risk assessments identifying CQAs, followed by DOEs, and understanding critical process parameters (CPPs) and then developing a control program are all "valid" processes. Process validation has moved back into process development and characterization, and confirmation runs are simply illustrating that at full scale the manufacturing process can run smoothly, without failures, on a regular basis.

The Role of Process Analytical Technology   PAT has been defined as "a system for designing, analyzing, and controlling manufacturing through timely measurements (i.e., during processing) of critical quality and performance attributes of raw and in-process materials and processes, with the goal of ensuring final product quality."[25] As the industry moves toward collecting and analyzing more process data (including continuous or online data), new challenges to these standards are requiring new thinking. Achieving QbD may involve the use of instruments more sophisticated than those currently used in manufacturing processes. Some of these instruments have been used for decades in other industries but have not yet been applied to pharmaceutical production processes. Some of the newer instruments available to general life science manufacturers make relatively simple measurements, while other instruments, such as near-infrared absorption, make much more complex measurements. For pharmaceuticals, in many cases, these instruments are capable of measuring CPPs and CQAs in real time. Such instruments generate large amounts of data that must be understood if the measurements are to be useful. PAT could be viewed as a facilitator of implementation of QbD by allowing for real-time (or near real-time) measurements of quality attributes and feeding the output to the dynamic control strategy so as to result in a more consistent product quality. Numerous publications that are now available utilizing such on-, in-, or at-line PAT applications highlight this concept.

14.3.6   Achieving Regulatory Agreement

Regulatory Strategy and Milestone Planning   QbD practiced properly applies to all stages of the product life cycle: development, scale-up, manufacturing (both for products in phase development as well as in-market products), and technology transfer of processes and products to other sites, and postapproval. In development, for example, the potential for an understanding of design space leading to robust manufacturing processes is perhaps the most widely understood aspect of QbD.

But QbD offers another advantage as well. Because development usually takes place over a long period of time and often involves many people, it can sometimes result in misunderstandings, errors, and redundant activity. QbD principles keep an understanding of design space in the forefront of development efforts, providing the coherence and continuity that trial-and-error approaches lack. QbD can also help achieve life-cycle development, the continued gathering of data after a product is already in production. Because only a limited number of dat accumulate during initial development, additional data, framed by the product's design space, can be helpful in deepening process understanding and continuous improvement of the process.[26]

One keyword to note here again is product knowledge. Typically, this is accrued over time and does not always contain continuous data. Much of the "sticky knowledge" that usually resides with the product champion can contain significant elements of information useful for identifying trends or causes of process variability. Process improvement initiatives must also be able to take advantage of this product knowledge together with newer data and other online measurements. Therefore, QbD requires an overarching infrastructure or a framework for managing the manufacturing process and enabling collaborative investigational analysis of the resulting data to improve the predictability and quality of operations and attributes of the final product. As a sponsor prepares to undertake preparation of the quality module for submission, one of the first and most critical steps is to engage a cross-disciplinary interdepartmental team whose members possess both the necessary technical knowledge and the ability to collaborate effectively. Establishing an effective team can be more easily said than done, but with such a team in place, the sponsor's likelihood of success can increase by countless magnitudes. As the quality team moves forward, a crucial requirement will be strong leadership (or organization infrastructure). For the team to accomplish its goals, the team must clearly understand and agree on what those goals are. In other words, what are the primary objectives? What are the weakest aspects of the data package, and what are the scientifically driven strategies for addressing those weaknesses? What are the immediate and long-term outcomes that the sponsor wishes to achieve for the program?

Building a complete quality program around QbD is an iterative process. Despite the magnitude of the tasks involved in preparing the eventual regulatory application, it is useful to remember that efficiencies can be built into the submission process. For example, a development plan can provide a foundation for a milestone meeting (pre-IND) briefing book. In turn, the pre-IND meeting document can serve as the basis for the eventual regulatory quality module (CTD Module 3). Thus, developing a clear, consistent message by the time the pre-IND meeting efforts begin is one way to maximize the efficiency of module 3 preparation.

If the team maintains its focus on the answers to these questions, the final CTD Module 3 documents will more likely be on target. The key is to provide not only the summary production data, but also the individual underlying data elements in a context that is natural to reviewers who may not be process experts. This improves the speed with which they can identify and understand underlying cause-and-effect relationships.

Designing the CTD Module 3: QbD Quality Module Module 3 is well defined[27] in Table 14.2 containing both the drug substance (active ingredient) and drug product

TABLE 14.2   Common Technical Document Module 3

Drug Substance (Active)		Drug Product (Formulation)	
3.2.S.1	**General Information**	**3.2.P.1**	**Description and Composition**
3.2.S.1.1	Nomenclature	3.2.P.1	Description and Composition of the Drug Product
3.2.S.1.2	Structure	**3.2.P.2**	**Pharmaceutical Development**
3.2.S.1.3	General Properties	3.2.P.2	Pharmaceutical Development
		3.2.P.2.1	*Components of the Drug Product*
		3.2.P.2.2	*Drug Product*
		3.2.P.2.3	*Manufacturing Process Development*
		3.2.P.2.4	*Container Closure System*
		3.2.P.2.5	*Microbiological Attributes*
		3.2.P.2.6	*Compatibility*
3.2.S.2	**Manufacture**	**3.2.P.3**	**Manufacture**
3.2.S.2.1	Manufacturer(s)	3.2.P.3.1	Manufacturer(s)
3.2.S.2.2	Description of Manufacturing	3.2.P.3.2	Batch Formula
3.2.S.2.3	Control of Materials	3.2.P.3.3	Description of Manufacturing Process and Process Controls
3.2.S.2.4	*Controls of Critical Steps and Intermediates*	*3.2.P.3.4*	*Controls of Critical Steps and Intermediates*
3.2.S.2.5	*Process Validation and/or Evaluation*	*3.2.P.3.5*	*Process Validation and/or Evaluation*
3.2.S.2.6	*Manufacturing Process Development*		
3.2.S.3	**Characterization**	**3.2.P.4**	**Control of Excipients**
3.2.S.3.1	Elucidation of Structure and Other Characteristics	3.2.P.4.1	Specification(s)
3.2.S.3.2	*Impurities*	3.2.P.4.2	Analytical Procedures
		3.2.P.4.3	Validation of Analytical Procedures
		3.2.P.4.4	Justification of Specification(s)
		3.2.P.4.5	Excipients of Human or Animal Origin
		3.2.P.4.6	Novel Excipients

TABLE 14.2   Common Technical Document Module 3 (*Continued*)

Drug Substance (Active)		Drug Product (Formulation)	
3.2.S.4	**Control of Drug Substance**	**3.2.P.5**	**Control of Drug Product**
3.2.S.4.1	Specification	3.2.P.5.1	Specification(s)
3.2.S.4.2	Analytical Procedures	3.2.P.5.2	Analytical Procedures
3.2.S.4.3	*Validation of Analytical Procedures*	*3.2.P.5.3*	*Validation of Analytical Procedures*
3.2.S.4.4	Batch Analyses	3.2.P.5.4	Batch Analyses
3.2.S.4.5	*Justification of Specification*	3.2.P.5.5	Characterization of Impurities
		3.2.P.5.6	*Justification of Specification(s)*
3.2.S.5	**Reference Standards**	**3.2.P.6**	**Reference Standards**
3.2.S.5	Reference Standards or Materials	3.2.P.6	Reference Standards or Materials
3.2.S.6	**Container Closure System**	**3.2.P.7**	**Container Closure System**
3.2.S.6	Container Closure System	3.2.P.7	Container Closure System
3.2.S.7	**Stability**	**3.2.P.8**	**Stability**
3.2.S.7.1	*Stability Summary and Conclusions*	*3.2.P.8.1*	*Stability Summary and Conclusion*
3.2.S.7.2	Stability Protocol and Stability Commitment	3.2.P.8.2	Post-approval Stability Protocol and Stability Commitment
3.2.S.7.3	Stability Data	3.2.P.8.3	Stability Data

sections, each containing the required presentations of drug technical information, processes and key parameters, and various justification supported by qualification and validation studies. These data and these reports provide the detailed evidence that a drug's quality attributes and characteristics are well defined and well controlled, such that one can assure that the next lot produced is essentially the same as the last lot. Manufacturing process control and reproducibility is the essential message that Module 3 must convey if agency reviewers are to conclude that a new QbD application merits approval.

Once development has finished their job and manufacturing has done their validation, how are you going to file all this information? In an ideal situation, Module 3 of the Common Technical Document (CTD) would be written once all of the requisite data were available. Unfortunately, the realities of modern drug development (including gaps in development) rarely, if ever, afford this luxury. Depending on the commercial opportunities, develop a global submission and standardize the content within the CTD to be used worldwide early on. Review the different granular sections continuously within Module 3 to say where you are really going to affect the overall license application.

Since efforts by the ICH have resulted in a unified dossier format for drug applications, regulatory agencies in the United States, Canada, EU, and Japan require the CTD, per content and format, when applying for IND and NDA (or equivalent) approval. This multiparty agreement facilitates the application process when regulatory approvals are being sought. The groundwork and preparation of the CTD is critical since it serves as the platform for regulatory filings. Regulatory authorities are not investigating [auditing the site(s)] at the investigational stage, but Module 3 should focus on the QbD documentation relating to substance and product quality. Providing the correct information in sufficient detail in this section will reduce additional delays and costs, providing a very simple value-added step.

The technical information submitted in Module 3 and the organization of the information are specified in detail in guidance documents.[28] Although the CTD Module 3 is now the preferred format for an application within the regions covered by the ICH, including the United States, CTD Module 3 does not in any way replace or supersede the regulations described for example in the U.S. *Code of Federal Regulations*. The CTD is an agreed-upon format for the presentation of summaries, reports, and data. Indeed, the actual content of the Module 3 must still conform to requirements and recommendations found in the regulations of FDA and EMEA guidance documents. Similarly, there may be particular components that are required by other ICH regions. Even with that stipulation, sponsors still have latitude in how data are presented and how important messages are formatted in the compilation of a CTD application. Although the content of this module is generally well defined, according to the various guidance documents referred to previously, considerable latitude for assimilating, discussing, comparing, and contrasting data is allowed and even encouraged, in particular within the module's conformance areas. Even though CTD Module 3 is typically only between one and two volumes, there are opportunities to be creative, to tell a story, and to craft cohesive arguments to help regulatory agencies understand the product. The granular format, with several layers of lesser or greater detail, allows for the presentation of the overall picture while making available all the supportive details. Prior to the CTD format, standard compliance sections served as an introduction to, and summary of, all the compliance data available on the product. Although these sections continue to be closely reviewed, and every section of Module 3 plays a vital role in supporting the ultimate approval of a new drug application, several sections now stand apart from each other in a few respects (see Table 14.3). Although each granular leaf of Module 3 has a specific function, the key areas for creative and informative content in Table 14.2 afford the opportunity to craft discussions, arguments, explanations and justifications, so that supportive data can be highlighted and less-than-stellar findings put in perspective. These sections can therefore influence the perspective of the reviewers more so than in the past, so it is preferable to tackle difficult potential issues head-on within these sections rather than waiting for regulatory reviewers to notice problematic data. These sections allow for integration of data between studies and the presentation of both the strengths and limitations of the data, giving the regulatory reviewer an opportunity to see the big

TABLE 14.3   QbD Compared to "Traditional" Approach

CTD Section	Traditional Content	QbD Approach Content
S22 and P33: Description of Process and Process Controls	Firm process description	Adaptive process description based on equipment differences or raw materials variability; unit operation interaction defined
	Tight process parameter ranges based on commercial scale production experience	Wider process parameters based on proven acceptable ranges; focus on critical process parameters
	In process controls and end product testing	IPCs instead of end product testing?
S25 and S35: Process Validation	The consecutive confirmation lots at set point	Continuous verification at commercial scale; validation of proven acceptable ranges
S26 and P2: Manufacturing and Pharmaceutical Development	Rational and history of the API and formulation process development	Rational for the design space and control strategy
		Risk assessments
		Process parameter and quality attributes defined; functional relationships discussed
		Linkage of critical quality attributes to critical manufacturing attributes
		DOEs
S41/S45 and P51/P56: Specification and Justification	Can include non-critical attributes	Focus on critical quality attributes
	Justification of acceptance criteria based on anecdotal evidence	Justification of acceptance criteria based on relevance to safety and efficacy

picture at any of several levels of detail. Clear and compelling presentations in these areas are critical to the success of the overarching QbD approach.

Manufacturing Process and Pharmaceutical Development   A few sections are of particular interest. Manufacturing Process Development (S26) and Pharmaceutical Development (P2) include the development work that supports the design space alongside the compliance data for the product, and are unique in that they intend to tell a story rather than simply being a collection of data. For most products, the manufacturing development program truly evolves, often such that substantial differences exist between a product early in development and that which is proposed for commercial approval. The challenge inherent in describing development changes is to convince agency reviewers that it is appropriate to consider and to integrate nonclinical and clinical data obtained at various points during development. This involves looking at critical attributes in the context of having studied drugs that might have been considerably different at these points.

Part of the difficulty in assimilating a cohesive and coherent Module 3 is the common situation that the generation of CMC data comes from various sources. Although sometimes all development is undertaken in-house, it is more common that the module must rely on the contributions of both in-house and outside parties. The pressure to generate batches of drug substance and drug product for nonclinical and clinical trials increases greatly as the development program accelerates. GMP standards are high, including documentation requirements for the analytical and stability programs supporting manufacturing. At the same time, technical experts in manufacturing are investigating more efficient process schemes and frequently looking to alternative contractors to reduce costs and to prevent being restricted to a single-sourced strategy, if feasible. All of these changes require documentation and evidence of control, if possible beginning at the initiation of the project and planned proactively as far out in time as possible. For purposes of putting together Module 3, it is particularly important to get it right from the start. It is extraordinarily difficult to have to go back in time to some primary source and try to reconstruct retrospectively, particularly if the people responsible are no longer available, or if other links and foundation approach are missing.

The most important approach to maximize the chance that the Module 3 is received favorably is to strive for clarity, to avoid exaggerations, and to discuss rather than hide negative findings and deficiencies. Avoid claims that cannot be substantiated, and keep in mind the age-old advice that if something is not documented, it is rumor. Current ICH, as well as local guidance, provides much assistance. However, more so now with QbD than before, in places there can be significant advantages to considering the "art" of the presentation as well as the science. These are the sections that are shown in italic type in Table 14.2. If reviewers look favorably on an application's content and presentation and can follow the trail from statement to documentation, there is a better chance for faster approval, and perhaps the full realization of a regulatory agreement.

14.3.7   Conclusions: Striving to Keep Pace

QbD within the regulations has received a lot of attention in the pharmaceutical community. As discussed, implementation requires a thorough understanding of the relationship between the CQAs and the clinical properties of the product, the relationship between the process and CQAs and the variability in raw materials and other analogous inputs. The approach presented here is aligned with existing regulatory guidance documents. Key developments continue to evolve. Regardless of regulatory relief or flexibility longer term, QbD fundamentals are a good thing. Sponsors can get a great deal out of the effort in terms of better process understanding and an elevated confidence level at the time of the submission (whether at the investigation and/or marketing application stage). Apply QbD principles to a major improvement and you may end up with a very robust, well-understood process, with data that allow you to understand issues if they occur. And having filed the proven acceptable ranges of the design space, there is a potential to move within them in a controlled fashion. Pressure keeps things moving forward at the pharmaceutical or biotech company in order to stay ahead of its competition, but this should not lead to rash decisions. The urge to learn everything at the late stage needs to be tempered with caution. The risks of proving product comparability and process improvements at this stage can raise inquiries.

Furthermore, there is a huge cost associated with *not* doing this in terms of nonconformance, execution of processes, and failure in processes. If you take away the regulatory flexibility, would we go forward with QbD? The answer is clearly, yes. Once design spaces have been established, by definition "you are able to move within that design space without reporting changes." You may still have work to do in the company to assess that movement, but it is not a regulatory change. As the regulatory authorities move to a more science risk-based process, they will rely more on scientific knowledge from product and process understanding obtained through QbD during product development as one of the key factors in determining greater flexibility in performing quality assessment. With higher-quality scientific knowledge about the product and the process, derived from product and process understanding, the product's performance can then be better predicted. Consequently, there is a lower risk of producing a product of inconsistent quality, and thus there is a corresponding lower risk of a nonapproval.

For many big sponsors, the commitment to QbD has already been made—and not just for the potential payoff of regulatory flexibility. As you get more people on board with the whole idea of doing more up-front work and understanding of the product and process, and as more QbD submissions are submitted, you are going to have to start paying more attention to the investigation (IND or equivalent) phase and the shift of review attention at this phase toward manufacturing and comparability issues as the QbD approach takes hold. Industry is going to have to shift to thinking more about what the agency needs to be seeing and understanding in the investigation phase to keep pace. Every sponsor should want to know its product, the quality attributes involved, and why its process runs where it does. This requires that sponsors open up a channel of communication early on, along with following good documentation practices. It requires solid strategy, looking at the risk areas, in conjunction with the Module 3 that has been built describing why the process operates where critical product attributes say that it should. These are basic, fundamental expectations, and well within reach of even the smallest company that wants to manufacture drugs in the twenty-first century. It is concluded here once again that although several of the concepts are being practiced by the industry, successful dialogue and partnership between industry and its regulators will be the key to successful implementation.

That is a powerful piece from Ed Narke that should lay the groundwork of under-standing for the technical aspects of modernization.

Now it is time to hear from someone working to QbD principles with a career at the heart of drug development, Sarah Callens. Sarah has worked in the SME environments for a number of years and has consistently attempted to maintain QbD principles as a guiding framework, without big pharma resources in support.

GUEST CONTRIBUTOR SLOT: SARAH CALLENS

QbD in Small and Medium-Sized Enterprises (SMEs)

It is difficult to convince management of a small or medium-sized enterprise (SME) to undertake a QbD approach, as it is perceived as costing more money and taking more time than conventional methods. Additionally, there has been strong aversion to three-letter abbreviations, and some of the concepts of QbD can seem mysterious and intimidating. QbD is often packaged as a new and novel concept that requires extensive training and a lexicon when it is really just providing a logical framework for development and manufacturing activities.

It is generally accepted that some extra work in the beginning phases of an investigational medicinal product establishing a design space and process understanding can save time, and perhaps money in the future. However, there are few, if any, examples of when this was actually carried out and shown to have benefitted an SME. Most of the examples demonstrating the benefits are provided by large pharmaceutical companies, and the benefits have rarely been displayed in financial terms but rather, as examples of how the process is better characterized and understood.

A small startup company aims to get to the clinic and may assume that once safety and efficacy have been demonstrated, the company may be purchased, the investors will be satisfied, and the process development and scale-up of the product becomes the responsibility of the buyer. Therefore, small companies often focus on generating enough material for clinical trials and release testing and may struggle to justify the expenditure required for scale-up to investors.

To date, using a QbD approach has not delayed time lines, but instead, yields more information within the same time lines. Due to the foresight that this approach has granted, various risks and unit operations resulting in process and product variation are understood. Tools such as FMEA allow us to focus our efforts on the most critical aspects of the process, from raw material procurement through to the supply chain, and to ensure that the limited resources of a small company are used appropriately. Additionally, through Ishikawa diagrams and compiling historical process knowledge, we have been able to identify which parts of the process are more flexible and can be altered to suit GMP operations. These activities have not required any additional capital and have helped guide the allocation of resources.

Sarah demonstrates here that modernization does not have to be about cutting-edge technology. The principles aim to support members of organizations in applying common sense to improve their and their company's lot.

15 Exemplar Thinking in Organizational Improvement

15.1 WHERE ARE WE NOW?

That is a good question! Nearly 60 years after Deming expounded his principles, the assessment in Chapter 11 indicates that we are still basically mouthing similar thoughts. In a sense, this is the universal dilemma for all improvement initiatives to date. For example, take principle 9: "People in research, design, sales, and production must work as a team". This is a recurring theme over the years—in fact, I will be saying it in the final chapter in relation to pharmaceuticals! This does not apply to companies across the board. There are companies getting benefit from adopting inclusive (concurrent) design processes and other improved ways of working, but not enough. Certainly, there are not enough, if any, in pharmaceuticals.

We are also still in this position with lean thinking and enterprise. The principles are there, but confusion still abounds as to how they translate into everyday actions that can inform ordinary people on a path to improvement. The tools and techniques are there, but how do they link with principles for the benefit of ordinary people on a path to improvement? We shine some light on that in this chapter.

A paper coauthored by John Sterman is a good starting point. The intriguing header for the paper reads "Nobody ever gets credit for fixing problems that never happened—creating and sustaining process improvement."[1] Hopefully, this will set the reader, if not already primed, to think systemically. John Sterman is Jay W. Forrester Professor of Management and director, of the MIT System Dynamics Group Sloan School of Management. Many will recall the Forrester effect, relating to demand amplification (or the bullwhip effect), which was named after Jay Forrester, who founded the group John now heads.

To get the systems message here, some explanation may help. A core tenet of systems thinking is that cause and effect are, more often than not, in totally different parts of the system. People being people, when faced with an effect, we tend to look around the parts with which we are in contact. Fires are fought and battles are won in the immediate vicinity. Unfortunately, as is the case with most fires and battles, if the underlying cause is not identified, fires become blazes and battles become wars. This is the spirit in which we progress in this chapter: how to identify approaches that can douse the fires and win the wars. They, no doubt, exist in much of the improvement work that has been documented over the years. Sadly though, in general use, the message gets diluted. A person's interpretation of the critical success factors become blurred and "initiatives" fail or flounder. This chapter is about what the marketing people term "staying on message." That is why the words of John Sterman above are so resonant. When faced with an issue of a systemic nature, experienced systems thinkers may well go off and solve the problem at source. It may be a delinquent supplier linkage, or a disconnect with the design team; or business partners who need more involvement in a specific activity. It could be anywhere, but the point is that the solution will probably go unnoticed because the issue just went away, apparently without anyone doing anything. These are the solutions we should seek. Some of my personal experience may help.

Observations, Views, and Experiences of the Author

My first job in the health care sector was as an industrial engineer in a manufacturing plant in Wales. Luckily for me, industrial engineering was a well-regarded discipline in the company (the head of materials management was a trained industrial engineer) and I was given almost carte blanch access to issues and problems that emerged. When I joined, an MRP I system had just been installed and implemented. There were many issues postimplementation and I was given the job of getting to the bottom of them. It was termed a systems survey *and was one of the most valuable experiences of my career—not for the fact that it was hugely successful (although it did unearth some useful corrective actions), but because at an early stage in my career, it drove home the wicked ways of the system. What I found through the investigations (using low-key interviews and simple IE tools such as high-level cross-functional process flow mapping) was that none of the issues seemed to be caused by anyone! Every person in the chain had done what the system had demanded of them. They had behaved exactly as you or I would have faced with similar circumstances.*

One of the recurring issues was that the warehouse staff kept recording the wrong quantities received against purchase orders for packaging items. Little wonder, because the new system required them to record a single item of packing (e.g., a label) as 0.001 rather than 1.000. This was because the unit of measure had changed to "one thousand," so, for example, 500 labels now had to be recorded as 0.500. If, as they had been doing previously, they recorded the quantity as 500, the computer system would believe that it had many more labels than it actually did have (500,000) and fail to recommend reorder of materials in replenishment. This would drive the planner crazy and end with demands for the warehouse manager's head on a plate. However, if you or I had missed the scant training available just before launch of the computer system, we would happily have gone ahead with our job totally unaware of the planner's misery.

This is only the start of it. If the enraged planner had taken herself down to the warehouse, she would have discovered this fact and relented, marching off to find those responsible for system training. She would learn that it was the computer system's people themselves who were responsible for the training, and on talking to them would find out that everyone had been invited but some did not turn up. Those damn warehouse guys again! Further enquiry would reveal that the staff who did not turn up were not on the list for training because the computer people had been sent an out-of-date list by the human resources department, which held the database. Sorry! And so it goes, around and around.

Steven Spear, author of *Chasing the Rabbit*,[2] gave an excellent video demonstration in his keynote speaker presentation at the 2009 LERC Conference. It started with a heartbroken father getting the devastating news in the hospital that his wife had died in childbirth. It proceeded through all the preceding events, highlighting the points at which the tragedy could have been avoided if someone in the drama had behaved differently. However, their behavior was perfectly rational given the circumstances. At the end, the culprit is a yellow sticky note becoming detached from a busy receptionist's paperwork. On it were details of the appointment the mother should have had with her gynecologist that was never made. That appointment would have prevented the entire event because it would have picked up an underlying problem that had occurred late in pregnancy.

The lack of an appointment was down to a failure in this small part of the *system*, weeks and weeks previous to their final loss. The mother's need for a last appointment before the due date was identified when she was in the gynecologist's office earlier in her term. The receptionist was at her desk in the outer office. All that needed to happen was for the doctor's appointment to be recorded in his diary and given to the prospective mum. Instead, it was written on a sticky note and given to the lady, who then put it on the distracted receptionist's desk, from whence it disappeared in a sheaf of paperwork. The rest is history.

Readers may be thinking that that's all very sad, but what has this to do with improvement? The message is this. The process of booking appointments was flawed, but not in a way that was obvious to those who were part of it. This is true particularly when the consequences of a mistake do not appear to be too dramatic. So we live with flaws in our processes. Those inside the system don't see the harm in it—but the *system* knows that they are there.

All this suggests one very important point in organizational life—there is no such thing as a "quick fix." That is not meant as a throwaway remark; it is a serious point. The improvement methods discussed in this book are very often seen as such. When espoused in meetings, the people in the room may declare clear agreement but then go on pursuing the quick fix. Similarly, the statement "forecasts are always wrong" invariably gets sage nods and reinforcing noises. Still, the supply chain folks measure forecast accuracy as if it were money in their pockets. "There is no such thing as a quick fix" elicits similar fervent agreement, just before people rush off to do the next kaizen event or their six-sigma black belt project without first checking the systemic impact that it may or may not have.

This is the focus of the chapter: seeking to highlight, from all the good work that has been carried out in the name of organizational improvement, those aspects that seem worth pursuing and building on them for the good of the system. We emphasize those approaches to improvement that really can and do make a difference, and we examine the barriers to effective organizational systems development that currently exist. This is what I mean by exemplar thinking in improvement and which I expand on below.

15.2   WHAT IS MEANT BY "EXEMPLAR"?

We begin this section by defining what we mean by *exemplar*. A search on the word unearths the work of Thomas Kuhn,[3] which provides a perfect explanation. Scientific practice alternates periods of normal science with periods of revolutionary science. In normal periods, scientists tend to subscribe to an interconnecting body of knowledge, methods, and assumptions (the reigning paradigm). In the search for answers to "puzzles" in the field, certain solutions become regarded as *exemplar*. This leads to what Kuhn termed a *paradigm shift* (although he did not coin the term). In that vein we examine approaches and discoveries that have purported to create a paradigm shift around designing, operating, and improving supply chains and the associated management processes. Of particular interest to us is which of the developments in the body of knowledge are genuinely exemplar and which are merely repackaging of an existing paradigm?

As we have discussed, the improvement disciplines have their genesis in the more controversial activities such as setting time standards and monitoring work output. In more recent times, the "us and them" approaches have subsided to be replaced by more rounded, all-inclusive improvement efforts. Probably the most current of these now are lean and six sigma, both of which have a methodology for problem solving (A3 Management and DMAIC; see Chapter 12) and a bag of tools. Associated with these is the term *continuous improvement*. For the sake of emphasis, as in Chapter 12, the concept of "continuous" will be removed. By doing so we also remove the constriction of Japanese kaizen as being the only way. Sometimes only discontinuous improvement will do, in the form of radical organizational surgery (see Chapter 17). From here on, therefore, organizational improvement can come from anyone, anywhere, in any guise.

15.3   A DIALOGUE ON EXEMPLAR IMPROVEMENT

The analysis starts with the words and insights of Javaid Cheema, a practicing expert in lean thinking and improvement and qualified in industrial and systems engineering.

GUEST CONTRIBUTOR SLOT: JAVAID M. CHEEMA

The Essence of Japanese Success in Production Systems

There has been an explosive expansion of research about Japanese companies and their phenomenal success in the global marketplace. In hindsight, only 30 years ago, even Japanese entrepreneurs wouldn't have anticipated their rise to the status of "management celebrities" around the globe. It is not uncommon to see a new book every time I visit a bookstore or Web site to see something new about Toyota, Sony, Mitsui, or similar Japanese industrial giant. Since a lot has been and is being about Japanese industry and management practices, it is not my intention to write a lengthy recap of literature already available, yet my intention is to explain some peculiar cultural values of Japanese society and how did they helped to enhance Japanese management practices. Living in Japan for a long time as a student, a professional, and an avid researcher of Japanese cultural evolution, *nihon shoki* I came across some unforgettable facts about small things in everyday life that evolve to have a huge positive impact on everyday working life. Although these values have been introduced to the West through literature published about the Toyota production system, but they are practiced more or less in every Japanese corporation.

For example, the Japanese perspective on making mistakes is entirely different from that of any other society in the world. In every non-Japanese society, the word *mistake* carries some kind of stigma not being able to perform according to established standards of a task or duty. Contrary to that, in the Japanese language, *mistake* carries a very benign meaning, and translated closely it means "a learning opportunity." This interpretation changes the paradigm completely; Toyota teaches their employees that a mistake provides 5 to 10 times more knowledge than a success. To make honest mistakes and learn from them is entirely different from adopting a "chronic loser's" behavior.

In Japan, be it in personal life or in the workplace; when people make mistakes, they really feel sorry about them and would regret and go through a rigorous self-reflection exercise or *hensei*. The Japanese as a society have a remarkable ability to learn from their mistakes and have long used this as a strategic advantage in the corporate world. After correcting a mistake, they do not forget the lessons learned. For example, all successful Japanese companies spend a lot of their time reviewing the past mistakes of their prospective suppliers and the lessons learned from those mistakes, or *kako tora*. In turn, *kako tora* becomes a major portion of the planning process for a new product or service. Going through many advance planning projects for Japanese companies, I have noted that no planning phase is complete unless all past failures have been accounted for, their remedies have been assessed, and risk mitigation strategies have been reviewed, a process traditionally called *kiken yochi*, *kiken* meaning "fire" and *yochi*, "planning in advance", so collectively implying avoiding sudden fires.

Since Japanese companies try to carry out exhaustive reviews of past failures and all possible alternatives to avoid them, the planning phase is usually far longer than such subsequent phases as design, development, production, and distribution. For example, in the automotive industry, almost all carmakers in the United States, Europe, and Asia use a five-Phase product development process: conceptualization, design, development, production, and commercialization. Most non-Japanese automakers divide their new product development programs into equal time periods for each development phase, whereas Japanese automakers commit 70% of their resources during the conceptualization and design phases, popularly called the *front-end loading*. [Author's note: Drug developers—heed these words.] During the conceptualization and design phases, risk mitigation is the highest priority. A study of Japanese history reveals that the country was often threatened with foreign invasion, particularly from Korea and China; in addition, they had long adopted a policy of avoiding any contact with the outside world. The policy of seclusion was abolished in 1868, but the practice has had the very profound effect of causing the Japanese to avoid risks.

Fear of a common foreign enemy for centuries has also helped Japanese society to develop collective strategies against competitors. It is probably a major contributor to the modern concept of consensus building, *nemawashi*. Internal unity is considered a critical factor in dealing with external threats; the Japanese did that for many centuries to avoid invasion and found it equally effective in the modern competitive business environment. Consensus building is generally a long and labor-intensive process. Although it is very similar to many decision-making tools used elsewhere in the world, there is a fine difference between *nemawashi* and non-Japanese consensus building tools. In typical non-Japanese collective decisions, if something goes wrong down the road, reluctant team members tend to dissociate themselves from undesirable outcomes by adopting an "I told you so" response. Contrary to that, in *nemawashi* are no reluctant worriers—each person bears a collective responsibility for the good or bad results of a decision, which makes it significantly slower than a non-Japanese decision-making process.

Another positive aspect of Japanese culture has been the tendency to accept mistakes and take responsibility for them. As Thomas Campbell once said: "Victory has a hundred fathers, but defeat is an orphan." Most people tend to take credit for their successes, but few people can publically accept their mistakes with dignity. In Japanese culture, this value is widely practiced and appreciated. Again, this is a rare social value which has helped Japanese businesses to evolve faster than their non-Japanese competitors, as making mistakes is considered a natural part of everyday professional life. In a typical Japanese company, responsibility begins at the top, regardless of who made the mistake and why. The highest-ranking member of a team holds the ultimate responsibility for the success or failure of a decision; generally, the attitude of looking for scapegoats is despised and discouraged.

Last but not least, another Japanese social value worth mentioning is the fanatical desire to be frugal in resource utilization. A lavish lifestyle was generally looked down upon in traditional Japanese society. Doing more with less and looking for improvements in the ways in which things are done is an integral part of Japanese society. Eating less, sleeping less, and spending less are considered virtues of a good person. A company where every employee has these virtues can be very competitive in the marketplace.

This wonderful exposition from Javaid should confirm that Japanese cultural heritage has been a huge enabler for the success of modern Japanese industry. Where does that leave non-Japanese companies wishing to compete? My aim in this Chapter is to shed important light on that question. Below digging deeper, readers should hear more from Javaid because his insights are awe inspiring. Below I have paraphased some communications that I have received from Javaid via the Internet.

I always joke that here in the United States, people (i.e., researchers and journalists) have made more money telling Toyota success stories through books and articles than Toyota made by selling cars. Having worked at Toyota for 14 years in Japan and as an avid student of *nihon shoki* (10,000 years of cultural history of Japan), I am taking the liberty of clearing up some misperceptions about the Toyota production system (TPS).

First of all, the very lean philosophy, of "doing more with less" is not a Toyota philosophy—it is a collective Japanese mentality (eating less, talking less, sleeping less, spending less) that defines a virtuous Japanese person. For example, Honda's NMR (new model release) process is far leaner and more efficient than TPS, and the same can be said of Nissan's PESE (process engineering systems excellence). Yet for some reason, Honda and Nissan did not create manufacturing showbiz around their core processes, whereas it is not uncommon to see a new book about Toyota everytime you visit www.amazon.com.

In fact, the most important factor in a lean enterprise is the human factor, which we in the West tend to overlook. In the contemporary literature about lean thinking, you will find that the practitioner who has emphasized the social side of lean more than anybody else has been Jeffrey Liker (professor of industrial and operations engineering at the University of Michigan in Ann Arbor). His three books, *The Toyota Way* (and Field Book), *The Toyota Talent*, and *The Toyota Culture*,[4] deal exclusively with Toyota's social model (TSM) because he is an anthropologist by education. Another great contribution to TSM recently has been the book *Extreme Toyota* by Emi Osono,[5] a book well worth reading or listening to.

Toyota's social model never succeeds by accident; there has to be a sequence of intelligent steps. I have used the following five steps with notable success before I started talking about the principles of lean enterprise at my client assignments:

1. Begin with a rigorous and passionate effort to develop self-esteem and self-pride in high-quality work, even if it means cleaning toilets on the shop floor.
2. Develop profound knowledge of the process and product, especially ways in which a person can positively or negatively affect a product or process.
3. Empower workers to practice their newfound values and provide instantaneous feedback.
4. Develop a system of self-control rather than external control. People avoid making mistakes not for the fear of external forces but because it damages their pride in their work.
5. Foster the ability to learn from mistakes, according to Toyota's social model; a failure provides 5- to 10-fold greater learning opportunity than a success. And plan ahead of time.

Last but not least, the technical side of lean transformation must not be overlooked; it is another critical workplace reality.

In one of my current consulting jobs, for a company that makes components for commercial aircraft, I am at step 4 in my list with most of the people, and the average rate of rejects has gone down from 8.5% to about 0.15% in about four months.

I think, that it is difficult to accomplish what the Five Principles espouse without a *solid social foundation*. In this regard I cite the NUMMI (New United Motor Manufacturing, Inc., Freemont, California) story from 1984 to 1987, the only successful joint venture between Toyota and General Motors [see Section 12.3.12]. The biggest success was Toyota's transformation of a hostile unionized (UAW) assembly plant into a highly focused and productive workforce.

This contribution from Javaid speaks for itself and will be drawn upon again in Chapter 17.

Next, we hear from Peter Hines, former chairman and professor of supply chain management Cardiff University's Lean Enterprise Research Centre, chairman of S.A. Partners, and coauthor of *Staying Lean: Thriving, Not Just Surviving*.[6]

GUEST CONTRIBUTOR SLOT: PETER HINES

Questions Regarding Thinking Lean

Throughout the last 15 years of applying lean thinking to organizations, I have consistently been asked a series of searching questions about its application:

1. Where do I start?
2. Is there a road map that I can follow?
3. What does lean thinking involve?
4. Who will I have to involve?
5. It is applicable only to the shop floor?
6. Is it only for manufacturing firms?
7. What will the benefits be?
8. Will it make me more profitable?

However, in the last few years the set of questions I am asked has widened, with a series of additional queries such as:

1. How long is it before the benefits start fading away?
2. Why do people here seem to have lost their enthusiasm for lean?
3. What is the secret of sustainability?
4. What is the difference between managing and leading a lean change?
5. How do we ensure continued buy-in from the workforce?

The focus on improvement has thus shifted from "Where do I start?" to "How do I make it sustainable?" In the *Staying Lean* book, my colleagues and I attempt to answer these questions and ensure that you don't just *start* a successful lean program in your business but continue to sustain and build on your early successes. For success, you need to focus on the visible or "above the water" features, such as the rigorous use of technology, tools, and techniques as well as a process-based approach. However, equally or, in many cases, more important are the invisible "below the water" features, such as strategy and alignment, leadership and behavior, and engagement. It is the contingent effective combinations of these visible and hidden features in sequential road maps that creates sustainable results. It is not just about the tools and techniques, as we see with so many so-called "lean" implementations.

So: further confirmation from a leading practitioner and academic that other factors are at play besides the tools and techniques.

To add to our knowledge, let's talk about improvement in the world outside Japan. To begin I asked Owen Berkeley-Hill to provide his perspective. Owen calls himself "The Lean Pensioner"! His tongue must be firmly in his cheek when he does that, but the fact is he has been able to retire from the rat race to pursue his personal interests, one of which is lean. Owen's words below were prompted by a question that, Peter Hines asked in an Internet discussion group: whether some modifications may be needed to the original five principles coined by Womack and Jones.[7] Seven alterative principles were suggested, and here are Owen's comments.

GUEST CONTRIBUTOR SLOT: OWEN BERKELEY-HILL

Do the Five Principles of Lean Need Modification?

The five principles (five P's) were a great step forward, particularly in the understanding of value and waste, systems and process thinking. Before lean, waste was anything my boss did not think benefited him, regardless of the value placed by the end customer or the customer of the work I did. There was, and possibly still is, a general lack of systems thinking above the snowline in most organizations. The 5Ps were sound but were open to abuse and often badly applied. How many leaders actually changed their philosophy? How many delegated the change to internal or external agents, with strict instructions that they were not to be disturbed? "Don't bring me problems; bring me solutions!" Why is lean struggling (after 30 years) to be understood by the leadership of the vast majority of organizations? Why is lean seen as the "all too difficult" alternative? Why do leaders happily choose outsourcing, offshoring, and yet another IT system?

Before addressing the five P's, I think we need a clearer definition of what lean is exactly. Lean vs. six sigma vs. lean sigma is a common subject of discussion in many forums, including this one. John Seddon[8] (a not-to-be-missed commentator on lean in the service sector and a fantastic speaker) is a systems thinker who distances himself from the "tool-heads" in the lean movement. The Toyota-tollahs will tell you that lean is a crude approximation of the Toyota production system (TPS). How does it fit with TOC, and why does it pay little regard to Deming? I think lean is hampered by its initial success, which has allowed it to be boxed into something called *operations*. From my experience, I prefer John Bicheno's inclusive and very large lean tent, as described in his various toolboxes.

Principle 1: Purpose   Jim Womack talks about purpose, process, and people, although I'm not sure that this was made explicit in the five P's. I think the importance of this principle will depend on how it can inspire leaders to engage in *hoshin*. I don't mean buying a strategy off the shelf from a consultancy, but developing one with the workforce so that everyone is "singing off the same hymn sheet." However, I doubt that many leaders have the skill to engage the workforce in explaining purpose.

Principle 2: Process   I agree that lean should apply to all processes and to the creation of value, not just the elimination of waste. Looking at the automotive industry, the Germans seem to be better at this (e.g., VW Audi, and the way they have revived or enhanced their brands, including Bentley and Skoda). In the days of greater certainty, if you had the money, Jermyn Street was the place to get your shirts made. How are the makers there coping with the likes of Boden? Will following Tesco (buy one, get four free) damage their brands?

Principle 3: People   Before I retired I developed a definition of quality: the measure of how well an organization delivers the customers' perceptions of value. As competition, technology, and consumerism are constantly changing customers' perceptions, quality becomes a moving target, and hence the need for *kaizen*. (You may detect the influence of Noriaki Kano.) Lean thinking has 31 references to kaizen, but there is a heavy bias toward kaizen "events," not about making kaizen into a pandemic that infects every employee with a positive form of OCD to fix problems. Ten to 20 improvements annually from every employee (including the CEO, CFO, and CIO) should be the aspiration—but not a target. There has been much talk over the years from the more socially minded about greater employee engagement. As far as I know, Mayo, Maslow, McGregor, and Herzberg were not Japanese, but have been largely ignored in the West because they were not of the "real world." On the other hand, can you think of a better synthesis of their work than kaizen?

Unfortunately, kaizen suffers from comparison with its bigger brother, *kaikaku*, and there is a natural bias toward the big, radical, and expensive changes even though these have a very poor track record of success. I still see examples of ideas from hourly workers being ignored, so this will be a tough one, as is recognized by previous contributions to this dialogue. "It won't work" or "we don't have the time to investigate it right now" are all too common.

In summary, I believe this to be the most important because true lean is different from all the other approaches (including six sigma) because in lean the workforce does it for themselves (kaizen); in any other approach, it is done to them by experts.

Principle 4: Pull   I have always felt that there was a strong relationship between lean, learning, and leadership (the subject of my M.Sc. dissertation). I'm reading Steven Spear's book, *Chasing the Rabbit*,[9] and agree that there is more to kaizen than problem solving. The issue here is whether the current leadership culture is able to encourage learning and to mentor and coach the workforce. As an aspiration, I believe a true lean and learning organization will have a Pareto 80:20 split in favor of growing its knowledge internally and not relying exclusively on external consultants.

Principle 5: Prevention   I am not sure why some people think that quality was ignored or downplayed in lean. Defects have always been recognized as waste, and I think lean brought *jidoka* to a wider audience, although I would agree that it needs a better explanation. Design for manufacture has been around for as long as I can remember, but I wonder if it is ingrained in every embryonic engineer.

Principle 6: Population   Ford, Matsushita, and the Toyodas: How many leaders think like they did and think of the benefits of their organizations to society rather than the tyranny of Wall Street, the next quarter, and the bottom line? When things get tough, today's leaders revert to command and control, which I believe is incompatible with lean, so this will be a tough nut to crack. There may also be a natural conflict between innovation and the green agenda. I cannot understand the need for either 4 × 4s or bottled water (shipped from the Massif in France) when tap water is perfectly palatable.

Principle 7: Perfection   Whether it is PDSA, or DMAIC or the five P's, I think these circular methodologies will stall at the top of the loop without the horsepower of kaizen.

In summary, the five P's greatest weakness is that they did not change leadership thinking in sufficient numbers to make lean the core management philosophy. I suspect this is partly the result of the ambivalent attitude of business schools toward lean, treating it as a speciality subject with little universal application. (How many deans have a visceral knowledge of lean?) In this connection, if we are examining the five P's, I think we should also be asking ourselves whether we can first redefine lean in the wake of all our experience. I would also suggest that there may be a need for an alternative to the MBA, the MBL (the master of business leadership).

There are many reasons why I included this piece from Owen. Almost the most important reason is to demonstrate the type of dialogue that is needed to move us forward toward exemplar. I do not necessarily agree with every point that Owen makes, but his desire to find the "truth" is plainly evident. We should all be doing that.

Next, readers should hear from Ian Glenday. Ian took me through his thoughts and philosophies one evening during a conference we both spoke at in 2005. He allowed me to summarize what he was saying and also allowed me to use large extracts from his workbook *Breaking Through to Flow*.[10] (for which Ian received a Shingo Prize in 2010).

GUEST CONTRIBUTOR SLOT: IAN GLENDAY

From Variability to Stability

Most people see the prime focus of lean as waste elimination and completely miss or misunderstand that leveled production (*heijunka*) is the foundation that is essential in creating the stability required to achieve sustainable improvements. This creates the phenomenon of economies of repetition and, along with root-cause problem solving, is how lean really works.

Economic order quantity (MRP I and II) logic is the foundation of nearly all planning and ordering systems, yet it causes both unnecessary variability (different plans every week) and firefighting (changing plans after they have been issued) as well as peaks and troughs (the bullwhip effect). The alternative logic is "flow," and let the stock float within limits—exactly the same logic as statistical process control (SPC).

Such views, I believe, fly against conventional supply chain wisdom and are indeed inflammatory to many people!!

Batch logic, or economic order quantity (as employed by MRP II), is the basis of most planning and ordering systems that one can buy. Yet this logic is fundamentally flawed for two reasons. First, it is responsible for causing the firefighting that is endemic in most manufacturing companies. Firefighting becomes inevitable if plans are changed after they have been issued. I will show why plan changes are *guaranteed* when using EOQ logic. It also causes unnecessary *variability* in what is planned and executed. Together, firefighting and unnecessary variability prevent a company with a stable foundation from needing to be able to sustain continuous improvement. Without stability, companies find themselves always running—just to stand still.

To see EOQ logic at work, let's look at an example from a large global fast-moving branded goods company. Figure 15.1 shows weekly orders from the U.S. affiliate company to the manufacturing plant in Scotland over a six-week period. The affiliate orders every week, on the same day of the week, but the orders vary between 4000 and 24,000 cases! Figure 15.2 shows the plant's planned production,

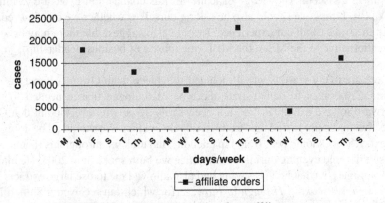

FIGURE 15.1   Fluctuating orders from affiliate company.

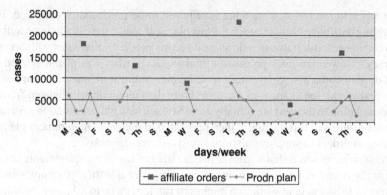

FIGURE 15.2   Production plans to meet fluctuating orders.

by day, to meet the affiliate's orders. Although production of the product is scheduled for each week, production volumes vary greatly, with production planned to run on different days each week. Figure 15.3 shows what was actually made each day or each week. On a week-by-week basis, each week's production was more or less what was planned. But actual daily outputs bear only a fleeting similarity to what was scheduled! In other words, the plan was never adhered to.

Overall, this supply chain was delivering what was required; the company was proud of its high customer service levels. But the degree of variability in affiliate orders, production schedules, and actual production was amazing, particularly when analysis of actual consumption of this product showed that it was relatively constant. Such a high degree of variability makes it extremely difficult (impossible?) to implement sustainable continuous improvement activities.

Managers' response is that they simply have to manage their processes and systems better. What they do not seem to see is that the EOQ logic in their planning processes actually generates this variability as *an integral part of the system* no matter how well it is managed. Why is this? There are two reasons. First, EOQ logic uses a

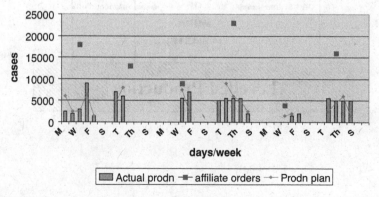

FIGURE 15.3   Actual daily production compared to the production plan and orders.

target stock figure to calculate what is required to be produced or delivered. If the underlying data have changed since the last plan was made, the calculation results in a different answer. But how often do sales forecasts predict actual sales with complete accuracy? How often does production make exactly what was planned? And how often do you come across inventory inaccuracies in the warehouse? When we look at the real world, the chances of the underlying data remaining unchanged from one plan calculation to the next are actually zero. So each new plan calculation generates a different result, and this change is then replicated in materials requirement planning, resulting in orders to suppliers also changing on a regular basis.

The second reason is that whatever the calculation says the requirements are, they are usually rounded up to create an "economic order quantity." Examples include pressure to fill a truck, to work to a minimum run length, or to fill an entire shipping container. These pressures introduce artificially higher demand, which then translate into artificially lower demand at a later stage in order to bring the stock back to the target level. The net result? Peaks and troughs in demand, otherwise known as the "bullwhip effect."

Production stability is fundamental to lean. So how did Toyota achieve such stability? I was fortunate to visit Japan in the 1980s to study under Sensei Yoshiki Iwata from Toyota Gosei, one of the first suppliers to be taught the Toyota production system. He showed me the TPS "house" as it was originally drawn by Fujio Cho of Toyota in 1973 (Figure 15.4). "Leveled production" forms the foundation of this house. As Iwata described it to me, leveled production is an evolution of steps.

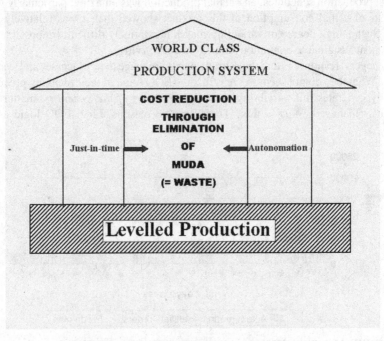

FIGURE 15.4   Toyota production system "house."

The initial steps are designed to create stability, which enables sustained continuous improvement, leading to better performance. Once better performance is achieved, it becomes possible to invest more effort in achieving greater flexibility and responsiveness to demand. This sequence of steps is vital. You have to create stability first. Then you can progressively match output much more closely to actual demand.

Iwata's diagram highlights another important point. To many people the prime focus of lean is to eliminate waste. People and organizations believe they are "doing lean" if they are focused on eliminating waste. Yet eliminating waste is in the middle of the diagram. All too often they completely miss the fact that leveled production is the foundation of lean. As a result, they find it very difficult to create a stable base to help sustain their improvement efforts. This failure to understand the significance of leveled production is one of the reasons why the gains made in many lean initiatives can be difficult to sustain.

Iwata's Beer Mat

Step 0: Batch Production   This is how Iwata described the steps of leveling to me. We were in a bar in Tokyo and he drew the following diagrams on a beer mat! First, he drew a simple diagram depicting three products with monthly demands of 100, 200, and 300 units, respectively. EOQ logic leads us to produce these products in the biggest batches and longest runs possible, to minimize changeovers and maximize line efficiency. So Figure 15.5 shows the ideal picture from the perspective of EOQ logic.

Step 1: Bimonthly Production   Next, Iwata drew another simple diagram (Figure 15.6). This time he halved all the batch sizes, which resulted in two identical cycles. This creates the same fixed sequence and volume of products in each cycle. This is known as *every product every cycle* (or *every product every interval*). Of course, in real life, factories don't have the capability to halve all batches immediately. Figure 15.6 sets a direction and a target. To achieve this target, people need to apply lean improvement tools and techniques in a disciplined way. To calculate what the changeover times *need to be* to achieve the identical twice monthly cycle, not what they *think* they can achieve in changeover improvement times.

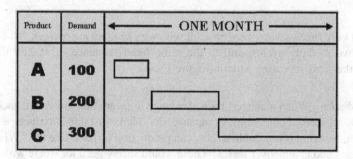

Product	Demand	◄─────── ONE MONTH ───────►
A	**100**	
B	**200**	
C	**300**	

FIGURE 15.5   Batch logic at work.

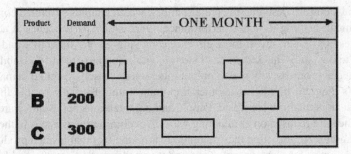

FIGURE 15.6   Every product every cycle.

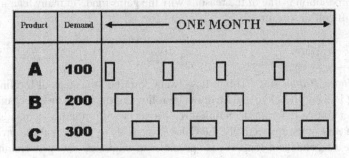

FIGURE 15.7   Every product every week.

Step 2: Weekly Production   Iwata then drew a third diagram where he halved the batches again. This creates the same fixed sequence and fixed ratio of volumes for each product type. It's called *every product every week* (Figure 15.7). This achieves faster cycles, but the main objective of the initial steps of leveling is to create a fixed *stable* repeating plan. Iwata told me that it was originally called "patterned production" at Toyota, but this term seems to have disappeared from the lean lexicon.

Why halve the batches yet again? It takes us one step closer to the ultimate objective of becoming more responsive to actual demand. Of course, again, it's difficult to do this. People need to apply the same improvement techniques to overcome the obstacles.

Step 3: Daily Production   Having achieved *every product every week,* the next step is to move to daily cycles, still in the same fixed sequence in exactly the same ratios—the same repeating pattern (Figure 15.8).

Why It Works   When managers trained in batch logic are first shown this succession, they raise all sorts of objections. Companies don't have just three products, they have hundreds. Demand is not stable so how can production be fixed like this? What about efficiencies and changeover losses? These would surely get a lot worse with shorter, more frequent runs, even if it gave stability. To their eyes, this alternative logic looks ridiculous. It is counterintuitive and flies in the face of conventional wisdom. That's

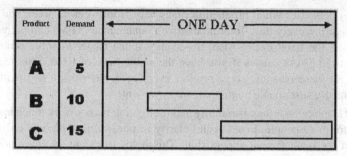

FIGURE 15.8 Daily cycles.

one of the reasons most people and organizations focus on the waste-eliminating aspect of lean. Yet Iwata insisted that this was the right path to take. Why?

By repeating the same pattern of *every product every cycle*, we generate a phenomenon called *economies of repetition* (EOR). People are often amazed by the improvements that economies of repetition produce. EOR works by building on two basic traits of human behavior. The first trait is the learning curve. When people do the same task repeatedly, they naturally get better at it. This isn't about applying improvement tools. It just happens.

The second trait is that most people like routines. Some people see this as being the same as learning curves, but our desire for routines is something different. To see it for yourself, go into your organization's restaurant at lunchtime. Draw a map of where everyone is sitting. Go in the following day at the same time and draw the map again. You will get practically the same map with most people sitting at exactly the same tables, mostly even the same seats!! People live their lives by routines. They like the stability, security, and predictability that routines give. They often find it stressful if their routines are disturbed. That's one reason why short-term plan changes demotivate people. If you give people routines, they will feel less stressed, more relaxed, and better motivated.

There's also a third reason why *every product every cycle* is so important: It creates an environment where standardization can flourish—and without standardization you cannot generate sustainable improvement. It is, however, very difficult to achieve standard work when short-term changes are frequent and the plan is different every week. In this environment, operators' natural response to standard work is: "Why?" It is much easier to accept the need for standard work in a stable environment of fixed sequence and volume cycles. In fact, fixed cycles encourage standard work because when people in teams do the same things in the same sequences, they naturally start to agree that it is the best way of working. When every day is different, this is far more difficult.

The benefits of these phenomena (of the learning curve, of stable routines, and standardization) are surprisingly rich.

- *Hard benefits.* Fixed cycles provide a base for the implementation of many other lean techniques. For example, it is almost impossible to implement just-in-time

(JIT) deliveries when production plans vary from week to week and there is firefighting every day. Total productive maintenance (TPM) can be built in as part of the fixed cycle. Also, it becomes much easier to solve problems by identifying root causes if you have the stable base of fixed, repeated cycles. For all these reasons, *every product every cycle* provides a key platform for genuinely sustainable continuous improvement.

- *Soft benefits.* Stopping variability and firefighting makes work much less stressful for most people. Fixed cycles clarify responsibilities, thereby reducing the need for management supervision. This helps to create an environment that fosters greater empowerment, teamwork, and motivation.

From Push to Pull   So far we have described the first three steps of leveling. These can and regularly do deliver levels of improvement beyond many managers' most optimistic expectations. But these first three steps are just a preparation for the next two. *Every product every cycle* is a rigid push system. But the real objective of lean is a flexible pull system that is responsive to real customer demand. The remaining two steps convert from rigid push into flexible pull.

Step 4: Fixed Quantity Production   In step 4 there is no longer a fixed sequence. Instead, we start producing all products in the smallest possible batch size. Iwata used the example of batches of 5. The daily demand for product A is 5, so we will aim to produce *all* products in batches of 5. So, for example, instead of producing just one batch of 15 C's in a day, we would make three batches of 5 spread throughout the day. This is called *fixed volume mixed sequence* production (Figure 15.9).

Why bother doing multiple setups in a day when one batch would do? Isn't this just a waste of time and effort? No. For two reasons. First, this is the next, necessary step toward the goal of perfect flow, making exactly what is required when it is required. Second, it is impossible to reach this goal of perfect flow without learning how to do multiple setups every day without wasting a huge amount of time and effort. Doing it this way forces people to learn; it forces them to apply the tools and techniques of continuous improvement. Without this learning, faster cycles simply aren't possible.

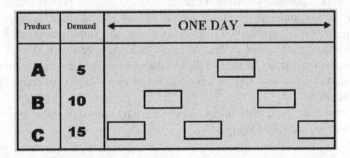

FIGURE 15.9   Fixed-volume mixed-sequence production.

Product	Demand	◄────── ONE DAY ──────►					

FIGURE 15.10   Batches of one.

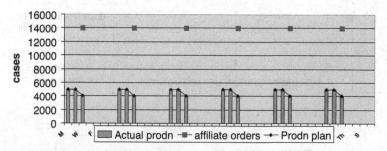

FIGURE 15.11   Affiliate orders and production after leveled production is introduced.

Step 5: One-Piece Flow   What is the next obvious step? Batches of 1 (Figure 15.10).

When people are used to making batches of 300, the idea of making batches of 1 looks like sheer fantasy. But followed properly, these five steps make it possible to make the dream come true. It all rests on the foundation of the five steps of leveled production, *every product every cycle,* and the stability and economies of repetition it delivers. Jumping straight to "pull," that is, responding directly to actual consumer demand without first achieving stability to provide the foundation for sustainable improvement that can be invested in faster and faster cycles, sounds like a recipe for disaster.

So how would our branded FMCG manufacturer organize production under this scenario? First, the American affiliate would order the same quantity each week, to reflect the underlying pattern of demand. Second, the plan would be to produce the same amounts on the same days each week (and production would retain this plan!) as shown in Figure 15.11. This uses exactly the same information as Figure 15.1. It just reorganizes the information to produce a stable repeating pattern that makes more sense.

Conclusion   This is all great in theory, but does it make sense in the real world? When they first come across it, most people and companies think not. If they had just one product with a stable demand, they might be able to do it, they say. But they are faced with many products and anything but stable demand. In this environment

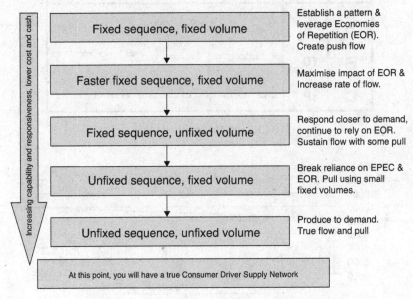

FIGURE 15.12   Five steps of leveled production.

it's just not practical. But Toyota makes many products with varying demand for these products and Toyota used this approach as the foundation of its famous Toyota production system and therefore for lean. Figure 15.12 summarizes the five steps of leveling that Toyota followed. Can your organization make this change?

The circumstances above, in my opinion, form the very basis of lean. I make that assertion from two vantage points. First, I experienced these issues firsthand from years of working with MRP I, MRP II, and ERP systems where functionality is based on mechanical rules of forecasting and scheduling that never reflect reality (and never could). These systems lead to changes being made when they shouldn't and changes not being made when they should. The resulting confusion and wasted effort can be immense.

What Ian says in principle is that stable production systems deliver fewer defects (better quality) and lower costs. Who would argue with that? We all know what routine and repetition (practice, in the words of Tiger Woods) do for learning and improvement.

The old school adherents will be thinking here that this is a production-driven mentality—we moved away from that to become customer driven! That is true up to a point. Mass production was the extreme as to lack of interest in customer choice. There had to be a move back toward center ground. What the customer-focused opposite end forgot, though, was that typically the plant did not supply the end customer, they supplied intermediaries; and the intermediaries distorted demand so that relatively smooth demand in the end market was subject to violent swings in the plant. This then led to the issues that Ian describes.

Whereas other companies have readjusted their approach, most pharmaceutical firms still use forecasts and MRP II to drive their facilities. Massive blister packers that take hours to change over are running orders for individual customers that take minutes to produce, all because the forecasts say so. We discuss this at greater length in Chapter 17. Now we move on to our next speaker.

Ranjana Pathak is a systems thinker living in the heart of pharmaceuticals. Dr. Pathak discovered systems thinking when it fitted clearly with her experiences in the world of quality and compliance, in which she is so proficient.

GUEST CONTRIBUTOR SLOT: RANJANA PATHAK

Systems Thinking and Compliance Within the Pharmaceutical Industry

So what is the connection between systems thinking and the pharmaceutical industry? As I was reading *The Fifth Discipline* by Peter Senge,[11] I began to see the relevance of systems thinking and its relation to compliance within the pharmaceutical environment. Before illustrating my point, I would like to explain briefly what systems thinking is. Scholars such as Ludwig von Bertalanffy, Peter Senge, Richard Scott, Charles Perrow, and Howard Aldrich have described and applied systems theory where decision making, the environment, growth, hierarchical order, dominance, control, and competition have been known to play an integral part within the system.[12] All these components are not unique to the pharmaceutical industry alone and play a critical role in the overall growth of a company and its people. However, these do not fall under the GxP controls but greatly influence compliance.

I would ask the reader to view the entire organization as a system with subsystems within it. For example, each unit is a subsystem (manufacturing, quality assurance, laboratory, finance, information technology, research and development, etc.). People are another subsystem within this bigger system. The decisions that people make in one part of an organization affect people in another part of the same organization. If there is lack of collaboration or consultation, the impact of these decisions can be negative or positive.

Processes, procedures, and policies are the tangible parts of the systems; decision making, personnel management, motivating employees, and influencing others are some of the intangible pieces. Yet they are intertwined where a person in one area has an impact on another in another part of the organization. Alternatively, action taken in part of an organization may influence another process in another department. Although this may seem obvious to many, it is not always the mindset of all decision maker, and decisions are made in a vacuum. This is where systems thinking can be taught, utilized, and applied.

The pharmaceutical industry is highly regulated and structured. The FDA expects compliance with all applicable regulations, and the patient expects companies to be socially responsible and do the right thing. A systems theory framework may be used to indicate how breakdown in one area affects another area within a pharmaceutical company. A *system* is defined as "a set of elements standing in interrelations"[13]. Any change within a system, such as a process, has an impact on other parts of the organization relative to the manufacture and distribution of products.

Problems such as concerns for quality, maintenance, sales, budgets, profits, and employment issues have required the urgent attention of executive leaders in most industries, as is the case in the pharmaceutical industry. These concerns may present administrative challenges for a manager who may experience career shifts every two years and who may not be able to evaluate long-term organizational needs effectively.

Kovner and Neuhauser[14] asserted that organizations are people and things combined together to achieve goals in an environment with limited resources which is constantly changing. Kovner and Neuhauser proposed: "Organizations create different internal cultures" (p. 132). So if the culture of an organization typically is to make decisions without adequate interaction between those who will be affected by the decision and those making the decision, it can have a spiraling effect that unbalances the organization. Such an imbalance can affect compliance.

As postulated by Von Bertalanffy,[15] systems can be open or closed. Physical systems that are isolated from their environment, such as reactions in physical chemistry, are considered *closed systems*. *Open systems*, such as society, are similar to living organisms. Systems theory is capable of dealing with these matters (as cited by Lin). The environment within this context is an open system.

Scott claimed that the structure of an open system is complex due to the variability of individual parts and participants and the connections between them (as cited by Lin). For these reasons, systems thinking is a good fit for the pharmaceutical industry, where activities to accomplish work can involve processing information between people or between people and information. Boundaries are set which are based on interdependent, interpersonal role behaviors and activities (as cited by Lin).

At its basic level, compliance demonstrates the desired state of adherence with the law, a regulation, or a demand.[16] An assumption may be that compliance is simply a measure of a standard, but compliance goes beyond basic and minimal adherence. The responsibility for proof of compliance rests on the entity is being regulated (Hutter, 1997). In our context here, within the pharmaceutical industry, compliance is affected by the failure of any of the subsystems or if the interactions between subsystems are not assessed as a whole.

Senge[17] noted that system thinking is a conceptual framework of events that are distant in time and space yet connected within the same pattern or that have an influence on each other. In this regard, there are no isolated parts within a system, and if viewed in isolation or as snapshots, the severest problems may never be resolved. This is what often happens in the pharmaceutical industry, often referred to as "one hand doesn't know what the other is doing." Process, procedures, equipment, environment, and people become a pivotal component of a system that relies on establishing an environment that will sustain compliance to federally mandated practices.

Senge postulated that businesses and other human endeavors are systems bound by invisible threads of interrelated actions whose effect can be felt after many years. Senge noted that those involved have difficulty seeing patterns change because the tendency is to focus on snapshots rather than the whole. "Systems thinking is a conceptual framework, a body of knowledge and tools that have been developed over the past fifty years, to make the full patterns clearer, and to help us see how to change them effectively."[18]

Among increased federal guidelines and FDA scrutiny of manufacturing and quality control processes, managers are doing their best to avoid regulatory notices. "Imperatives that must exist within an organization include senior management's philosophy, commitment, and follow-through; staff-level commitment and follow-through; training and documentation, correct materials and workflows, and finally compliant equipment and utility systems."[19] Organizations are influenced by the interactions of all components that have an overall effect on the whole from a systems perspective.[20]

For example, if the person responsible for purchasing, purchases material from an unqualified vendor, this decision jeopardizes the vendor certification program that is in place. If this unqualified material follows the manufacturing stream, the final product is made using this material, and the product gets released for distribution, it puts the company at risk for having released a lot of product that was manufactured using unqualified material, which in turn affects the compliance state of the company. This is a case of not using systems thinking.

The feedback mechanism suggested by the gurus of systems thinking is to see the reality by seeing what the influencing factors are and then to address the root cause of problems—in this case, compliance. Senge (1990) postulates that in using systems thinking the flow of influence should be traced to see if a pattern exists and if this pattern is repeating itself. This feedback mechanism is essential to individual pharmaceutical organizations. This feedback allows the pharmaceutical professional to understand what is working and why and assess that if something is not working, it should be corrected, rectified, or changed. Reinforce what is working and balance what is not!

Howard and McKinney[21] viewed systems theory as an organization in which individual subunits of a broader system are interdependent of other system units, and the functioning or malfunctioning of one affects the other. The system strives to achieve balance as it adapts and changes. In the pharmaceutical industry, changes in regulations, technology, and personnel are frequent, and these changes make it challenging to remain complaint. Systems thinking can increase awareness within people to show how one part of a system affects the other and hence must be considered when making changes.

Dr. Pathak has been able to leverage her interest and knowledge of systems to great effect at her company, Endo Pharmaceuticals—something for us all to emulate on a continuing basis.

15.4   AN APPROACH TO SCM BASED ON SYSTEMS THINKING

15.4.1   Basic Principle on Systems Dynamics

It is beyond the scope of this book to attempt to develop an exemplar approach to production systems—there are enough experts working on that as it is. What can be presented here, however, is some practical way of working that would help pharma-ceuticals move forward based on what has gone before in this and earlier chapters and what we cover in Chapter 16. The framework will be based on systems think-ing as the only true way to create successful supply chains that deliver competitive advantage. The suggestions will be targeted at ways of using knowledge of systems dynamics to inform action, including preventive and corrective actions (relating to any organizational challenge). It will not be any more exhaustive a treatment than is required to inform the transformational ways discussed in Chapter 17.

We begin with an understanding of the high-level concept of systems thinking based on my personal experience.

Observations, Views, and Experiences of the Author

Some years ago, I had a problem whereby I was prone to a stiff neck on my right side whenever I exercised or did any lifting. My GP, after some investigation, suspected that it was something to do with the muscles in my shoulder. I was prescribed anti-inflammatory tablets, which fixed the problem while I was taking the tablets—but guess what happened when I stopped. After a few further unsuccessful attempts by the GP to find a solution, she referred me (under private medical insurance coverage, luckily) to an orthopedic surgeon who specialized in shoulders.

From my appointment and brief consultation with the surgeon, I was sent for an MRI scan to help the diagnosis (that was not a cheap diagnostic). On the follow-up appointment, the specialist informed me that the news was good—no need for surgery. That was somewhat surprising to me because the prospect of surgery had never entered my head. There was wear and tear in the shoulder, but nothing more. I was dispatched to a local physiotherapist.

After three sessions of physio and no apparent improvement, he began to use chiropractic techniques on me. His opinion was that this would be more appropriate and referred me to an experienced practitioner in chiropractic. This was only partially successful and I was resigned to living with the problem for life (as I had been advised if the last-ditch attempt did not work).

So I did just that. Until I saw a new sports massage clinic advertised by the local hospital. The physiotherapist there, who looked as if she didn't have the strength to manipulate a mouse let alone a full-grown adult, took my through the diagnostic. This is what happened from there.

First, it was deep friction work where the pain was occurring. It was excruciating at times but felt as if it was doing some good. I than had to use ice packs to continue to get the inflammation down. Once it was settled down over the course of some days, she strapped my shoulder back with some standard hospital tape. It was a strange arrangement whereby the plaster hooked on to the end of my shoulder and pulled it back. It was doing something that the muscle had stopped doing. A few more days like this and I could feel my shoulder muscle was beginning to work a bit more.

A replacement of the tape and a few more days left the shoulder feeling as if it was doing things that it had not done for some time. To cut a long story short, she then worked down the major muscles of my back and eventually identified the culprit. Correction involved exercising a muscle I didn't even know I had. I still don't know what it is called, but it lay in the front of the pelvis and is the first muscle that is supposed to begin the engagement of the stabilizing muscles when exertion is to take place (apologies in advance to all physios for the description). That is what leads to the stabilizing muscle in the shoulder pulling the entire thing into alignment so that the major muscles take the strain. Mine was not working, so I was using the smaller muscles in my shoulder and neck, and hence the pain and stiffness. Problem solved!

Well, not completely, because on reflection I remembered a small injury I had when rowing in the gym years earlier. The GP had again given me an anti-inflammatory for the pain. The discomfort left after a few days, but the problem was not solved (in hindsight). My body had remembered that was a weak spot and began to compensate. This was the root cause of the initial problem. If I ever start to feel it these days, I know exactly what to do,

This demonstrates how problems (pain) can have their roots in very distant places; also, how remedial work has to occur in totally unexpected places before sustainable solutions are found. It is so easy for improvement efforts to pinpoint exactly the wrong areas and potentially make things worse.

Another factor involves how causes of problems can resist diagnostic processes even when they are carried out by experts. Sometimes, the solutions are held by those much closer to the problem, yet seemingly less qualified. The physio, although not an orthopedic surgeon, had learned to follow the systemics of the human frame from an intimate knowledge of the muscle and ligament linkages. Unfortunately, although the principle holds for any systems, production systems are infinitely more interconnected and subject to noise than is the human frame. So how does one go about dealing with more complex systems problem?

First, then, a recap on systems dynamics is in order. A system is made up of inputs to a conversion process to create outputs. It is an open system if there is no adjustment to allow for changes. For example, a central heating system would be an open system if there were no thermostat. Without a thermostat sensing the ambient temperature and correcting for differences from the desired temperature, it would be freezing in winter and boiling in summer. A temperature-controlled heating system is a closed system, where there is feedback and comparison of actual versus desired. Inputs to the system are then adjusted based on the gap to be closed.

Under controlled conditions, the system will tend to maintain a steady state. Control theory often models a system's response to a step change (a step response) applied to a system for it to achieve a new steady state. The speed of response depends on lags (time delays) in the system, and this affects the degree to which the system may overshoot the new state before homing in. This is the measure of the system's instability. Long-time lags are not good to have in systems.

That was a brief, layperson's explanation of systems dynamics. It will not be necessary to delve any further for the needs of this book. We have established some basics on systems. That is not the end of it because as we know, organizational systems are not that mechanistic; but the principles are helpful. Expanding from a single system to joined, interconnecting thousands of sub systems that make up an entire system, some open, some closed, suggests the scale of control and coordination required. Ways of working must respect the particular constraints of systems in terms of the need to maintain control and make allowance for human failings.

Attention now turns to a potentially game-changing approach.

15.4.2 A Practical Model

From here on, the focus is on pharmaceutical products as outputs from production systems. The inputs are the various materials, people, and resources used by the systems of conversion. The conversion systems (including laboratory prototypes) are the end-to-end arrangement of facilities, machinery, and equipment, and the associated information flows. The output from a production system is determined by the nature of the inputs and conversion processes. The converse is therefore also true. The output demanded of a production system determines the nature of the inputs and conversion process. In other words, you get what you ask for. By limiting what we ask for from clinical trial supply chains, the production system suffers accordingly.

Below is a suggested alternative. Please remember that the terms *production system* and *end-to-end supply chain* are treated as the same systemic entity. Also, there is nothing new here; it can all be taken form the approaches that have been taken since the days of Deming in the early 1950s.

1. *Be clear on the required outputs of a system. Effective* supply chains and productions systems can only be designed through a deep understanding of the outputs required. That includes close engagement with end customer's (patient's) needs. This is the point also made in the first principle of lean. It is also made in many other approaches, such as TQM, WCM, and six sigma. It is not always well understood, however. In fact, this is where these approaches are often insufficient compared to the strategic marketing methods explained by Malcolm McDonald. Understanding customers is much more than "delighting the customer," because that in itself makes a one-size-fits-all assumption. The relevance of this for pharmaceutical supply chains is that this idea of getting close to customer segments has produced consistent business success. It may not work every time, but those who try are more likely to make a success of things.

2. *Focus the organization on delivery of the required outputs as specified by end customers.* This is the equivalent of concurrent engineering in other sectors. Readers may research further into how this has led to dramatically improved results. The sources cited throughout this book should be a good starting point. For pharmaceutical companies, this means doing a strange and daring thing. It means including those, traditionally at the end of a process, at the beginning. That doesn't sound too scary, though, does it?

3. *Organize the conversion processes around product families.* This involves putting more emphasis on patient value and arranging processes to deliver. In simple terms it includes such things as joining up production machinery and equipment,

making closer supplier relationships, simplifying business processes, and introducing stability into schedules.

4. *Make production workers (value adders) central to purposeful activity.* The rationale behind this is that the value adders are responsible for creating the physical product in the end customer's hands. Their activities are therefore converting latent value into realized value. That value is otherwise known as cash in the bank. Everyone else should be behind them in making that happen.

5. *Build effective supporting linkages along the end-to-end supply chain.* This comprises all the activities of the SCM holistic; it builds a business process support framework for production systems to operate effectively. This aspect often takes a backseat in lean workings, but it is critical to have all this in place for success.

6. *Develop stable schedules that respect natural constraints.* This involves taking the supertanker effect from Chapter 1 into account. Supply chain systems contain natural lags (delays) and responses that work against changes. The level loading method described by Ian Glenday aims to reduce those lags by increasing cycle frequency. If that work has not been done, those lags can be significant and destabilize the system in delivering the end result. The use of master production scheduling is one good way to set a road map to stability, in advance of true stability leading to pull scheduling.

7. *Produce inventory so that it flows through the system constraint.* Make inventory travel through the supply chain at a rate consistent with end demand. Hold inventory in sufficient quantity to maximize the OEE of the constraint. Synchronize all other operations and equipment with the constraint. Remembering TWT, long lead times necessitate higher inventory holdings. This is a fact of life that cannot be changed.

8. *Strive to minimize the time required by the system to complete a full cycle.* A vitally important contribution to production systems made by Taiichi Ohno was to highlight the importance of minimizing the time between receiving and satisfying a customer order. This means, that if I arrive at a supplying company's door, and the last remaining product has just gone to the preceding customer, how long do I need to wait for the next? This is, in effect, working to the principles of level production as described by Ian Glenday.

9. *Manage the system as a whole.* This brings us back to Deming and all the other commentators making the point forcefully that improvement can only be made at the level of the entire system. The discussion above covers the system mechanics. In Chapter 16 we cover the organizational and cultural aspects.

Before moving on to that, let's enjoy a success story on the nutty noggins front.

A Helpful Metaphor

Dad was indeed delighted with the results from his lean training. When he extended his product lines to delicate dough balls and puffy puddings, his first instinct was to fill the kitchen with faster mixers, bigger proving/baking ovens, and automated packers. This would, in theory, allow him to get his ingredients through into products at maximum speed and efficiency. Having been warned of the failings in the process village way of working, he decided that forewarned is forearmed.

What Dad did then was to arrange his equipment in sequential operations so that all the nutty noggins went down one line, the delicate dough balls another, and the puffy puddings a third. The equipment was roughly the same for each, except there was a proofing oven stage for the dough balls. Instead of buying massively expensive equipment to run at high speed, he used his existing stuff and also bought some second hand. One or two new brand new pieces were purchased, but these were selected for quick changeover rather than absolute speed.

He then made sure that the variety of products within each family could be accommodated by the setup. This he did with some simple spreadsheet calculations based on anticipated demand from end customers (takt) and demonstrated capacity. Next, he worked on setup times so that he could change from one product to another as quickly as possible (remember Shingo from Section 12.3.12?). He found this tough, but on giving Ian Glenday a call he was charged with renewed vigor and made massive strides; also, he made sure that there was a total productive maintenance program in place and operating. Any failures now and the entire supply chain would come to a halt.

When business began, customers would draw from the shelves, and when inventory levels were getting low, a signal was sent to top up the reservoir to keep within a min–max tolerance. It all worked like clockwork! Life for Dad was rosy as it also was too for Mom and the kids.

16 Building a Foundation for Sustainable Change

16.1 FOCUS ON THE INDIVIDUAL

This chapter begins with a quotation:

> Our deepest fear is not that we are inadequate, our deepest fear is that we are powerful beyond measure.
>
> It's our light, not our darkness, that most frightens us. We ask ourselves: Who am I to be brilliant, gorgeous, talented, and fabulous?
>
> Actually, who are you not to be? You are a child of the universe. Your playing small doesn't serve the world. There is nothing enlightening about shrinking, so that other people won't feel insecure around you. We are born to make manifest the glory of the universe that is within us. It's not just in some of us: It is in everyone. And as we let our own light shine, we unconsciously give other people permission to do the same. And as we are liberated from our own fear, our presence automatically liberates others.[1]
>
> —Marianne Williamson

The quotation above sets the scene for the chapter. Many readers will be familiar with these words, often quoted in relation to personal and spiritual development. The originator of the words, Marianne Williamson, became widely known following an appearance on the Oprah Winfrey show. She really is an inspirational being and her book, *A Return to Love*, is a recommended read.

Readers may be wondering why a book on the apparently mechanistic topic of SCM starts in such a manner. The reason is this. Supply chains are run by human beings and as we all know, to a greater or lesser extent, each human being is an emotional and spiritual entity. If humans are at the helm, then the study of them and their inherent unpredictability must be included. There is also another reason. Marianne Williamson's belief in God is profound and undeniable in all her writings and through her various communication media. None of it, though, smacks of being founded on religious dogma. It is one person's lifelong learning on the way that things work naturally according to forces we know little about.

Observations, Views, and Experiences of the Author

I do not subscribe to any particular religion, but I do believe in the existence of some kind of universal "way." What strikes me from my limited knowledge of Marianne Williamson's beliefs is that she follows a universal truth that does not depend on the dictate of a specific religion. Her ways seem to get at the right and sensible ways to be in the world. Read her work and see what you think. I bring it up here because I truly believe that we have developed "religions" in our efforts relating to running customer serving organizations and their supply chains. There are so many camps, marshaled under canvass, that claim to be the answer to all our woes. We have lean vs. agile—what is that all about? How can a supply chain be agile given what we have learned about the length, complexity, and interdependencies involved? Yes, it is possible to design a supply chain system to be responsive to certain defined levels of variation at the customer face. Dell, for example, has proved that this can be done by configuring personal computers to specific customer requirements. We are kidding ourselves, though, if we believe that there is no supporting supply chain below that top level that needs stability and a level of inherent predictability to perform. The way to achieve this stability is described by Ian Glenday in Chapter 15, but surprisingly few in the religious faith that is lean make that connection.

So we also have six sigma and lean sigma (not sure who invented that combination?), just in time (or "just too late" as many heretical nonbelievers dubbed it), optimized production technology (OPT), total quality management (TQM), theory of constraints (ToC), world class manufacturing (WCM), and business process reengineering (BPR). All of these are perfectly valid and appropriate ways of dealing with aspects of running successful supply chains and production systems. The founders and developers of the approaches have been equally insightful in developing fresh ways to view and solve problems.

The problem only emerges when followers become fanatical about finding an answer in the faith, to the exclusion of alternative approaches. In effect, they stop learning by doing what seems right in favor of following a set of prescriptive rules. This is therefore the starting point for a chapter on creating and sustaining change for the better. This builds on the exemplar systems–based approaches discussed in Chapter 15. Let us all keep open minds and speak up when actual outcomes from a particular "religion" do not yield to expectation; also, let us recognize that supply chains do conform to certain "universal" laws that should be the pursuit of all those with a stakeholder interest and teach each other what these are.

So, starting with those inspirational words of Marianne Williamson and the thoughts above, the underpinning theme of this chapter is the human being, otherwise known as a person or an individual. Use of the term *person* or *individual* may seem an irrelevant detail, but in my opinion it is fundamental. So often the word *people* is used in the context of human interaction in business. We use terms such as *people skills, good or bad with people, people management* and similar phrases. We forget that *people* is plural and accordingly leads to a focus on people in aggregate. This can be totally unhelpful, since it gives the impression that there can be a set of simplifying assumptions that can inform ways of working with humans as an amorphous "blob." This draws focus away from individuals toward teams, groups, and organizations. While these are all important topics, the building blocks are individuals.

A Helpful Metaphor

In the same way, a chemical compound is made up of atoms joined together to form molecules joined together to form increasingly complex chemical structures, such are organizations. Scientific progress in chemistry would never have been made without the discovery and deep understanding of atoms. The concept of the individual is similar, although not identical, since for every atom type there are trillions that are exactly the same, or so it seems to us humans at our current level of knowledge. Who knows, though, maybe an atom has a personality to set itself apart!

The point of the metaphor is to establish the concept of the individual person as the underpinning building block of all work on culture, leadership, management of change, teams, and group dynamics.

Observations, Views, and Experiences of the Author

My original degree in production engineering was termed a "sandwich" degree, which meant combining study with practical experience in industry. It was a "thin" sandwich, requiring spells at two different companies. The first was for six months learning the skills of engineering "on the bench" at what was then the British Steel Corporation (now Corus). The second was at a company supplying rack-and-pinion steering gear to a wide range of automotive manufacturers (now part of TRW). It was through these experiences that I changed the focus of my degree to specialize in industrial engineering, having realized how fundamental the human component was in the world of organizations.

What I had discovered in the world of real work was that we all seemed to acknowledge but still behave as if we were not aware of the human element. People are often irrational, emotional, self-seeking, competitive, and fearful. They can also be sensitive, caring, unselfish, collaborative, and committed to the greater good of all. The early conclusion I came to was that a person needed to be a clinical psychologist to maintain a successful career in any organization. Getting hold of even the simplest piece of information from someone in another department was often like pulling teeth. Why do you want it? Who asked you for it? Who will you give it to? Why is it your business? These question were not always raised directly—in fact, rarely were they raised—but the looks and pauses gave away the silent musings every time.

For this reason, I decided to start the chapter with the individual. Remarkably (and some may say I would say this, wouldn't I), after starting the chapter I looked over some of the work of Deming that I had included in the draft and was reminded of his identification of the individual as a prime focus. Great minds think alike, I thought! Whatever the truth, he and I agree on this point. In fact, it is hard for me to think of any of Deming's work that I don't agree with. The puzzling fact is why the world went on to study his star pupil(s) rather than the tutor!

Now to move on to some important frameworks from the world of organizational development and change. Nothing heavy, just enough to relate the world of academic progress with the practical realities of building, managing, and improving supply chains.

From the foregoing, the premise is that for improvement to take effect, leadership, group, and organizational performance must ultimately permeate to the individual level. Organizations are made up of separate people working together toward an end goal (hopefully!). Leaders are individuals, managers are individuals, production operators are individuals, chemists are individuals—the list is endless.

This has huge implications for those working in and studying culture and leadership in organizations. The vast amount of literature on the subject is predicated on the fact that, eventually, individuals will think and behave differently. True, individuals behave differently in groups and varying cultural settings, which should be understood. However, that behavior can alter only if a person decides that it will. Leaders as individuals can be immensely influential in creating the right environment. That in itself needs the leader, "as individual," to act in a particular way. So as the chapter traces through groups, teams, cultures, management styles, and other organizational aspects, retain the notion that it is "we," as individual human beings, that hold the magic ingredient.

This should motivate readers to research the area of personal development. There are plenty of books that cover personal development and influencing skills that are worthy of exploration. There are also many that are a waste of time. Here are a few areas worth exploration from my experience.

Observations, Views, and Experiences of the Author

These are some of my favorite books on personal development:

- Dale Carnegie: *How to Win Friends and Influence People.*[2] *This book drives home the all-important message that the only route to influence is by taking a genuine interest in others. It is very easy to read and can seem to some as "pop psychology," the underlying serious messages are a million miles from lightweight.*
- Steven Covey: *Seven Habits of Highly Effective People.*[3] *With a focus on timeless principles by which to run one's life, this is right on the money. A particularly powerful point made for Western society is the emphasis on taking time to build and nurture relationships.*

- John J. Emerick, Jr., *Be the Person You Want To Be*[4] This in the best treatment and demystifier of neurolinguistic programming that I have come across. It really helps explain how certain effective ways of behaving can be developed even if they do not come naturally.
- Eric Bernie: *I'm OK, You're OK.*[5] This book covers transactional analysis and the relevance of strokes and discounts (rewards and penalties) in everyday life—although that is a vast oversimplification of this an important work.
- Benjamin Hoff, *The Tao of Pooh.*[6] You have to read this to appreciate it! It's a wonderful exploration of Taoism in relation to life in the West. Pooh is portrayed as the original "uncarved block," the one who asks the stupid questions that are not always quite so stupid.

Readers are encouraged to start anywhere, as long as they build an increasingly better understanding of how they fit in and perform in the world and develop accordingly. Don't be fooled, however, into thinking that this is the answer to organizational effectiveness. It is just a part. Deming made it clear that organizational systems design and operation was the major factor in things going wrong. Part of this includes the impact of group dynamics (conscious and unconscious politicking), which can override the best intentions of the individual. The personal development of individuals is about recognizing that and working with others to make the right corrections required to stay on course whenever possible.

Another important commentator on the topic is Peter Senge, who has a personal development message in his book *The Fifth Disciple.*[7] It is termed *personal mastery* and is one of the five disciplines, along with systems thinking, mental models, building shared vision, and team learning. Senge's messages are very consistent with mine, although his come from far deeper research in an academic sense. His assertion is that these five areas must be present for effective organizational functioning, or to become the learning organisation.

This section on the individual ends with the words of Deming and with my personal experience of the work of Peter Senge. Deming first[8]:

> The first step is transformation of the individual. This transformation is discontinuous. It comes from understanding of the system of profound knowledge. The individual, transformed, will perceive new meaning to his life, to events, to numbers, to interactions between people.

> Once the individual understands the system of profound knowledge, he will apply its principles in every kind of relationship with other people. He will have a basis for judgment of his own decisions and for transformation of the organizations that he belongs to. The individual, once transformed, will:

> Set an example;

> Be a good listener, but will not compromise;

> Continually teach other people; and

> Help people to pull away from their current practices and beliefs and move into the new philosophy without a feeling of guilt about the past.

Human beings in the Western world certainly often find these traits difficult to cultivate. Being a good listener can be taken as not standing out for further promotions. Teaching others is about sharing knowledge and information without fear of losing a power base. Shaking off old ideas and beliefs can mean admission of failure, often regarded as a sign of weakness.

Personal Observations, Views, and Experiences of the Author

I was fortunate enough to attend one of Senge's workshops in London in 1995.[9] There was too much content to recount here, but there was one section that focused on the role of dialogue in the learning organization. The entire audience of nearly 200 delegates was asked to take part in the exercise. It involved just one person speaking at a time without being interrupted until they had finished. There was no judgment of the contribution, just receptivity. It went on until fewer ideas were contributed as thoughts started to dry up. Then silences started to occur. There was to be no shame in silences. Individuals in the audience waited until the next comment and contemplated each thought. Senge contrasted this "dialogue" with "discussion," which he aligned with percussion, a kind of collision of views.

I have since had the experience of working for a Japanese company, and in conversation with Western colleagues observed the tendency in groups for this type of absence of competitive speaking. Often, meetings would be silent when there was no more to be said on a topic. Is this food for thought for us here in the West?

Now it is time to move on to individuals occupying specific roles in organizations.

16.2   INDIVIDUALS AS LEADERS

To start this section, we hear form a leading expert, Donna Ladkin.

GUEST CONTRIBUTOR SLOT: DONNA LADKIN

Leadership in Supply Chain Management Roles

Hedley will make a strong case in this section for the importance of organizational leadership in mobilizing meaningful change within supply chain management and in organizations generally. Here, I'd like to reflect on the kind of leadership that might make the most effective impact within the context of the specific needs of SCM.

One of the problems with the word *leadership* itself is that it often conjures up images of heroic men on white horses charging in to save the day. Of course, every once in awhile, situations call for that mode of leading (e.g., when there is a "life or death" situation at hand). But within the context of SCM, when the people who are being "led" are often expert professionals in their own right who may consider themselves to be leaders in their own fields, heroic leadership can often get people's backs up rather than mobilizing meaningful change.

So what are leaders of such situations to do? One thing that might help in answering this question is considering a different positioning of leaders within constellations of people engaged in collective action. Whereas we often think of leaders as occupying the top of organizational hierarchies, from which they spearhead initiatives, perhaps within the supply chain context it might be more helpful to think of leaders as occupying the center of a hub of interconnecting relationships. Rather than overtly directing, the leader's role becomes facilitating conversations between key people and professions. In this way, rather than directing, the job of leading becomes one of connecting people with different expertise, experience, and contacts in order that they can work together to achieve jointly recognized goals.

"Leading from the middle" turns on its head many of the traditional concepts associated with the concept. For example, instead of necessarily providing a vision, such leadership requires having a perspective about the interconnecting aspects of the organization and the many stakeholders who need to be involved to obtain the most effective ways forward. Rather than spending a lot of time communicating their own message, the leader needs to spend much more time listening to the many different priorities, agendas, and concerns that will support, or thwart, new initiatives. Perhaps most important, instead of providing the right answers, leading in this way requires asking the right questions, questions that will get to the heart of issues which will enable synergies within supply chains to be realized.

This style of leading poses a number of challenges for those who can see the benefits of taking up the role in this way. It requires the ability to work with emergence rather than working to a plan. It requires the capacity to listen to many different views of a situation and competing commitments and discern which priority really needs attention. It also requires shedding attachment to any egocentric understanding of leading, and in its place attending to the purpose toward which leadership as a collective endeavor can flourish into effective organizational realities.

There is so much to pick up on in those few paragraphs; where should we start?

First, for some readers, the realization may be that they are leaders and did not even realize it! Joining up the strands that lead to necessary connections and outcomes is positive leadership behavior. Since it is not always done with vested authority, these ways of behaving can be stopped in their tracks. Old-fashioned leaders often see this as threatening behavior to be curtailed at once. Their authority lever will allow them to do it. This is where the concept of the individual returns. The individual as leader, in the traditional management system, behaves as you or I probably would be tempted to behave given the value system around us. High-performing subordinates plotting positive connections can divert the limelight in unwelcome ways for bosses. Hands up anyone who wouldn't feel a twinge of the little green monster; but Donna's comment on shedding attachment to the ego is the key starting point. Many organizations must address the ideas held about leadership in order to advance.

Then there is also the personal challenge for the pathfinder of listening and questioning, often in environments where there is intense pressure to move forward, or taking other views into consideration when time is tight. This can often be perceived as weak behavior, and it takes courage to hold firm ground. Often, even that is not enough if your job is on the line.

There is much more in all of this and, again, individuals should research the work of Donna and others in this field. Just one more point that is implicit in Donna's contribution here. She talks about leadership in SCM. This leads nicely to a critical aspect of leadership: the contingency dimension. There are situations that *do* require a very directive style. Things need to happen quickly and the leader has a full grasp of what needs to be done to steer the situation to a successful conclusion. The emergency services attending a road accident would be one situation. Similarly, in situations where the way forward is clear and the leader has most of or all the answers, the directive approach is often the most appropriate. Setting up a new production department (especially where good manufacturing practices are present) may be such a situation, where operators need to learn the correct methods and ways of working and there is only one best way of achieving the final result. This concept, known as contingency theory in leadership texts, is recommended as an area worthy of exploration for budding leaders of industry.

16.3   INDIVIDUALS AS MOTIVATORS AND THE MOTIVATED

Some individuals appear more highly motivated to achieve outcomes than others. That is a fact of life. What is not a fact is that they were born that way, or that is how they are in all aspects of their lives. Who doesn't have an example of an individual in a routine, unremarkable job who has major achievements in their out-of-work activities? In personal terms also, sometimes we find ourselves in situations that make us come alive and others where we are mind-numbingly bored. There are extremes, of course, where some appear to "buzz" most of their waking hours, whereas others seem to live in almost constant hibernation. Somewhere in between is where most of us reside, and this is where knowledge of the two sides of motivation is important.

Much has been written on this topic, and the work of pioneers such as Maslow and Herzberg is well documented. Maslow spoke of a hierarchy of needs[10] and Herzberg of hygiene factors[11] (those that can make you unhappy but not get you going) and motivating factors (those that give you a reason to wake up in the morning). The work of both should be in the reader's armory. To some extent as well, Elton Mayo's Hawthorne experiment informed the world of motivation in an industrial setting. But we are not looking here to build on the theoretical body of knowledge that exists today. The main aim is to examine some practical evidence and thoughts of mine mixed up with some input from guest contributors. The aim is to allow individual readers to factor some positive actions and behavior into their everyday attempts to motivate others and to remain motivated themselves.

We begin with a guest contributor. Before we hear from her, I should mention that she provided me with some (free) business advice through the auspices of the Welsh

Assembly Government.[12] On reading my first attempt at a newsletter, I heard from Ruth Rowe as follows.

I have just had a good look at both the brochure and the newsletter and Web site. What can I say except that I am very, very impressed. Everything looks really professional and perfectly in tune with your experience/credibility and market position.

In no particular order, I loved:

- The layout and colours
- The clarity, eloquence, and emotive nature of the language (e.g., revolutionary results—very powerful, I thought)
- The benefits, which are really clear and leap off the screen at you
- The case studies and testimonials—fantastic! Full of impact but not too long.
- The boxes with arrows!

The only things I was a little unsure about were:

- The use of "we" and then "Hedley," as opposed to "we" again or "PharmaFlow" when talking about work completed.
- American spellings (e.g., specialty). (I think that's probably just me!)
- Maybe a few too many testimonials? I can't decide on that one really.
- "Credentials" as a heading—I think I would use something like "experience" instead.

Hope this is useful. If I can be of any help, please do not hesitate to get in touch.

On the face of it, that may seem to be fairly straightforward, but when I got it, starting with its "blast" of positives, it really perked me up. That made the negatives much easier to read and accept as candidates for change, especially since the negatives raised questions as opposed to making statements of fact. The changes were made quite readily. Looking back now and from working further with Ruth, it is obvious that this is just one of her many motivational strategies.

GUEST CONTRIBUTOR SLOT: RUTH ROWE

Motivation in Business

As a business adviser it could be said that my primary function is to help my clients achieve their commercial goals. Target setting, business planning, and determining strategies based on solid market research are all therefore very important tools in my armory. None of these, nor an encyclopedic knowledge of Maslow's hierarchy of needs or any of the myriad other models that can be used, however, is as crucial as having the ability to actually motivate someone; to spur them into taking life changes won't help unless a client has the desire and determination to put theory into practice when no orders are coming in and the phone seems to have stopped ringing. The above use of militaristic language is no coincidence either, as all great warlords know that rhetoric is effective only if one understands the hearts and minds of one's troops and share a common goal.

The only way to help people to help themselves, in my opinion, is to follow the advice of the Spice Girls and ask them to tell you "what they want, what they really, really want." You will then need to listen carefully to the answers and look closely at the way those answers are delivered. Understanding body language and tone of voice is vitally important if you are to determine the truth and discover what truly makes someone tick.

Listening properly involves much more than just good eye contact and the occasional sage nod of the head; it should involve asking searching and pertinent questions based on what has been said. These should both check and demonstrate your understanding of the answers given and hopefully, by use of an occasional interjection of wise words based on your experience, your client will appreciate both your empathy and your skills. This is crucial, as they must not just listen to your advice but act upon it if their situation is to change, so acting as devil's advocate can be very useful, as it will help you to see how committed they are to bringing their project to life. If you are genuinely interested in people, this behavior is likely to come naturally to you; if you are not, then perhaps it is time to have a long hard think about whether a role where you are required to motivate them is right for you. The skills you will need can be acquired by studying and putting your newfound knowledge into practice. I don't believe it is possible to motivate people unless they believe that you want them to succeed, however, so unless you are the next Daniel Day-Lewis or Emma Thompson, it will be extremely difficult to demonstrate this passion unless it is genuine.

Ruth is a person who takes a deep interest in other people from a genuine will to do the right things. Personal development personified!

16.4   INDIVIDUALS AS GROUP MEMBERS

Next, it is the time to look at groups, and helping us to do this is Elisabeth Goodman.

GUEST CONTRIBUTOR SLOT: ELISABETH GOODMAN

How People (Individuals) Are Integral to Business Process Improvement

Jeffrey Liker, in *The Toyota Way*[13] gives a wonderfully in-depth account of the origins of what we now call *lean*, and of Toyota's strongly human-centric approach to it, something that Western practitioners of lean and six sigma often lose touch with. He suggests that the application of lean is only 20% about the tools, but a big 80% about reflection.

As a practitioner of lean sigma myself, mainly in pharmaceutical R&D, but in both scientific/clinical and business support functions (such as HR, IT, and finance), I have some firsthand experience of just how important what we bring as people is to any business process improvement activity. I will explore this people-centric perspective further through the role of individuals within business process improvement teams.

The Role of Individuals Within Business Process Improvement Teams   Key assets that individuals bring to any work within teams are their knowledge and their own way of thinking, of tackling problems, and of making decisions. I have written in my blogs[14] about the importance of left- and right-brain thinking, intuition (and bias) vs. facts, and the role of "clevers"[15] in relation to problem solving, decision making, and innovation vs. process improvement, and will expand on them here.

1. *Left- and right-brain thinking, creativity, and problem solving.* There is a concern that lean and six-sigma workshop participants often voice when following the DMAIC (define, measure, analyze, improve, control) structured problem-solving approach. They worry that the essentially linear process of identifying the problems (or undesirable effects), then the root causes, then the solutions might only give them the solutions that they would have thought of at the start (i.e., nothing very new), although this approach does have the benefit of building greater cross-team appreciation of the issues that each member faces in his/her work, consensus about the right solutions to adopt, and data to back up the team's recommendations to managers and sponsors.

Lean and six-sigma tools seem to place a special emphasis on left-hand critical/logical thinking. Although there is an opportunity for creative right-brain thinking at various stages, it may not be quite enough. This is why incorporating some form of "blue sky" thinking at some point in the workshop can be very valuable. It is an approach that I have adopted, and it has resulted, not surprisingly, in some new ideas as well as corroboration of those that come up in the more linear process. Participants in workshops that have included blue sky thinking have also demonstrated a greater level of comfort about the opportunities for creative thinking.

2. *Intuition (and bias) vs. facts in problem solving and decision making.* Many management techniques, lean and six sigma included, put a lot of emphasis on taking a structured approach to decision making, as in:

- Identifying the criteria against which some options are to be evaluated
- Prioritizing or weighting the criteria
- Scoring the options to be evaluated against each criterion
- Adding up the scores and declaring the option with the top score to be the option of choice

Each step allows for a certain amount of subjectivity, but because this type of exercise is often done in a group, there is some apparent objectivity in the outcome.

However, someone will invariably speak up and say either "Why did we bother doing that? I could have said which option we were going to choose," or "I just can't agree with the outcome." So sometimes a group will end up going with "gut instinct" anyway.

My experience, and that of many other practitioners of lean and six sigma, is that there is a definite role for intuition alongside fact-based analysis of problems and root causes, in the evaluation of potential solutions, and in decision making. The following points from Malcolm Gladwell's book *Blink*[16] are, I think, particularly worth considering:

- There seems to be a particular role for intuition:
  a. When encountering very new or different options for which known criteria are just not valid.
  b. Where decisions based on intuition just cannot be explained in a logical way (although Malcolm Gladwell gives some very poignant examples of how experts can learn to interpret their intuition).
- Conversely, there are circumstances where it would be quite risky to rely on one's intuition:
  a. When under tremendous stress (to a certain extent this could sharpen our decision making, but there is a point beyond which we would make very bad decisions).
  b. When there is just too much information to be digested and we would do better to go back and identify the few critical criteria.
  c. Where our subconscious "houses" prejudices of which we are not conscious, or we are otherwise adversely affected by external factors. This is the most difficult to deal with, because we are not conscious of what is affecting our decisions!

Ben Goldacre's book *Bad Science*[17] elaborates further on this last point:

- *Our brains are conditioned to look for and "see" patterns and causal relationships where there may be only random noise.* Goldacre gives examples of random sequences of numbers that, when presented to people, reveal clusters and patterns where statistical analyses would show that none exist. The ability, rapidly and intuitively, to spot patterns of activity and causal relationships between them, may in the past have been an important survival mechanism for humans, but today can be very misleading in process improvement, where, for example, we want to make sure that we focus our efforts on addressing the truly significant problems. Approaches such as Pareto analysis, quantification of issues (or undesirable effects), and matrix diagrams can help us to review data more objectively and thereby focus on the right things.
- *We have a bias toward positive evidence.* We are much more likely to pay attention to findings that prove our theories than to those that do not. Our natural

bias toward positive evidence is also why process improvement and change management exercises such as force-field analysis, SWOT (strength, weakness, opportunities, threats) analysis, FMEA (failure mode effect analysis), and Six Thinking Hats can be so powerful. Knowledge management practitioners also make a point of capturing "deltas" or "what could be improved" in learning reviews. These tools, when applied to process improvement and decision making, encourage us to think about what might prevent our solutions from succeeding rather than getting carried away by how wonderful they are! They also help us to present this understanding more clearly in our dialogues with our stakeholders (sponsors, colleagues, and customers).

- *Our assessment of the quality of new evidence is biased by what we believe.* If we are aware of this potential pitfall, we can aim to be more receptive to opposing views. In a team of people that have been working together for some time, common beliefs may be more predominant than instances of opposing views. An effective team leader could look out for and encourage differences of opinion as a potential way of overcoming the team's bias in assessing new evidence. Discussions with customers, suppliers, and other stakeholders could also be very powerful for this. In addition, as change practitioners know, we value resistance from stakeholders, as this highlights potential areas for consideration to which those implementing the change may be blind. It seems that we should also value resistance from stakeholders as a counterbalance to the risks of intuition.

3. *The role of "clevers" in innovation vs. process improvement.* Goffee and Jones' definition of *clevers* includes people at the forefront of innovation, such as R&D scientists in the pharmaceutical industry. Many will argue that the role of clevers should focus on innovation rather than on processes, process improvement, or efficiency. My experience of running lean and six-sigma workshops for research scientists in pharmaceutical R&D indicates that effective teams have an iterative dynamic between the two. They develop new models and assays, add them into their screens for new drug candidates, continuously review and improve these processes, and innovate some more.

Final Thoughts on the Value of Knowledge Management Practices in Business Process Improvement Practices more commonly attributed to knowledge management, such as after-action reviews at key milestones, learning reviews or retrospects at the end of projects, and peer-assists at the start of them, are really valuable ways of encouraging reflection and of drawing out and sharing individual knowledge and perspectives across the entire team. Another way that people connect with others beyond their formally assigned teams is that described by knowledge managers as *communities of interest* or *practice*, and in social sciences as *social networks*. By encouraging and supporting (but not formalizing) people's participation in these informal networks, organizations can further enable important reflection, learning and development, innovation, and ultimate input to business process improvement.

To Conclude   The individual members of a team bring their own people-centric slant to the work of the team. It is an astute team leader who not only recognizes the diversity of his/her team, but actively encourages and makes use of it to get the best results beyond the prescribed use of lean and six-sigma tools.

This piece by Elisabeth stands alone as a learning opportunity. One point to reinforce is the iteration in innovation of which Elisabeth speaks. The history of pharmaceutical discovery research and development does not exhibit such an approach in any meaningful sense. It goes back to the "throwing it over the wall" approach that was so characteristic of the design–production interface in mass production through the 1960s and 1970s. Exemplar companies moved away from that and started to design concurrently so that at the critical point for innovation (the concept stage), consideration was also given to the harsh realities of production (a mix of left- and right-brain thinking). Elisabeth's piece speaks wonderfully to the blend of individuals and teams required to achieve that. This is the challenge ahead for real quality by design approaches.

16.5   INDIVIDUALS AS PARTICIPANTS IN CULTURAL CHANGE

At this point the plot begins to unfold. Organizational culture is often defined as "the way we do things around here." It therefore drives the way an organization and individuals within it behave and act. This makes it a very important topic because ultimately the way an organization acts results in either satisfied or disappointed customers, motivated or downbeat suppliers, pumped-up or brain-dead employees.

In my opinion, any work on culture has to begin with the work of Ed Schein. He is a prolific commentator and author on the vitally important softer (human) side of organizations. If readers only ever get the chance to enquire into one source of knowledge on this topic, it has to be *Organizational Culture and Leadership*, by Edgar H. Schein.[18] There is so much tremendous insight there it is not possible to do it full justice here. As a starter, though, some of the points are outlined below.

Schein's work defines three levels of culture: artifacts, espoused beliefs and values, and underlying (basic) assumptions. The first two levels are observable and tangible but are not easy to make sense of, as they relate to the heart of an organization. Walking around any plant or office building, for example, there may be performance monitoring charts on the wall, banners shouting "The Customer Is King," and mission and values statements positioned in strategic locations. In my experience, these bear little relation to what actually goes on in an organization day to day. Reality may paint a totally different picture. Attitudes toward quality, for example, may belie the messages on the wall.

This is the cultural level that Schein terms *basic assumptions*. This is where culture lives and breathes. This is the unseen, unspoken level that is the script by which the players act; and one of the important lessons from Schein's work is that change can be sustainable only if it gets at the root cause of behaviors—basic assumptions. We explore this further with a personal example.

Observations, Views, and Experiences of the Author

Since my professional work comprises a mix of consultancy and interim management assignments, I experience culture as a "newcomer" on a regular basis. I have seen it written that the best source of information on the existing culture of an organization is to talk to a new arrival. Those steeped in the culture have long since failed to recognize it. They aren't aware of the forces that act on them.

As a newcomer, actions and behavior contrast immediately with experience of other organizational cultures. You find yourself asking: Why are they behaving like that? Doesn't make any sense. The reason is obvious, of course. They have been conditioned to act that way by the past (and present, vicariously) leaders of the organization through their ways of behaving and acting. No blame or credit to those involved; it must happen to us all if we are to survive for any meaningful period within an organization. Those not resonating with the culture, at least to the minimum extent required, will find themselves on their way, seeking new pastures. The culture will see to that. This is the way that culture reinforces itself, drawing in those that fit and casting off those that don't.

This is why leaders are so important in change; because they form culture over time through their actions and behaviors in response to the challenges of running the organization. If they do not change, the culture won't; and if the culture doesn't, the company performance won't. Let me give an example of how leaders form culture to form behavior patterns within the entire organization. This is based on a previous client company where I was carrying out an interim assignment to build an outsourced supply chain infrastructure. The CEO appointed me and I joined the team as a newcomer who "knew how to make fire," so to speak. At my interview for the role, it was explained that this was a tight-knit outfit; people were supportive of each other; decisions were made quickly; it was an "open culture."

When I started, it certainly was an open plan office arrangement. The CEO had his desk out in the main office. Yet he spent much of his time peering into his PC screen with an imaginary sticker saying "Do Not Disturb" pinned to the side of his head. On the one occasion I attempted to disturb him with a question, it was clearly an irritation—I avoided doing that again. When it came to booking the conference room for meetings, the CEO always got first pick; even if others had booked it previously for their meetings, he would kick them out because his were more important.

In the regular weekly meetings, he would announce that we would make mistakes along the way, but would learn from them. That was just before he would interrogate and berate one of the unfortunate team members who admitted a delay or issue with his or her project. People had long since stopped owning up to mistakes. I quickly realized that they had developed their own coping mechanisms, which basically boiled

down to "looking after number one" so as to survive the interrogations. This meant
preparing a plausible story before the meeting. Luckily for me, I had the secret of fire
and did not have aspirations to stay longer than absolutely necessary. Even then, I
could never get used to people being shouted at for things that were not really their
fault. Those that stayed were the ones that could put up with it. The sensible ones
moved on, or never joined in the first place.

Rather than continue with what could be a long tale on similar lines, I should
get to the moral of the story. That is, within organizations, there are artifacts (open
plan office, potted plants scattered around) and espoused values and beliefs (mission
statement, company values). However, an open plan office does not necessarily mean
an open culture. One has to be around for awhile to distinguish that. Charts on the
wall and MS project plans don't always mean that employees are really concerned
with their performance. It takes awhile to distinguish that also. But after that magic
bit of times, the basic assumptions start to emerge.

In the example above, the leader, in drawing people over the coals for project
delays, will lead to a basic assumption, if it is repeated, that will become ingrained. The
assumption will be something like: If you own up to mistakes, you get kicked—always
cover them up. Another example would be where the importance of customer service
is an espoused belief. If, in practice, the leaders of an organization distance themselves
from customers, such as in the case of banks closing branches and moving to call
centers, this can create a basic assumption along the lines: Customers need to be kept
at arm's length and only need to know what we tell them. Not the best recipe for
customer relations! Clearly, then, to have healthy organizational cultures, there must
be positive basic assumptions. When they exist, they scream out.

From here on, the analysis of culture is based on a documented case study in which
I was personally involved, studied and reported by the UK Advisory, Conciliation and
Arbitration Service (ACAS)[19] as one of four best practice case studies in industrial
relations in Wales in the 1990s. The report was compiled in 1993 by a working
party led by Brian Chaney, convened by ACAS (Wales), representing the companies
concerned. My thanks go to Paul Morris, then head of personnel for Miles Ltd.,
who was the management representative involved; also thanks go to the ACAS head
office for agreeing to share their work with others who could benefit greatly from the
insights. The report is reproduced by kind permission of ACAS.

16.6   CASE STUDY: MILES LTD., BRIDGEND, GLAMORGAN

Ownership   Miles Ltd. is a subsidiary company of Miles, Inc., Indiana, which in
turn is part of the German multinational company Bayer. Miles was bought by Bayer
in the late 1970s as a way to penetrate further into the U.S. market.

Employees   The company currently employs about 270 employees, mainly operators, engineering workers, and lab technicians.

Unionization   Three unions are recognized: the TGWU, AEEU, and MSF. Union membership is close to 100%.

Products   Miles is a pharmaceutical company whose main businesses are as follows:

- *Diagnostic products:* treated strips used for diagnosis of such things as blood sugar levels. This makes up approximately 60 to 65% of the business.
- *Self-medication products:* for example, Alka-Seltzer. This makes up approximately 25% of business.
- *Parental products:* such as sterile vaccines for the treatment of allergies.

All the products produced by Miles are sold within the Bayer Group, both UK market and export.

The Need for Change

Over capacity   Miles had plants in various European countries and some of these duplicated existing Bayer capacity. This duplication increased with the purchase of another company, Technicon, which was bought by Bayer to give increased access to the diagnostic products market. By the late 1980s there was an obvious need for rationalization. Miles at Bridgend had a bad image within the group in terms of costs, customer satisfaction, and industrial relations. These factors made the factory a possible candidate for closure.

Organization   At the end of the 1980s Miles at Bridgend had a steep hierarchical structure; for example, the existing chain of command in the production area was:

- Plant director
- Department manager
- Superintendant (in some cases)
- Supervisor
- Charge hand
- Leading hand
- Operator

This contributed to poor communications and managers who were remote from the shop floor. Management style was one of control: Employees were clocked in and out, money was lost for lateness, and permission had to be asked to leave the line for toilet breaks. Managers indulged in "empire building" and units were operated as separate entities with little lateral communication. Much of the factory was poorly laid out and did not fit the image of a modern pharmaceutical plant.

The Impetus for Change

New Plant Director   In 1989 a new director of plant operations took over the Bridgend plant. He quickly made it clear that if the plant was to survive, drastic changes were necessary. In March 1990 he communicated to the works committee the principles and characteristics that he believed should be present in a progressive plant environment. These became known as "The Vision" and may be summarized as follows:

- Beliefs about people
  - Treat people as mature adults who, if expectations are defined, will discipline themselves as a group to follow rules.
  - People want more than just money from working and would like to grow and develop and contribute their ideas.
  - The majority of people enjoy working in an environment where they are challenged to acquire new skills which are reflected in a progressive compensation structure.
- Organizational structure
  - A simple flat structure with the minimum number of levels, with a simple and effective communication system in place
  - A minimum number of job categories
  - Decentralized budgeting and decision making
  - Clearly defined roles
  - Senior managers who act as coach and counsellor, thinking and planning up to a year ahead
  - Managers who think and plan up to three months ahead, solving issues in a proactive manner
  - Operators who solve day-to-day issues on the line, know and are committed to weekly line expectations and are aware of and involved in future improvements and plans for the plant
- Administrative systems
  - Decentralized administrative responsibility with operators writing standard operating procedures and involved in filling batch manufacturing records
  - Well thought out and consistently administered training programs for all employees in group dynamics, project management, group problem solving, and quality expectations in the pharmaceutical Industry
  - Well-managed and administered progression system with no more than three levels
- Physical facility
  - Logical material flows
  - Minimum work in progress

- Built-in surge
- Flexible lines with easy changeover
- Pharmaceutical standards applied
- Meaningful operator-administered preventive maintenance

The director asked for views on the principles, but they were not open to negotiation. He was convinced that they were necessary for survival and that many existing managers did not have the knowledge and experience of the type of reorganization being proposed that would be needed to make an input at this stage. Acceptance of the need to change arose partly from the predicament of the plant, but the director's strength of personality played a major part.

Instituting Change

The Works Committee   A works committee existed before the changes were made, but according to members, dealt mainly with trivial matters. The plant director determined to turn it into the major forum for discussing and communicating decisions to the workforce. The key people in the organization, from both the management and trade unions, were on the committee. The plant director convinced them that the principles and measures he was proposing were the correct ones, and the committee became the driving force behind the changes.

Communications   A full and frank discussion of the proposals took place at the plant level and at works committee meetings. The plant director addressed the entire workforce, split into small groups, setting out the need to change and explaining the changes proposed. This was designed not as a consultative exercise but to enable employees to consider whether or not they could work in the new environment. A new simplified communications system followed naturally from the changes made to the management structure. Information from works committee meetings is passed directly to the shop floor by committee members at department meetings. Information from senior manager meetings is passed on to department managers, who communicate it directly to the workforce at the same meetings.

De-layering   The major initial change was to de-layer the management structure by removing all the supervisory levels. This happened throughout the factory but was particularly noticeable in the production area, where most of this structure was to be swept away, leaving only the department manager between the production manager and the operators. Some junior managers were promoted to fill senior posts that became available. Only two existing senior managers survived the changes. The plant director judged that some managers would not be suitable for the new environment, and they were offered generous severance terms. This had the effect of removing the ideas and influence of the old regime and helped acceptance of the new philosophy.

Severance Payments   A generous severance payment package was also made available to those employees who felt, for whatever reason, that they would not be able to live with the new philosophy. A small number of staff who were considered unsuitable but who did not leave voluntarily were dismissed.

Investment   The staff savings made during the reorganization released money for investment in plant and machinery. Much of the machinery was replaced with up-to-date equipment. In addition, the building was refurbished, providing much better working conditions. This had the effect of demonstrating to staff that there was a commitment to maintaining and developing the Bridgend site. Not only was the investment targeted at new machines, but offices, canteens, and rest areas were brought into the twentieth century. The refurbished building gave a more favorable impression to representatives from other parts of the Bayer Group (customers for Miles products and significant decision makers on product sourcing policy).

Multi skilling   Under the previous management, operators say that they were not expected to think. For example, if a machine broke down, they would report it to the supervisor and wait idly for it to be fixed. They were now to be responsible for their own supervision, and a training program was introduced as part of a multiskilling package. Separate multiskilling programs were to be devised for the production, engineering, and quality assurance workers and negotiated with the unions. In the production area, a working party known as the multiskilling group was set up to work out the program. Four levels were agreed to:

- *Level 1:* consisted of new employees for a probationary period.
- *Level 2:* covered basic skills (existing job functions plus analytical troubleshooting training
- *Level 3:* covered intermediate skills for routine operations (skills broadly equivalent to those of charge hands under the previous management structure)
- *Level 4:* was the top multiskilling level and had a certain amount of flexibility

Five groups of skills, known as *grids*, were defined:

- *Grid 1:* administration
- *Grid 2:* machine–mixing operation
- *Grid 3:* material receipt and handling (for the goods in/dispatch staff)
- *Grid 4:* computer operations
- *Grid 5:* truck

To be multiskilled, employees had to be capable of performing grids 1 and 2 together with two of grids 3 to 5. Employees were paid a "journeyman" rate at the intermediate level, which attracted an extra £13 a week. Reaching the multiskilled level attracted a further £17 per week, making a total of £30 over the basic rate. Operators were trained to train others and were provided with new training facilities.

Autonomous Working   The multiskilling program helped employees to become responsible for their own supervision. As they acquired the necessary skills, operators joined the rota for "the desk," which was the control point of the operation. Here they performed supervisory duties such as controlling batch cards and allocating work. Production workers also regularly held their own production meetings, where production problems, faults, and mistakes were discussed and corrected. Faults and problems were written on white boards in each production area so that it could be seen that they were being addressed.

Employee Reaction to Multiskilling   Initially, many employees were apprehensive about multiskilling. Typically, they had been performing the same routine job for many years and doubted their ability to learn new skills, such as operating computers and driving forklift trucks. Some admitted to being very worried during the early stages of the program and to suffering sleepless nights. However, as skills were learned, a real sense of excitement developed and employees became aware that they had abilities of which they were previously unaware.

New Management Style   Management have changed their style from one of control to one of enablement. Clear signals of the changed style were sent by abolishing "clocking" and letting operators take breaks without asking permission. However, more significant changes have taken place on the production line, where management now intervenes as little as possible and operators are empowered to take fairly major day-to-day decisions that could potentially cost a considerable amount of money in lost production. Most employees have reacted well to this new responsibility, but there are still a few who feel that "managers are being paid for sitting in the office doing nothing."

Relations Between Managers and Employees   The plant director made it a deliberate policy to raise the status of production workers. As the employees who actually produce the goods, he sees them as the most important workers in the plant. This has helped to give them a real sense of pride in their work, and it is evident that the old "them" and "us" attitudes have been broken down. Operators speak of the old days when they would look at the floor as they passed a manager, knowing that their presence would not be acknowledged. Now it is evident that managers and operators speak to each other in an open and friendly manner.

Conclusions

A Great Success   Miles at Bridgend has been through three years of fundamental change which has transformed an underproductive, threatened plant into one that is vibrant, pleasant to work in, and has an assured future. The transformation from an old-fashioned, traditional, strongly hierarchical, rigid organization to a modern flexible plant is impressive by any standards. The commitment of the workforce is admirable, as is the way the production operators have learned new skills and have become largely self-directing. There is a sense of excitement and adventure at Miles which bodes well for their future success in a world becoming increasingly competitive. There are some questions raised in these conclusions about the success of some aspects of the change, but these must be seen in the context of the quite remarkable success of the project as a whole.

The Vision   A good deal of money has been spent on the plant and machinery, and it would be difficult to determine how much the improved performance is attributable to this. However, the most powerful factor in the process of change was probably the initial vision of the plant director. That vision laid the framework for the new management structure and organization and also asked employees for their commitment to the ideals that lay behind it. The beliefs about people contained in the "Vision" document are not mere slogans but really do guide the behavior of managers and all employees. Time and again operators refer to their agreement to act and be treated as mature adults. Production operators are convinced that these beliefs and the consequent reorganization and changes in attitude are far and away the most important factors in the facilitation of change.

Banners and Slogans   Many of the ideas and practices that formed the vision are often promoted under banners such as empowerment, quality circles, QWL, TQM, and BS 5750 (now ISO 9000). These terms were deliberately avoided so that the organization could concentrate on what was actually going on and being achieved. There was a view among some senior managers that banners and slogans are counterproductive. As an interesting aside, the quality assurance department, which checked the quality of incoming pharmaceutical supplies (a legal requirement), had noticed that the quality from some suppliers who had achieved the BS 5750 standard had actually deteriorated upon certification by BSI.

The Plant Director   Although the ideas that formed the vision were fundamental to the success of the changes, the drive and determination of the plant director cannot be overestimated. He is looked up to by managers and shop floor workers alike, knows everybody in the factory by their first names, and will see and be seen by everyone whenever he is on site. He has been a prime factor in maintaining enthusiasm and motivation when doubts arose, especially in the early stages. Although the success of the changes was based on the ideas in the vision, they were undoubtedly pushed through by his force of personality.

Changed Status   Production workers have had their status raised by the change process, and this has certainly lifted their morale. However, some groups, mainly skilled workers, have seen their status fall as a consequence, and this has caused a certain amount of resentment. Skilled workers have been slower to agree to multiskilling and believe that they are being asked to add more in the way of skill and knowledge for little extra reward. They complain that production operators can earn an extra 20%

whereas only 10% is available to them. Although most groups accept that previously, production workers were undervalued, there is a feeling now that the pendulum has swung too far the other way. Although this problem should not be overemphasized, its solution would help the plant pull together as a single team.

Consultation   Communication on day-to-day issues at Miles is now much improved. However, there are those who might criticize senior management for their failure to consult in framing the broad change strategy. Acceptance of the vision was necessary for all who wished to stay, and although there was a full discussion of the proposals, there was no real consultation on its substance or content because the decision to implement had already been made. It may be that at Miles the "do or die" strategy was correct and that genuine consultation would have diluted the approach and led to a less effective result. However, in other circumstances it might be preferable to develop the initial vision on a joint basis with employees and their representatives in order to gain their commitment.

Job Losses   It is arguable that some staff who left or were dismissed could have been retained if greater initial consultation had taken place. The company was able to work very rapidly toward a smaller, more committed workforce, and the doubting Thomases and those with a negative view of the changes were not allowed to influence the process. Such an approach is not without its dangers, and in other organizations could induce a feeling of insecurity among those staff that remained, which might have hindered the changes. To some extent this was avoided by the demonstration of commitment to the future of the factory shown by the investment in the plant, but the approach could easily have backfired.

The Future   The success of the changes made by Miles, especially in motivating staff to self-development, may carry with it the seeds of new challenges. Operators are developing an appetite for greater responsibility, and some are already talking of greater responsibilities in the future (although not the immediate future). At present there are no plans to allow development above the full multiskilling level, and the flat management structure means that there will be few promotion opportunities. It will also be a very big jump for operators to move straight to the next level of department manager. Some ambitious operators will doubtless move elsewhere, and this is probably both necessary and healthy, but some of the expertise developed by the best operators will be needed and thought will have to be given to how they can be retained.

Having recently read Steven Covey's foreword to his son,[20] I could not help drawing a comparison. Covey recounted the words of Henry David Thoreau: "For every thousand people hacking at the leaves of evil, there is one striking at the roots." The plant director in this case study, John O'Neill, was that 1 in a thousand, although the scale of the assault on "evil" made the figure closer to 1 in a million. The impact of the change was also to engage individuals in such a way as to achieve the state that Covey goes on to describe as "instead of compliance, the focus is on optimization through developing an ethical character, transparent motivation and superb competence in producing sustained, superior results." This would be a laudable goal for the pharmaceutical sector: less emphasis on rote compliance, more on building supply chains to be proud of.

As mentioned, I was intimately associated with that change, having been one of the junior managers promoted to a senior management position (site head of SCM). In fact, the reason that I have been able to write this book is due in no small part to the educational and development opportunities afforded me during the change. As a result of one of those opportunities I was able to study the specific issue of de-layering in the organization, which in turn meant studying the dynamics of this cultural change program.

At the time of the change, management thinkers had been heavily focused on reducing the number of levels, in organizational hierarchy. Fueled by successes of companies such as GE and the emergence of concepts of organizations as networked, orchestra-like, clustered, boundaryless, and self-directed, the entire ethos of hierarchy has been called into question. The layperson could be forgiven for concluding that organizational effectiveness was inversely proportional to the number of levels in hierarchy. However, much of the literature suggested that there was far more to de-layering than changing the structure of an organization. Reducing levels of hierarchy merely by taking slices out of an existing structure does not guarantee the success of a de-layering process. As I carried out a brief review of some of the work on hierarchy, I found a few interesting perspectives on the subject.

Elliot Jaques[21] argues that hierarchy is essential in organizations of meaningful size, and far from inhibiting the potential of people, if structured optimally can release massive potential. He asserts that the key issues in hierarchy are of accountability and skills, and it is these factors, rather than the absolute number of levels, that determine the effectiveness of the hierarchy. The corollary of this argument is that the success of recent de-layering initiatives should be attributed to a more appropriate distribution profile for accountability and skills rather than reduction in levels of the hierarchy per se. (We see in the case study the incredible impact that redistribution of these factors had.)

This would also seem to contribute toward an explanation of the apparent success of the Japanese system of management, despite having typically taller, more formal structures than their Western counterparts. This would support the proposition that successful de-layering is a far more complex operation than merely reducing the number of layers in an organization.

Keuning and Opheij[22] support this multidimentional aspect to de-layering by arguing strongly that achieving results involves more than structural readjustment. They identify six key areas that must be addressed to make the process productive:

1. Leadership
2. Performance information
3. Reward system
4. Budget allocation
5. Staffing
6. Culture

All of these considerations are contained within the case study above, although applied intuitively by the plant director. Lack of time prevents further exploration of this topic, so the section is finished with some personal findings on possible ways to deal with three important aspects of delayering.

1. *Dealing with the skills gap.* How does an organization plan for the loss of key skills during transition to a flatter structure, and then establish a meaningful redistribution of skills consistent with the needs of a leaner and fitter enterprise?
2. *The managerial span of control.* How can managers operating in a flatter structure be helped to remain productive and adopt management styles supportive of the revised organization?
3. *Management development.* What can be done to maintain a motivated and appropriately experienced management staff when there are fewer positions in the hierarchy to provide an opportunity for promotion and development of managerial skills?

I studied these questions to identify the main factors employed to help and applied my own assessment of the dynamic, based on theory and practical experience, which is outlined below for each of the three areas for examination.

Dealing with the Skills Gap   First, let's look at the key initiatives employed in the case study.

Retain displaced personnel on-site to hand over skills. The people identified as occupying redundant positions were offered a much enhanced severance package, with the request that they remain on site to assist in the transfer of work over a six- to nine-month period, after which they would be expected to have found alternative employment. Outplacement was provided over this period. None of these people were offered alternative employment within the plant, on the basis that this would provide too high a risk of passive resistance remaining.

Work units with rotating leadership. The work of the supervisor was replaced by introducing an administration function into the already existing work units. This function dealt with things such as computer transactions on output, usage, and inventory movements and also covered the allocation of work in discussion with the planning department. All this work had previously been carried out by the supervisor.

Multiskilling program. This program laid the foundation for operators to acquire the skills necessary to undertake the supervisor's duties. Much of the design and implementation work for productive operatives was completed by the union convenor of the TGWU and as such received a high degree of commitment from the membership.

Plantwide training in troubleshooting skills. A company specializing in problem solving and troubleshooting training (Kepner-Tregoe, a U.S. consultancy company well known for work carried out with the NASA space program) was engaged to provide plantwide training in the techniques of identifying and solving both technical and organizational problems.

Upgraded induction programs. The personnel-driven half-day induction was replaced by a full week of structured basic training and in-depth information provision run by the line managers and in-house trainers.

Observations, Views, and Experiences of the Author

Anticipating the skills vacuum. *The urgent need for change meant that the business was unable to do any meaningful up-front planning for potential loss of key skills. There were three suppporting reasons for this: (1) the change process would require that the way in which many skills had been employed would alter in emphasis and even possibly cease to be required; (2) it would be unrealistic to expect a severely disadvantaged group to contribute willingly to a planning process that would lead to their certain demise (no one willingly plans themselves out of a job, do they?); and (3) skills interact in a complex way as a business restructures (systemic effects). It was considered to be virtually impossible to forecast the exact value-adding skill mix requirement as the business responded to change. In practice, the supervisors helped somewhat in the process, but it was left to the operators to devise skill grids and organize on-the-job training to meet the skill requirements of which they were aware. This resulted in a six-month period where the business was exposed, resulting in two mislabelling incidents where a limited product recall was necessary. The response of management to this was to introduce equipment that effectively "de-skilled" many aspects of the process operation, but this took a period of months to implement. In hindsight, it should have been possible to anticipate the benefits of this as a potential contingency approach.*

The apparent lack of planning in this approach was linked with the history of bureaucracy at the plant. The plant director was concerned that a complex project could emerge which would never be implemented. In fact, a very detailed implementation plan was prepared by some members of the works committee. The plant director was resolved in his opinion that this level of planning was not feasible and the plan was carefully consigned to the filing cabinet.

The implementation was, in reality, heavily dependent on a strong belief in the existence of a natural process something akin to the force that causes air to fill a vacuum. This required a huge act of faith and was based on the plant director's opinion that (1) there was a highly skilled workforce at the plant awaiting the opportunity to become empowered, and (2) much of the work of managers and supervisors was self-perpetuating and non-value adding. However, even with this being the case, clearly business-critical skills were being exercised that could not easily be identified. The main strategy employed was to buy time for the organic regeneration of skills by providing a political umbrella over the necessary period. This appears to have been very astutely effected by the plant director through a process that can only be described as 'selling the benefits' to those in a position to intervene.

Limited uptake of problem-solving training. *The plantwide training program cost a significant amount of money, with little apparent carryover into the work environment.*

The application of the skills was patchy, at best, and never became a part of the routine working pattern. A possible reason for this may have been the absence of any direct, tangible reward, combined with the highly structured approach demanded by the techniques. One aspect of this which appeared to work very well, however, was the process of involving most of the plant in a common activity involving group sessions with a variety of people. This brought together personnel who had not worked together before; also,'there was a degree of symbolism in allowing production operatives to get involved in this type of activity. The effect on morale was very positive, which was not anticipated, and this contributed significantly to the critical mass lending support to the overall change process.

Varying-speed introduction of multiskilling. *The multiskilling program was taken up enthusiastically by the production operators group, with a consequent broadening and deepening of the role of production operatives. This created an amount of animosity with other areas, such as engineering, quality, finance, and administration. It was as if a step shift had occurred in the relative perceived positioning of the production function in relation to the rest of the plant, emphasized by the change in the reward system. These other functions were given the opportunity to adopt their own scheme quite soon afterward, with the effort of providing impetus for multiskilling to spread throughout the plant, but an underlying sense of resentment remained in some areas, associated with gaining agreement to equivalent levels of difficulty in comparison with the production operators' scheme (notably in engineering). This latent tension appears to have remained to date.*

Providing the leadership role. *The skills grid included the need to take on a leadership role during the desk work, but it was clear that some staff took to this better than others. Consequently, there appeared a need to consider what happens when a less competent person is on the desk. The tendency for more able employees to develop quasisupervisory positions was observed. Since these roles were not overtly recognized by the company, it required far more skill on behalf of management to balance the legitimate structure with operation of the informal structure.*

Pitching the difficulty level of multiskilling status. *An initial concern with the multiskilling approach was how to make it sufficiently challenging without making the skill levels required prohibitive. It was the opinion of management that one of the key factors in the success of the change process was to achieve a critical mass of employees benefiting from the change. The extra reward associated with multiskilling was perceived as an element in creating a "feel good" factor. In practice, since the difficulty level was pitched with the full participation of those involved, there was a general agreement that a fair level had been established. One interesting aspect was in the area of access to skills training. Multiskilling resulted in many people skilled for duties they probably would never carry out (e.g., forklift truck driving, materials handling). It was found to be difficult to target skills acquisition and more effective to use a "scatter gun" strategy on the basis that it raised the probability of all areas being accounted for. The unexpected upside of this was that it instilled a general feeling in the workforce that an opportunity had been given for employees to grow and develop, irrespective of any immediate tangible benefit to the company. This had the effect of demonstrating a congruence between the newly espoused beliefs and actual managerial actions, raising the level of trust felt toward the entire change initiative.*

Pressures on the role of trainer. *Some problems arose in this area because by virtue of the position of knowledge, the decision to award the status of fully multiskilled lay with the trainer, yet there was no hierarchical difference between the trainer and the employee being assessed. Over a period of time, this power invested in the trainer became a source of pressure, as peers sought to invoke a kind of moral allegiance as an argument for being less than stringent in assessment standards. This resulted in a dilemma for the trainer in deciding the level of personal accountability that should reasonably be given to this voluntary role of trainer.*

Experienced workers' attitude toward improved induction. *It was a surprise to realize that initially, the process of taking new employees through a full-week structured program was resented by experienced employees because they had not received similar high-quality information and training. Schemes had to be run for the existing workforce to provide equivalence.*

Catering for high achievers. *A small percentage of operators very quickly attained the requisite skills and competencies and then looked for the next stage of development, even though there were no obvious additional skills to be acquired. These were individuals who would probably have been promoted to the next level of junior supervision in the earlier structure. This problem is covered later under the heading "Management Development."*

The Managerial Span of Control   In this category the following key initiatives were employed in the case study.

Selection of individuals with natural coaching and counseling approaches. The remaining managerial positions were filled, wherever possible, with persons who had demonstrated a natural ability to employ a coaching and counseling style.

Top-level support for Theory Y assumptions. The plant director made it crystal clear that the preferred managerial approach was based on mutual trust and on valuing the contribution of each person. This belief was reinforced in practice by such things as abolishing clocking and detailed recording of breaks, giving computer access to a much wider population, and making strategic information available to the works committee.

Problem-solving and decision-making training. All managers and staff were taken through techniques in complex problem-solving and decision-making routines. This type of training is referred under the heading "Dealing with the Skills Gap" and was provided by the same organization.

Observations, Views, and Experiences of the Author

Adjusting to the new expectations. *The revised role of the manager was broadly defined as coach and counselor, but within that broad umbrella lay a multitude of possible interpretations. Neither the surviving members from previous managerial positions nor the new cadre of managers had any direct experience of what this role entailed, other than to model the plant director or follow others who appeared to be doing it right. It was also clear that "macho" management was the familiar way of operating for many, and even in the knowledge of the approach preferred, they found it difficult to change. There was evidence of personnel suffering role ambiguity, and a number of early appointees were redeployed or left the company. This is one area where the company could have helped by adopting training initiatives focused on helping individuals to obtain increased role clarity. Much of the difficulty seemed to emanate from personal value systems which had developed over years of exposure to the old ways. Assistance in lending credence to a more people-centered approach was required to help new values emerge.*

Predicting managerial potential. *The ability of individuals to manage in a less directive mode was assessed, almost totally, through the plant director's judgment. This was necessary because of the accelerated time scale of de-layering. The outcome showed clearly that intuitive judgment was not always an accurate gauge. As an aid to the selection process, a more structured instrument may well have been utilized.*

Providing an empowered infrastructure. *The groundwork in terms of multiskilling and teamworking was an absolute necessity in enabling the increased span of managerial control required to function effectively. However, with rotating team leadership in the form of the administration desk, the quality of leadership tended to vary according to the confidence and ability of the person running the desk. In some cases the most able operator could be seen to supplement the work of a weaker colleague. The logical progression here was that eventually, a small group of the most able operators acted as a quasi-supervisor for the entire department. This then required that the department manager become increasingly effective at managing the informal structure of her group.*

Adopting the appropriate thinking horizon. *There were clearly articulated guidelines for the thinking horizons with which managers should be working. Department managers should be thinking three months ahead and functional managers, 12 to 18 months ahead. The aim of this was to reverse the managerial focus from the day-to-day routine of the business. This demanded a readjustment of thinking patterns throughout the plant and was heavily facilitated by the senior management team removing themselves (with the encouragement of the plant director) from routine decision making. It would be interesting to speculate as to how successful this would continue to be should the plant director lessen the degree of encouragement that he currently gives. Without a sound conceptual underpinning of the necessity for this approach (and this has not been provided explicitly), and with little opportunity in a flatter structure for lower levels to develop a longer thinking horizon (see the next section), there seems to be potential for an irresistible force to draw managers back to the comfort and familiarity of the day-to-day routine.*

Coping with numbers of people. *Some managers suffered from the inability to stay in sufficient contact with staff due to the physical difficulty of making time. There were also greater emotional demands created by the propensity for transactions with people throughout the working day. This remains a very real problem in a flatter environment.*

Management Development   The final key initiatives that we'll look at follow.

Problem-solving groups. The suggestion scheme was abolished on the basis that it discouraged people from openly investigating problem areas and sharing information. Focused problem-solving teams were formed within the work units, assigned to identify, investigate, and present recommendations on potential solutions to senior management. These groups acted as a vehicle for exposing employees to business issues and the difficulties associated with achieving high-quality solutions to problems. For most of those involved, this was a novel and valuable development opportunity.

Cross-functional project teams. The business (normally the plant director in consultation with senior functional managers) detailed cross-functional teams to deal with projects requiring complex coordination of effort and resources. The structure of a team was dependent to a large degree on the critical success factors of the project. For example, if there was a major logistics implication in a successful outcome, the project leader would probably be drawn from the logistics group. Often, these were well-profiled events with a relatively junior but high-potential person in the leadership role. There was a conscious effort to limit the membership of senior managers.

Horizontal transfers. A number of horizontal transfers between functions were made to give the additional challenge of managing in a different environment.

Observations, Views, and Experiences of the Author

Problem-solving groups. *The initial success of these groups was remarkable, both in terms of solving problems and in providing development opportunities. A major factor in this was the high visibility afforded the presentation of findings: One group presented to the CEO of Bayer Diagnostics and to a board of directors member for Bayer AG. However, activity slowly tailed off, some reasons given for this being (1) that the burden of leadership tended to fall on the same personnel; (2) that pressure to produce became greater as the business success created extra work; and (3) the system of overtime payment was a negative influence on ideas as to producing efficiency improvements. The positive outcome from this experience is the knowledge that given the appropriate degree of cooperation and exposure, a significant broadening of workforce involvement can be achieved. This fact also reveals, however, how easily gains can be lost if the elements cannot be maintained in the correct balance. These groups must be nurtured continuously to ensure that the issues described above are controlled, so as not to impede progress.*

Hierarchical considerations. *Development opportunities that cut across the existing hierarchy caused uncertainty and in some cases led to subversive resentment. For example, if a junior manager was given leadership of a cross-functional project team, with a consequent high profile, higher-ranking managers within the same function were visibly confused as to how they should relate to the new situation. There were several examples of senior managers inviting themselves to project team meetings to provide unsolicited input, using information that was gleaned through channels only available to the senior manager by virtue of his position.*

Meaningful reward systems. *The earlier structure lay great store on rewarding promotion with pay. With fewer opportunities for promotion, and hence pay increases, in the flatter structure pressure could be expected to build up for pay rewards through other channels. The company believed that it was not possible quickly to introduce a meaningful system to address this problem, and was living with the underlying tension this caused in some employees. The rationale behind this is that a hurried and arbitrary method may do more harm than good. Part of the solution would be to break the natural association of immediate reward with additional responsibility, fostering a longer-term attitude to competency development. A structured system of competency-based performance management is one possibility that could be explored.*

Observations, Views, and Experiences of the Author

The case study we have been studying was left toward the end because for me it represents the core of meaningful improvement based on principles, not methodology. Almost everything that has gone before in the book was present during the transformation, but applied in a commonsense way without labels. Individuals were respected, production lines were joined together and level-loaded, important competencies were developed, setup times were reduced, and strong induction programs were introduced—I could write a list as long as my arm. We all knew intuitively that these were the right things to do, but we also knew how difficult and complex it was and that no amount of studying the case would help anyone do it for themselves. Why not, you may ask? Well, the principal reason is that many invisible things went on in the way that change was effected. From my personal involvement in the case, I could see John had strong working relationships in important areas that needed to support change, such as with the union leadership and his immediate boss. He used to model the behaviors he expected from his reporting staff. He insisted that our job was to keep out of day-to-day issues and focus on developing others. The weekly one-on-one meetings were about harnessing people's best efforts teams and making improvements stick. There was a lot more besides, but it would be impossible to put it down on paper. That is why I believe the deep examination of Toyota as a specific company has helped only partially in the West. The invisible parts are not on show. These lie heavily around the leadership executing on principles without compromise. This is what I believe all successful companies need—leaders who apply sound principles in these systemic organizations in which we operate until the right behaviors are ingrained into the fabric of the organization; by leaders I mean those at the top of the tree of change (e.g., Taiichi Ohno). It cannot be anyone else to start—the others are followers until the path is set. Then leaders emerge at lower levels in the tree. And so it goes on.

The scope of this topic is enormous and has not been given full justice here. We must, though, now focus on applying these 16 chapters to improvements in pharmaceuticals.

17 A Cure for the Pharmaceutical Supply Chain

17.1 WHAT IS THE DISEASE STATE?

In earlier chapters we expressed concern about the malaise that currently pervades pharma supply chains. The author has a name for the condition. I have termed this "serendipity-induced chronic disconnectedness accompanied by change inertia" (SICCI = *sicky*; please excuse the awful pun). The serious meaning behind this is that the frantic search to discover blockbuster drugs has resulted in a disconnected industry which in turn is disconnected from its supply chains. This, together with the continued belief that serendipity can form the basis of a sustainable business model, kills the will to change.

Pharmaceuticals has always been a fragmented industry, with no single company ever holding more than a single-digit market share. This fragmentation grew into full disconnectedness when pharmaceutical companies began to re-trench into the opposite ends of the business: discovery research and marketing. In metaphorical terms, the brain kept its head and legs and threw away its body, with arms attached. The body is now in no-man's land, making do as best it can with little meaningful contact with its previous fellow body parts.

That metaphor aims to highlight where we are now. The head and legs are pharmaceutical companies spearheading the drive to discover and register drugs to cure unmet medical needs and build a market for them. The disconnected body parts, the engine room of drug development, manufacture, and supply, are sitting in the land of outsourced services. In this land it is survival of the fittest; and the fittest know how to manage commercial contracts for maximum benefit.

There is also more to this disconnectedness. The marketing part of the head is not engaged with patients, as we demonstrated in Chapter 2. The discovery research part of the head has now entered the disconnection game by outsourcing its work to small and medium-sized companies, known as biotech or virtual drug developers. These are typically companies with insufficient critical mass to undertake the vital early stage work required for modernization, discussed in earlier chapters.

So this is the disease, and the symptoms are not difficult to see. Patients not in need of breakthrough drugs, but who could be better served by existing drugs, are rarely

Supply Chain Management in the Drug Industry: Delivering Patient Value for Pharmaceuticals and Biologics, By Hedley Rees
Copyright © 2011 John Wiley & Sons, Inc.

a focus of management or marketing. Even if they were, marketing is disconnected from research and development and in no position to influence matters.

Counterfeit drugs can enter the disconnected distribution channel under the nose of the pharma companies that should have made them. Contract researchers and manufacturers have little incentive to "sharpen their pencils" for patients because *their* customers are interested in gaining license approvals at almost any price. Need we continue? If we did, there would be a long list of symptoms. As any GP would probably conclude, the patient certainly needs treatment in the form of an effective medicine!

17.2   WHAT IS THE LABEL CLAIM FOR THE MEDICINE?

The potential to transform supply chains in pharmaceuticals may seem a dramatic "label claim" for this book. However, this is what the claim is, as long as the patients take the medicine as directed. This is a medicine made up from tried and tested ingredients from another part of the world where the beneficial effects have been demonstrated. The medicine is already available and waiting to be used. This book is intended as its "Instructions for Use."

This medicine does not come in a bottle. It comes in the form of programs of change which we discuss next. To this point, the book has been factual, reflective, and analytical. Now it is time to carry out a searching critique and make some concrete recommendations. If the medicine is taken, I believe that there is a real possibility of forging a pathway to transformation of this industry's supply chains. Like any prospective medicine, though, it must be taken to have any beneficial effect. That is outside the scope of the book!

If the reader has not already guessed it, the medicine is twenty-first-century modernization. However, the guidelines, as laid out by regulators within the critical path initiative and ICH Q8 to Q10 are only a start to the solution. They must be applied in concert with sound organizational commitment to modern ways of working in the supply chain. This includes development of SCM competencies to rival and even exceed other sectors. The instructions for use contained in this book are meant to explain how that might be achieved.

An initial question that a potential patient might ask is: Under what principles have these instructions been developed? My answer is: evidence-based Instructions. The evidence of my own experiences and that of the guest contributors will help us diagnose the condition and develop prospective treatments.

To start, it should be recognized that the business world is littered with examples of radically improved ways of working, but these are normally prompted by external pressures, especially competitive activity, dictating the need. There is evidence of a changing environment in pharmaceuticals, but it is slow to make a difference. For the most part, the limiting basic assumptions (see our discussion of Ed Schein's work in Section 16.5, Chapter 16) highlighted in earlier chapters still exist. Until these are broken and replaced by new assumptions, nothing is likely to change. We therefore talk here about radical ideas, not tinkering on the fringes. We also look far outside what are traditionally regarded as the boundaries of SCM. This is necessary because we have studied the systemic nature of organizations and realize that problems in one part of a system can arise from fundamental concerns in areas apparently totally unconnected. This means that patients' experience of pharmaceutical drugs intended to treat their conditions can be influenced from the earliest stages of research and development.

This is not a new concept in the world of satisfying customer needs. Returning to Nick Rich's points in Section 1.6.3, successful organizations achieve that status by connecting their supply chains up to early stage design. Remember again that the customer experience is based on what the supply chain delivers: no ifs, buts, or in betweens. Researchers and developers should therefore be fanatically interested in seeing their discovery delivered to customers in the form in which it was intended, and so should the entire stakeholder community involved with the provision of safe and effective medicines to patients.

17.3   WHAT WILL LIFE HOLD WITHOUT THE MEDICINE?

Unfortunately, the answer to this question is: attrition rates, as described in Chapter 1. This means that those of us in drug development are wasting most our time working on expensive failures. Who can be satisfied knowing that their life's efforts are going to waste? What of the resources used up in producing those failures?

The issues now plaguing the industry, such as cost escalation, compliance failures, supply chain shortages, counterfeiting, and adulteration, have their roots in life without the medicine. The patient's resistance to infection is low and the effect is clearly evident. Stakeholders (including regulators, payers, and patients) are losing patience with an industry that is failing to respond to current treatments. Taking none of the medicine is not a route worth pursuing for companies wishing to survive in this new stakeholder environment.

For those still of the opinion that the pharmaceutical sectors occupies a place in the past, the battle is lost. For those readers remaining, we move on with this exciting new medicine.

17.4   WHAT IS THIS BETTER WAY TO DEVELOP DRUGS?

This "better way" is based on achievements in other sectors that were explicitly and implicitly referred to in Woodcock's words in 2002 – which became embodied in tewnty-first-century modernization: the critical path initiative and ICH Q8 to Q10 (see Section 14.1). These were about adopting the same approaches as those adopted in sectors and companies demonstrating success. These are sectors where competition had created the necessary head of steam to make change the only feasible option. Supply chains in these sectors are designed to perform against quality (as measured by the absence of defects), cost, and delivery performance measures. That design starts as early as feasibly possible: at the concept stage.

An exploration of what is possible starts with a metaphor regarding a scientist behind a concrete wall.

A Helpful Metaphor

Occasionally, a scientist emerges from behind the door in that wall and lays a tiny baby in a basket on the ground. The scientist leaves the baby and walks back, closing the one-way door behind him. A watching scientist in the second room approaches the baby and finds, tucked under the blankets in the basket, the baby's passport and a letter from the parents behind the wall. It reads: "Please look after our baby. We do not have time to look after it as we have so many hungry mouths to feed in here. It has a pulse, is breathing, and seems to be able to cry for hours on end, so it should be able to look after itself. We have scribbled some notes down about the baby's background on a piece of paper included with this letter. We didn't get to know it very well, though, because a fairy came along (or was it a wicked witch?) and told us that crying babies couldn't be allowed to hang around; they had to go out through the one-way door."

The metaphor takes us back to the birth of the baby and tragic death of the parents in Chapter 14. Drugs are discovered through intensive "birthing" processes and then handed over to a totally new set of "parents" to continue the upbringing. The issues with this approach can be explained through the metaphor. Parents (especially mothers), from their pre-birth and early day experiences, know things about that small child that no one else could. Even if they spent months writing detailed accounts, they still would not do the child justice in explaining it to others. Yet we hand over a compound to a new set of scientists in a basket with a passport and supporting documentation.

The point here is that childhood development is always most successful when there is continuity of parentage (ownership), focused on the long-term good of the child destined for adult life. Why, then, is there this early divorce which leaves the child with foster parents? Why, then, do the foster parents cosset the child through childhood by protecting it from the realities of adult life?

This flies in the face of the successful approaches developed in other sectors, where a deep understanding of their customers is the unwavering starting point. They start with the end in mind, an end that is defined by the utility that product will have in the hands of customers, known as patients in this sector. There is a body of evidence through the book that pharma does not do this very well.

This is therefore the first target for curative medicine: to move the research and development line of sight beyond the regulatory body's approval process on to target the patient—for life. Without this, quality by design (ICH Q8) is a pipe dream if we accept the fact that the intention behind QbD is to design for commercial manufacture and supply. To design for commercial manufacture, one has to engage with those undertaking commercial manufacture, which in turn has to engage with the patient. Presently, this does not happen in a meaningful way.

If we adopt this target for medicine, correcting a "sight" problem, the mode of action will have a number of effects, which we examine next.

17.4.1 Reinventing R&D

The shared mission will be to design drug prototypes where safety and concept have been proven, that are designed for manufacture, and that can be produced on a commercial scale. The term *prototype* is used purposely to emphasis the common received wisdom in other sectors that prototypes prevent expensive future failures. As we said in Chapter 1, failure is never far away. Many industry veterans will throw their arms up in despair at this naive comment. But is it naive? I really don't know—do you?

The next effect relates to development teams. There are far too many people working in drug development who do not even realize that they are helping to build supply chains, let alone knowing anything about proper management of supply chains. This comment is not meant to be derogatory, because I work closely with people in the field and know how talented many of them are both scientifically and managerially. However, most are not educated or trained to think in terms of end-to-end processes.

Science is a vitally important discipline in which, as Peter Checkland[1] puts it, "the highest value attaches to the advancement of knowledge." To do this, scientists are trained to use reductionist thinking: running experiments and drawing conclusions from them. Checkland compares this way of working with the mindset of an engineer or technologist, who "prize most highly the efficient accomplishment of some defined purpose." The two are, of course, equally valid human endeavors.

Checkland makes an important distinction between science and technology. He provides an example of his work in a science-based industry. His team was charged with developing synthetic leather to seize a market opportunity. A research scientist gave the project a negative response. Checkland reports his comment: "The three-dimensional matrix of natural leather is so complex that it cannot at present be accurately described; therefore we cannot hope to simulate it." He had assumed that the question was about furthering scientific knowledge. The observation from Checkland was: "Had he [the scientist] assumed the question to be a technological one, he would have asked not 'can we copy leather?' but 'can we imagine a material which will perform satisfactorily in end users hands in which natural leather is now used?'" The search is then totally different. It is about finding an alternative solution to an end user's problem. That is a vitally important distinction when developing products. How many companies are studying their molecules and materials rather than developing solutions for patients?

This leads us to the second area to be affected by "the medicine."

17.4.2 Design and Technology

This discussion is not to discount the value of science; it has more to do with securing the gains made from scientific pursuit. To achieve this, science should be "pulled" from the technology of developing products for markets. If technology does not demand it, then science shouldn't pursue it. Again, there will be hands in the air from industry stalwarts claiming all sorts of need for "blue sky" science; and of course there is a need for that. In commercial organizations, however, the cart must position itself firmly before the horse. No income means no money to pay for blue sky research. Currently, the cart appears to be well ahead of the trusty steed.

This goal can only be met by abandoning much of the science for science's sake. Situations in which scientists are not working on projects to support the technology should be appraised and, if necessary, redirected. This will only happen if the design effort switches emphasis from science to technology in a purposeful way; and to achieve this monumental task, the relative importance of technology must be emphasized, as it is the route to paying the bills. What would this involve?

Initially, as with all the medicine recommended here, the most senior levels in the industry should recognize the need. This could then lead to a demand for:

- Teaching, in universities, our future drug researchers and developers the technology and processes of bringing products to market. Therefore, in the same way that undergraduate engineering students would have operations, manufacture, and design on the syllabus, so would pharmacists, chemists, and biochemists.
- Training those who are currently in R&D. The urgent need is for them to understand the opportunities afforded by quality by design, PAT, and ICH Q8 to Q10. Without this, the future is grim for modernization.
- Building a technology interface between the design function and its stakeholders.
- Spending effort in finding low-cost optimization approaches at early stages such as preformulation.

This brings us to the next effect.

17.4.3   Design and Stakeholders

This involves design personnel seeking out those with whom they must work on getting products to patients to build trust and loyalty. The starting point is patients, to understand their various needs. If the future predicted by Pricewaterhouse Coopers in their report is to become a reality, the one-size-fits-all approach must change. Target product profiles will have to become far more specific to segmented groups of patients. Design will need to be formed around approvals for much smaller patient populations with more specific needs.

One possible way to begin to improve the situation would be to start with an extended target product profile (TPP) developed by pharmaceutical companies themselves. The regulatory requirement for a TPP is fit for the purpose for which it is intended. It is not, though, sufficient for a professional design and manufacturing company to develop their commercial products for sale to customers. This extended profile would include details on patient needs, from which practical factors such as target dosage form(s) can be established. Reverting to the words of our speakers in

Chapter 2, these details currently warrant scant attention. If the compound in question is handicapped for a particular dosage form, is there a similar molecule that would be better suited? The divorce we talked of above presently works against this type of dialogue.

To achieve this goal means adopting and institutionalising quality by design, risk management, and quality management systems as part of normal-day business. These should be interpreted in organizational terms in addition to the technical aspects of the guidelines themselves. For example, risk management is not just about carrying out a failure mode effects analysis (FMEA) to have on file (see Martin Lush's contribution in Section 14.1). For a start, an FMEA has limited utility in complex development and supply networks. Theses exercises target only the very highest risks, leaving the rest unmitigated. Often, it is the smaller risk that eventually causes a problem; also, FMEAs are extremely labor-intensive, so tend to be done once and then forgotten. An approach taken from the automotive industry has proven to be far more effective. Here it is explained by Tim Williams. I happened to be chatting to Tim one day about his experiences as a project manager with a tier 1 supplier to Toyota. Since Tim was not from the pharma industry, I explained to him that members of pharmaceutical development project teams do not always appreciate the impact that their actions have on the supply chain. The point often missed is that for every chemical and biological material specified, contract manufacturer identified, analytical method designed, or process instruction written, there are ramifications for risk in the supply chain. Many of these risks are not mitigated easily because departments tend to work in isolation and are therefore not fully conversant with more than one aspect of the supply chain. This can mean that the cross-functional team does not work effectively in keeping risk under control. Tim then told me about his way of working as a practicing project manager in the automotive industry.

GUEST CONTRIBUTOR SLOT: TIM WILLIAMS

Managing Supply Chain Risk

I wish to advocate an approach to supply chain risk management founded on practical experience gained in the supply of safety-critical components in the automotive sector. The overriding premise is that the entire development team has collective responsibility for managing risk, and the process is incorporated into project leadership and planning. Of the two methods of risk assessment contained in ICH Q9, I propose fault tree analysis (FTA) as the simpler, more effective of the two.

Figure 17.1 shows the basic steps of risk management in phase I of a clinical trial. In the early part of the phase, the project team is established to map out the supply chain, carry out an FTA, and list the actions necessary for mitigation. During phase I, regular meetings are held to review the status of each action. Finally, the lessons from phase I are formalized and noted before the risk assessment process begins again for phase II. This assessment of risk is vital to the management of

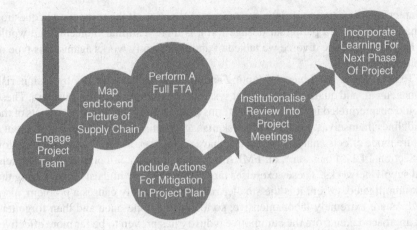

FIGURE 17.1 Basic steps of risk management at start of clinical trials.

any new project, and it should extend to all phases of a clinical trial. As a trial is an iterative process, it is paramount to consider the time and resource constraints placed on project management practitioners, and consequently, the inherent risks to the supply chain. To do little or no risk assessment throughout the life of a project is to jeopardize both the supply chain and therefore the trial as a whole. This is because a project manager needs to address the impact of the change to the final supply chain at every one of the many changes to the material or manufacturing method. Only then can the new risks be addressed and suitable corrective action be taken by the project team and respective suppliers to mitigate them.

Zero Risk From an ethical point of view, the target amount of allowable risk for any safety- or health-related product must be zero. In practice, zero risk is virtually impossible to achieve. Zero risk is, however, a credible target, as this is the only target that genuinely allows project teams to mitigate and plan the necessary corrective actions to guarantee that sufficient resources have been assigned to provide the project with the best chance of success.

Risk is the result of an unknown future, but unknown outcomes may be mitigated if studied with the right tools and the right team. Good planning at the project outset can also help to avoid project delays. For example, if a test has a high probability of two possible outcomes, two plans may be put in place to take action based on the actual result. Activity and resources may therefore be assigned earlier to keep the project running smoothly.

FTA versus FMEA A guideline for quality risk management is given in ICH Q9. This guideline includes two well-known industry methods: fault tree analysis (FTA) and failure mode effects analysis (FMEA). A comparison of the two methods is outlined in Table 17.1.

TABLE 17.1   Comparision of FMEA and FTA

FTA	FMEA
Visual	Written
Intuitive	Needs full concentration
Simple	Complex
One page	Many pages
Less likely to miss unknown risk	Less likely to assess all risks
Full picture in less time	Does not always get the full picture in the time available
Excellent for assessing existing and new pojects	Good if there is carry over from a previous full FMEA with minimal changes
All risks have actions and therefore mitigation is assigned	Actions are prioritized based on an accepted risk priority number threshold
Team can participate easily	Sometimes an individual, last-minute activity

Toyota Camry Example   The technique of using FTA for risk assessment was implemented successfully for the launch of the 2006 Toyota Camry passenger vehicle, Toyota's first "one car for all markets" and its all important entry into the booming Chinese marketplace. To supply nearly 1 million passenger protection systems to four separate locations around the world, one Toyota supplier faced its newest and biggest challenge. This was not a technological, but a supply chain challenge. The global Camry project team was responsible for delivering an identical product, designed in Japan and manufactured in four separate locations around the world. Before this landmark project each location would have designed, developed, and manufactured its own system to individual specifications using local suppliers. The global project manager needed a full risk assessment in order to launch a single global product that would be launched in the United States, Japan, Australia, and China. In particular, the team needed to establish a global supply strategy that acknowledged fully the risks in the supply chain. Having little knowledge of the particulars of each local site's risks and their impact outside the local country, an FTA session was held in Japan between the local project managers and members of their respective teams. Three days were spent reviewing known risks and investigating new ones. The result was a comprehensive risk assessment and a list of actions that provided a solid foundation for project risk mitigation on a global scale. Due to the visual nature of an FTA, the project team members could understand the associations between the risks identified and act accordingly at the local level after returning to their home country. An added benefit of the FTA session held in Japan was that each contributing team member felt attached to the risk assessment and became more committed to achieving the goals and targets of the project. The first product was delivered to Toyota successfully in January 2006, on time and on budget. All four locations around the world produced products to the same build and quality standards. Table 17.1 shows that there are many advantages to using the FTA method. It uses fewer resources to complete a full risk assessment, places actions against all risks, and allows all team members to participate and take responsibility. As

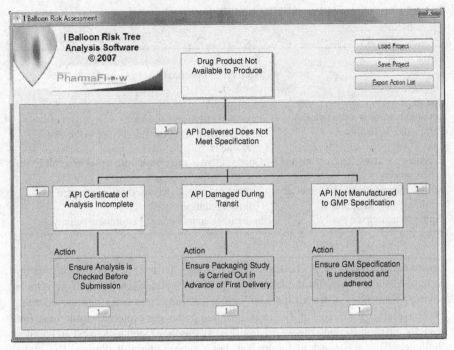

FIGURE 17.2   Excerpt from a fault tree analysis exercise.

the FTA is done at the start, resource can be assigned to complete all actions with a minimal amount of additional resource and effort. This, in turn, makes the concept of zero risk a realistic target. An excerpt from an FTA example is shown in Figure 17.2.

This contribution from Tim leads to the next effect of the medicine.

17.4.4   Project Management

The implication from our discussion above is that project management is for the life of a compound, not just through one or two phases. It should certainly be targeted well into commercial launch. Since the case has been made for early efforts to plan with the end in mind, project managers will need to have a technological rather than a scientific focus. Their skill sets should reflect that. Project management must become akin to program management that occurs in other sectors. The programs will be about taking drugs to market. Design activities will then be carried out concurrently wherever possible and the program will include making the transition from design into production. There is a massive implication here for training in program management competencies.

17.4.5   Interface Between Design and Production

Production personnel (responsible for taking a prototype to market) will sit down with design personnel and discuss a process of ongoing collaboration in getting to market, not just making a handover. This should, again, be a dialogue with the focus on building a world-class supply chain based on the principles discussed throughout the book. Production must be satisfied that the prototype is sufficiently developed to act as a starting point. The two areas should then work closely together around the interface until there has been an appropriate sharing of knowledge. Experimentation with the process should be kept on a small scale until answers has been found to outstanding questions. Drug should not start travelling around the globe between manufacturing sites until confidence levels are high.

In suggesting this, I can visualize wheels turning in industry brains to the effect that some things cannot be established at such an early stage. The point is, though, that if you don't try, you will never find out. The other point is that twenty-first-century modernization demands such an approach. Otherwise, how can quality be designed in?

The regulators have a critical role in making the action described above happen. The bar must begin to be raised at the IND/CTA stage of drug development. At present, this industry only really responds to *dictates* from regulators, so guidelines must eventually start to become regulatory requirements. Also, in the same way that product quality cannot be inspected in, regulatory filing quality cannot be inspected in. Review of a filing is, in fact, an inspection process; it is after the fact. It must be incumbent upon the producer of a filing to adopt processes that have quality built in. This requires effective quality management systems and risk management approaches (discussed above and included in ICH Q9 and Q10). This is where regulators can make a real difference by directing a piercing spotlight onto the resources and processes that sponsor companies put into their filing product. This again has to be carried out at the IND/CTA stage.

Observations, Views, and Experiences of the Author

Working with drug development companies, I find it amazing how many embark on development work without a quality system in place. I have come across chief scientific officers (CSOs), clinical project managers, and others signing-off on development protocols where they had no idea of the technicalities involved. Certainly, they would be in no position to approve such a document. A proper quality system would define the competency set required to sign-off on such a document.

I have also encountered a legal counsel being a sole signatory to a quality or technical agreement. Again the signatory had no competency in drug development. I have concluded that these cannot be isolated incidents, and judging by the limited critical mass of many drug development companies these days, that is almost guaranteed to be the case.

In these cases, the reason why it happens is clear. The competencies do not exist within the company. Reliance is placed on the CMO to have done their work correctly. In most cases they probably will have, but the ultimate responsibility does not lay with the CMO, as we know. In Section 5.5.2 Marla Phillips explained how things can go awry here.

To me, this is evidence that competent authorities should redouble their efforts to inspect the effectiveness of company quality systems in assuring that proper drug development is taking place. Ranjana Pathak, who contributed to Section 15.3, is an expert on such things. As vice president of quality and regulatory compliance at Endo Pharmaceuticals, she is highly experienced in the world of virtual pharma and has practical experience with FDA expectations. Endo had a four-day FDA inspection in 2006 and that led Dr. Pathak to make the following comments.

A quality system for a virtual company is a subject close to my heart. A virtual company needs to have the systems in place which can enable them to ensure that the product distributed will be safe and effective. In filing with the FDA, companies must ensure that the data supporting the application are authentic; also, ensure that there are systems in place at the virtual site that will continue to monitor data generation. Therefore, a rigorous record review program, including change control, must be in place. An effective and meaningful audit program must also be in place. A complaints program should also be in place whereby the CMO informs the sponsor of all the complaints and adverse events are handled in a timely manner. The sponsor must ensure that the validation program is carried out in a timely manner (cleaning, process, equipment, etc.). Once the drug is approved, the company must set up an annual product review program.

Her words should help smaller companies embarking on drug development to appreciate the scale of the undertaking.

The requirements noted above for a quality system clearly must be properly resourced with the right mix of technical and scientific competencies. This is a key part of any assessment and in the author's opinion should be included in the IND/CTA approval process. Along with this should be clear guidelines as to how the production supply chain will be assessed and constructed using the principles of SCM described throughout. The opportunity to get this right evaporates if it is not completed early on. In practical terms, this means adopting a strategic procurement approach for materials and CMO services. It means defining the value stream in alignment with patient segments. It means proper risk management. It means all the things that have been presented throughout the book.

The next effect of the medicine deals with regulators.

17.4.6   Regulators and Quality Systems

The aim of regulation is to follow the words in that well-known song "It Ain't What You Do, It's the Way That You Do It." Therefore, if the development company did not hire a pharmaceutical technologist (the ones at the CMO don't count), how can they assure their CMC data? How can they move forward with the quality by design principle of developing a design space?

The overall conclusion from this is that competent authorities have an opportunity to make some preemptive strikes on behalf of modernization. The IND/CTA stage is the time to do it. At the moment, the CMC data requirements are limited at this stage. This is understandable in some respects. However, when this means that a company has done little or no work to characterize a compound and does not have processes and people in place to do that, why press on? Failure is likely to occur along the way. Additionally, as we have determined, once a submission to run clinical trials is approved, there is great inertia in the way of change. As discussed earlier, the reason for that is the unwillingness to rock any boats that may jeopardize an approval. The counter to that is for regulators to demand a starting point that is at a higher level than that used currently. To make this happen from a sponsor company viewpoint, production would need to be involved with the IND submission, which would be based on the prototype developed. That would mean that the CMC data in the IND would, by definition, assure that the product is manufactureable.

This completes the analysis for design. We now move on to an examination of further potential for the medicine. For things to really change sustainably requires continuation of different working practices throughout all disciplines affecting the supply chain. This could be catalyzed in one simple way.

17.4.7 Regulatory Affairs Engagement

There is a natural aversion to change in the world of pharmaceuticals, and regulatory affairs teams are no different from the rest of the industry. For QbD/PAT to be effective, regulatory submissions must change to become more fulsome, with data relating to process capability, edge of failure analyses, input material characteristics and so on. When these teams start demanding data from the various disciplines, a wave of action should start in response. This will again depend on companies' real understanding of the aims of modernization. The process aims to take the competent authorities further out of the day-to-day loop of making changes. No longer should the regulators be used as a reason why changes for the better cannot be made. That is the message, and it should be the role of all regulatory affairs teams to make that message clear and to champion the cause of modernization. It is in every stakeholder's interest.

17.5 FULL-SCALE PRODUCTION OF DRUGS

17.5.1 Abandoning the Ways of Mass Production

It is difficult to envisage how change will be catalyzed without the competitive pressures that other sectors experienced from the 1960s onward. The industry appears to be somewhat in denial, like an alcoholic who does not want to admit to a problem. However, acceptance is the first step toward recovery, as we all know. So, given that acceptance emerges, what happens next?

17.5.2   Production Linkages with Design, Marketing, and SCM

Production personnel must meet at the table with design staff, accompanied by marketing and SCM. The respective roles should be defined to foster a concurrent approach to product development and market launch.

17.5.3   CMC in Design and Production

CMC in design will be focused on building a body of knowledge that can be used by production to construct a robust supply chain by supporting the PAT and QbD approaches. This will be the point where experimentation and main process definitions take place. This must happen well before clinical trials are contemplated. Preformulation activities could form a basis for this. This team would be responsible for developing the CMC package for IND/CTA based on QbD/PAT principles.

There are resource implications in this, but in the new world of modernization, competencies must be redistributed from traditional functions such as quality control to those areas that target the root cause of defects. This should also be far more interesting work scientifically than catching slip-ups. Those in drug development who enjoy this kind of work should join design. The rest should join production. There would then be no distinction between a clinical trial supply chain and a commercial supply chain. They would be one and the same thing—a single entity on a continuum of improvement.

Design wouldn't necessarily need to understand supply chains, but would need competency in the characterization of compounds from inception up to prototype stage. This would also involve having a deep understanding of the requirements from production before they accept a drug as "producible." By the same token, those in development taking the production route should give up experimentation and work at building an interface with design that allows them to take the product right through to patients in the market by following world-class supply chain management principles.

17.5.4   Quality Is Everyone's Job

This builds on the point made by Marla Philips in Section 5.5.2. *Quality is not the police anymore.* Supply chains can only perform if all players deliver quality (the absence of defects) ways of working. Having a body with the word *quality* in the title does little other than create a huge responsibility whereby individuals are responsible for things they may not have the power to control. For example, in the EU, when a qualified person releases a batch for sale, he or she may have all the documentation at hand, but that is all they have. The entire release process is dependent on those creating the documentation to have operated in a "quality" fashion. That is what we should be concerned about, making sure that people work within a quality system. This is the only way to keep a handle on the systemic issues that arise in supply chains that affect compliance (see Dr. Pathak's contribution in Section 15.3). A robust quality system will drive for root-cause solutions. From previous chapters, it should be clear that those solutions may span organizational boundaries and so deter a problem investigator from pursuing a proper closure. The quality system should empower problem investigators to search for the truth.

Again, there is a regulatory angle in all of this. It may be one of those unintended systemic happenings that can sometimes have a strange impact. The common technical document (CTD) refers to Module 3, CMC, as the "Quality Section." So the word *quality* is taken as being synonymous with the word *manufacture* from the term *chemistry, manufacture, and controls*. This is reinforced further by GMP regulations holding the quality unit ultimately responsible for outputs from production.

In fact, Module 3 is about manufacture, analytics, and the associated end-to-end supply chain. Quality product is the outcome of compliant manufacture and supply chains, and this is the responsibility of everyone operating in the supply chain. At the moment, operations (production) produces and quality inspects. This is an outdated notion which is inconsistent with the principles of twenty-first-century modernization. A critical corollary to this is that modernization requires a shift of organizational accountability from quality control to production. How this is done is not the subject of this book, but to follow the success of other sectors in driving defect rates down, it can be the only way to move forward.

There is pressure, then, to keep CMC off the development critical path. This means important technical trade-offs can be made to move trials forward quickly. These can seriously affect future performance of the supply chain. Often, time is not taken to fully understand a compound's characteristics at the preformulation stage; or difficult-to-source materials are selected for the sake of time expediency. Supplier relationships are often arm's length and do not encourage exchange of information. There is a tremendous amount of secrecy linked to commercial sensitivities (e.g., drug master file information available to sponsor companies) that would not exist if proper commercial relationships were established. The net result is that sponsor companies carry out GMP audit inspections that give a false sense of security. It is the overall working and business relationship that can make or break the supply chain, not a once-off audit.

17.5.5 Proactively Building, Managing, and Improving Supply Chains

This step follows from the order of events above. In fact, without those prior events, this step has a metaphorical banana skin on it, so it is best avoided. Given that the groundwork has been done, we set about incorporating exemplar thinking in pharmaceutical production systems and SCM. It means going back to Chapters 6 to 12 and Chapters 14 to 16 to understand what this means. It also means taking due heed of the words in Chapter 5 on why supply chains do not perform. Some of the key imperatives are:

- Design for manufacture (the pharma equivalent is QbD/PAT).
- Adopt strategic procurement at an early stage for materials and outsourced services.
- Involve suppliers and contractors in design.

- Review outsourcing practices where critical assets cannot be engaged for competitive advantage (e.g., in development of new innovations).
- Source in-house where relevant; build strategic relationships where relevant.
- Design supply chains proactively.
- Incorporate scenario modeling and risk management into supply chain planning.
- Organize end-to-end around product families; cease dependence on volume.
- Build stability and learning through leveled schedules (Ian Glenday).
- Source smaller, easy-changeover equipment aligned to throughput efficiency, not machine speed.
- Manage contractors as part of the business of production. Don't let contractors manage you. Create shared destiny relationships where appropriate (Dan Jones).
- Manage risks and change according to sound principles, build on guidelines from regulators, but don't follow the guidelines blindly if they can be improved.
- Develop a deep understanding of organizational needs to support change for the better (see the Miles Ltd. case study in Chapter 16).
- Think systemically, act systemically, follow systemically, and above all, lead systemically.

The list above is not meant to be a prescriptive solution to our problems in supply chains. It is more an agenda for dialogue and the development of something that works for a particular organization. What has become clear from the various initiatives that have been tried out over the years is that ownership and commitment to the entire enterprise is absolutely fundamental to success, from the highest level on down. It is no coincidence that successful organizations almost invariably have single-minded leaders at the helm driving supportive cultures.

17.5.6   SCM Competencies

The goals stated above can only be achieved if the necessary underlying competencies are developed and applied. The realization and acceptance that supply chains have been neglected is important but is only the starting point. Also required is action based on sound principles of SCM, as discussed throughout. The one saving grace is that many, if not most, companies suffer from deficiencies in SCM. The opportunity exists for pharma to leapfrog ahead, especially given the vast intellectual base working in the industry. This is where we arrive at the challenge for change.

17.6   WHAT ARE THE BARRIERS TO CHANGE?

Many readers will probably have at least a mental list of those aspects of current industry structure and business models that may act as barriers to change. Those that follow are some suggestions of important areas to be resolved but by no means constitute an exhaustive list.

17.6.1 Mindsets

A change in mindset is easy to propose but difficult to achieve. The prevailing industry mindset is characterized by the following, where each point leads to the next.

- A chase for blockbusters (colloquially known as "seeking unmet medical needs")
- A search for marketing approval from regulators for the ultimate prize (approval to sell)
- Hugely differentiated, captive markets
- The concept of the customer as the regulatory body, the product as the regulatory filing
- Endpoint thinking (thinking only to the next stage of regulatory filing for trials)
- Minimum time taken at the early stages ("need to know first if we have a drug")
- Scientific and technical trade-offs to move forward in the clinic
- No focus on supply chain quality, cost, and delivery performance
- *Supply chains that underperform dramatically*

The underpinning midset can be expressed:

If we get an approval, patients will demand it, so why worry about quality (as defined by the absence of defects), cost, and delivery performance?

This mindset leads to supply chains being ignored until the last minute.

Also part of the prevailing, unhelpful mindset is the fact that many scientists, who are used to dealing with complex issues and relationships, underestimate the difficulties of SCM. One R&D director said to me some years ago: "Once the white powder is there in the bottle, you are home and dry." Little wonder that development teams under that type of leadership are tempted to make compromises for the sake of expediency.

17.6.2 Historical Dependence on Regulations

Regulations are, of course, vitally important but should not be the sole determinant of behavior. Laws and regulations are there to provide a minimum standard of right and wrong. This industry has gotten used to looking toward regulators for their (minimum and safe) standards, even though it is mature enough to decide for itself. Being mature means steering a course way past minimum. In my opinion, that is what modernization is aiming to achieve. At the moment, many larger pharma companies are spending money on the technology of QbD and PAT without recognizing the common sense business practices behind it. Most smaller companies are steering clear because of the perceived costs involved.

17.6.3   Tactical and Inappropriate Outsourcing

The wave of tactical outsourcing that has swept the industry now makes it very difficult for producing license holders to control their cost base and improvement activities. Most, if not all, relationships with CMOs and CROs are short term and contract priced (with swingeing provisions for scope creep and cost escalation). Although there is posturing around risk-and-reward-based agreements, they are very much in the minority in the industry. There are also signs that some companies have began to notice this. A report at In-Pharma Technologist.com[2] described how Lundbeck (a pharma company focused on central nervous system disorders) had taken action. The report, dated October 20, 2009, described how Lundbeck had acquired a French-based contract manufacturing organization. This was positioned as a strategic move "to gain greater control over costs and increase production flexibility." I have spoken to others in the industry whose companies have in-sourced activities such as analytical development to regain control over their project time lines and costs.

Not only is it the tactical nature of outsourcing that is at issue, it is the original decision to outsource that must be questioned. What other sector has outsourced the development of its products in the way that pharma has? CROs operate in preclinical and clinical *development*, although the word *research* is in the title. This means two things. First, the skills and competencies required to move forward are in the hands of third parties (part of the disconnected body and arms). Second, sponsor companies and license holders have to allocate cash to the pursuit of innovation. That was never the case with vertically integrated pharmas. Drug development was contained in-house, where priorities could switch without further injection of cash resources being required.

Much more attention to this topic is needed, but we have no room here to go into that further. My plea is that pharmaceutical companies wake up to potential issues here and reappraise accordingly. A starting point would be to study the work of Andrew Cox discussed in Section 9.5.2, as he gets to the real issues of power and dependence in supply chains. (Professor Cox is also Chairman of the newly formed International Institute for Advanced Purchasing and Supply—IIAPS).

17.6.4   Thirst for Volume

The entire supply base is geared up for blockbusters demanding massive volumes. Machines and equipment are built for speed. They are often hugely expensive and inflexible when it comes to changeovers. The impact of product variety has been slow to permeate equipment manufacturers. With moves to greater variety as patient segments become more targeted, this will soon become more of an issue, especially where prototyping is required in the design arena described earlier.

17.6.5   Sourcing Decisions Based on Financial Principles

Much of the sector decides sourcing strategies based on maximization of fiscal (economic and monetary) benefits. Fiscal aspects are obviously important, but to decide purely on these grounds disempowers the supply chain practitioners that operate in the sector. The same can be said of low-cost country sourcing that leads to more complex and convoluted supply chains.

17.6.6   Patients Divorced from Producers

The now vastly powerful buyers and sellers of pharmaceutical products, drug wholesalers, have no meaningful relationship with the pharma companies that are developing and manufacturing the drugs. Although they have the products in common, there is little flow of important market and patient satisfaction data between them. Even for pharma companies to get the basic minimum information on sales volumes and patterns they have to pay organizations such as IMS Health,[3] a third-party collector of information on their (pharmaceutical company) customers and selling it back to them! The problem, of course, is that the wholesalers have all the information, as they own the products they have bought from the manufacturers.

The other issue with this is a potential key to explaining the counterfeiting, that we now see on an ever-growing scale. It is the manufacturers who know (or should know) the pedigree of the product up to the final packaged product. Once it leaves them, however, the connection with the product is lost even though there may be some nominal attempt to provide identification on the packaging. This is never enough—counterfeiters are very clever at defeating attempts to find them out. So we have pharmaceutical products traded within a channel, where the ethical intentions of the vast majority of the players cannot be questioned, but where the system works in favor of the minority wishing to inject inferior products under their noses. What other sector's distribution channels are so remote from their producers?

These are some barriers, and possibly the mindset barrier is the one that once breached will open the flood gates on the rest. Let us hope so.

17.7   WHAT ARE THE POTENTIAL BENEFITS OF CHANGE?

Benefits are there to be taken, although that may not be obvious. They lay in the evidence from other sectors. Prior to the Japanese revolution, the perception was that if quality went up, costs would have to go up correspondingly. This is still the mindset in pharma. The misperception, of course, is founded in the concept of quality. In this sector, quality is synonymous with the standard "we work to high quality around here." This is only one side of the quality factor, and it relates to the specifications. If a higher-grade material is specified in preference to a less pure alternative, this is the specification decision. There is great pride in this industry in using high-quality materials (even sometimes when lower-quality specifications would still be fit for purpose).

The other arm of the quality factor is the ability to produce the specifications repeatedly within predefined limits. This is the area where the Japanese proved that there was an inverse relationship between quality and cost. When quality (the absence of defects) went up, costs went down. The reason is, as we learned earlier, that production systems, as all systems, become massively destabilized when defects interfere with flow and predictability.

To envisage the potential benefits, readers will have to look toward other sectors. To realize that potential, we must believe in the art of the possible.

17.8   DEFINING THE ART OF THE POSSIBLE

17.8.1   What Could Be Possible?

What is possible can only be envisaged by melding real-world evidence with long-term vision. Production systems working successfully in other sectors provide ample evidence that sustainable business models can be built, but in every case, *without exception*, they are built on the sound principles discussed throughout the book. Ambivalence toward paying customers is not one of them.

I remember a case in the UK in the 1960s relating to crisps (potato chips to our U.S. colleagues). Smith's Crisps had been a predominant brand for years. They came in large tin boxes that the retailer kept behind the counter. Each paper bag included a salt packet that every child (and many adults) found it good fun to pour on top of the crisps and shake up. It was a well-established brand that hadn't changed for years. They did have one drawback, however. They were prone to becoming stale and soggy after a few days in storage. The tin box and paper bag together did not offer much protection against moisture. This had gone on for years and was accepted as the way of life for crisps.

A company called Golden Wonder came along in the early 1960s. In 1964, their UK factory became the largest crisp producer in the world. They introduced "stay fresh" packaging and an entire range of flavors. Smith's lost their market dominance almost overnight. This competitor had studied their customer and addressed issues that the customer was not really aware of until an alternative appeared. They then loved it, and there was no turning back for Smith's. They were eventually taken over by another aggressive competitor, Walker's Crisps, in the late 1970s.

The vision should therefore be about the potential to build a sustainable business model through satisfying *target* customers needs for solutions to their medical problems (yes, that includes me and you). These could be fulfilled by prescription-only drugs, drugs in or out of patent, over-the-counter medications, medical devices, diagnostics, herbal remedies (clinically controlled), food supplements, and even good, straightforward, commonsense advice. I am not the first person to point this out; there are also companies trying to make it happen. However, there is little real sign of it working in any meaningful sense. Drug companies still let products go when they are out of patent, even though they could make a valuable contribution to the company bottom line (given cost-effective supply chains) and, of course, to patients. The ensuing rush of companies to be the first to pick up those profits (albeit substantially reduced) leads to an unhelpful explosion of players in the supply chain. This leads to many of the issues to which Chris Oldenhof refers in Section 5.5.1.

They also operate financial thresholds below which candidates for drug development are not advanced, even though there may be a reasonably profitable market for it in some patient segments. These are often acquired by smaller drug developers hoping to make their futures in drug commercialization. This again leads to the supply chain issues of complexity discussed earlier. Thus the answer to the question of what could be possible is that it could be possible to engage with specific patient populations, to build mutual understanding and loyalty that converts into predictable revenues and margins. Serendipity then takes a back seat and the medicine has started to work; and supply chains start the process of reconnecting with the eventual beneficiary of their work.

17.8.2   How Can the Possible Be Realized?

The answer to this question is simple—reread Sections 17.3, 17.4, 17.5, and 17.6. I have been willing to take a stab at it as a stimulus and starting point for change. But the industry must define the art of the possible for itself.

17.8.3   An Industry Second Opinion

As we conclude, it may be appropriate to request a second opinion from someone who should know, Jennifer Miller. The author worked with Jennifer on a webinar co-produced by Pharmaceutical Technology[4] and FDASmart.[5] The owner of FDASmart, Ram Balani, placed Jennifer and me in contact. The webinar was a joint presentation on current product development models and improvement suggestions. It aimed to give a perspective from a big pharma executive with a mandate to drive improvement together with a practicing consultant specializing in supply chains. We then talked about change. I have paraphrased Jennifer's words here for the sake of brevity.

GUEST CONTRIBUTOR SLOT: JENNIFER MILLER

Meeting the Challenge of Business Excellence at Pfizer

I was happy to join Hedley in presenting this topic because it is of extreme relevance for me personally and for my company. We have certainly identified the importance of drawing science and technology into the world of supply chain development, where previously the area had been regarded as a separate entity. Figure 17.3 is a diagram that I use to help people understand the issue. In early-stage development it is difficult to "see" problems, but if and when they are identified, they can be fixed relatively easily. Left undetected, those problems can become ingrained and lead to issues down the line that are immensely costly to rectify given all the manufacturing and related infrastructure that has surrounded the product. This is an important insight and, of course, in full support of Hedley's comments throughout the book.

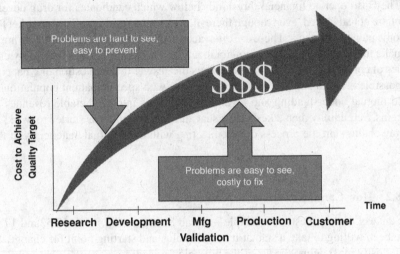

FIGURE 17.3   R&D vs. manufacturing problems.

As part of the presentation, I put together a slide that described my personal agenda for the work I am doing. Some of the points are reproduced below.

Skill Sets

Supply chain as a discipline: introduce value chain thinking and competencies at an early stage

Program management: managing the project throughout the life cycle

Risk-based approaches: applied to target resources at critical areas

Internal Processes

Well-defined procurement processes with properly negotiated supply agreements

Alignment with clinical development; improved clinical trial supply chain processes

Transparency into internal financial and political connections and issues

Subjectivity elimination: increasing objective data-based decisions

Sponsorship and Change Management

Driving change properly and systematically

Moving from the "quality always catch it" mindset to operator accountability

Creating and leveraging flexibility

Encouraging value stream owners, not silos

Moving to a more collaborative organizational environment

Recruiting and retaining top-tier managers proficient in supply chain strategy

Investment Flexibility

Design of product and processes

Value the option to stage investments and use it to your advantage

Customer Insights

Customer-driven business unit model

Objective analysis of customer need

These points are not solutions as much as our best knowledge of what needs to be a focus as we move toward more patient-centric supply chains and products.

Neither Jennifer nor I is a trained scientist. Yet here she is, successfully occupying an executive position, responsible for significant change in the biggest pharma company in the world. More food for thought, don't you think?

17.9   ENDING WITH THE BEGINNING

To draw this work to a conclusion, we return to the beginning, where the aims and aspirations for the book were articulated. We postulated four key milestones. The first was to produce a *practical* guide that could act as a reference for those operating in the pharmaceutical sector so that they could make a valuable contribution to improving supply chain performance. As far as possible, I believe that this has been accomplished. The second milestone was to engage with those outside the industry with SCM competencies by providing them with information on how the sector operates and inviting them to join up. I believe that this has been achieved also.

The third milestone was to help catalyze change in this industry, and hopefully, the book has sparked a desire to *contemplate* a better way to develop and run pharmaceutical supply chains. In my opinion, that change can happen only when there is a massive redefinition of business models, as discussed above. This, in turn, should drive toward patient-centric supply chains founded on sound SCM principles. If the third key milestone were to come to fruition, the author believes that the fourth would be an eventual outcome—those in the industry would start to realize the importance of SCM and become passionately interested in moving the profession forward.

With some very personal words from me, the book concludes.

Observations, Views, and Experiences of the Author

As I was contemplating my final remarks in this chapter while sitting in the Central Tube Line going into London on a client assignment, a thought struck me. It referred me to the words of Janet Woodcock relating to the twenty-first-century initiative explained in Section 14.1:

> *Janet Woodcock's desired state:* "A maximally efficient, agile, flexible pharmaceutical manufacturing sector that reliably produces high-quality products *without* extensive regulatory oversight."

That thought rightly informed me that this *is the ultimate goal. To achieve that goal, the systemic argument must win the day. Currently, in the language of my "pain-in-the-neck" metaphor from Chapter 15, the industry is massaging the neck and shoulders to rectify problems. We should be working down to the location where the source of the issue resides—the stabilizing muscle down near the industry's metaphorical groin, otherwise known as early-stage development. Let's get those hacking at the leaves of evil to join those with hatchets at the roots, and begin hacking our way to a better future for patients – that includes you, me, families, friends and loved ones, and the whole of humankind.*

End Notes

Chapter 1

1. U.S. Government Accountability Office, New Drug Development: Science, Business, Regulatory, and Intellectual Property Issues Cited as Hampering Drug Development, Report GAO-07-09, available at http://www.gao.gov/new.items/d0749.pdf, accessed Nov. 2009.

2. Bioscience Innovation and Growth Team, Bioscience 2015: Improving National Health, Improving National Wealth, available at http://www.bioindustry.org/bigtreport/downloads/exec_summary.pdf, accessed Oct. 2007.

3. A. Smith and E. Cannan, *The Wealth of Nations*, Modern Library, New York, 2000.

4. M. E. Porter, *Competitive Strategy*, Free Press, New York, 1985.

Chapter 2

1. Robin Jaques, Partner at S. A. Partners, http://www.sapartners.co.uk, Mar. 2010.

2. Lewis Carroll, Alice's Adventures in Wonderland and Through the Looking-Glass, Oxford World's Classics, 2009.

Chapter 3

1. John Bicheno, *Cause and Effect Lean: Lean Operations, Six Sigma and Supply Chain Essentials*, Picsie Books, Buckingham, England, 2000.

2. A. Walker or R. Johnson, contact at Alactria LLP, http://www.alacritaconsulting.com, 2010.

3. http://www.ich.org/LOB/media/MEDIA484.pdf.

4. http://www.ich.org/LOB/media/MEDIA3303.pdf.

5. http://www.fda.gov/downloads/RegulatoryInformation/Guidances/ucm129524.pdf.

6. http://www.ich.org/cache/compo/502-272-1.html (S4-S8).

7. http://www.fda.gov.

8. http://www.ema.europa.eu.

Supply Chain Management in the Drug Industry: Delivering Patient Value for Pharmaceuticals and Biologics, By Hedley Rees
Copyright © 2011 John Wiley & Sons, Inc.

9. http://www.ich.org/cache/compo/276-254-1.html.

10. A. Walker or R. Johnson, loc. cit.

11. http://ec.europa.eu/health/documents/eudralex/index_en.htm, accessed Sept. 2010.

12. http://ec.europa.eu/enterprise/sectors/pharmaceuticals/documents/eudralex/index_en.htm.

13. Regulation 2003/94/EC, *Official Journal*, L 262, oct. 14, 2003, pp. 22–26.

14. http://www.fda.gov/downloads/RegulatoryInformation/Guidances/UCM1299 04.pdf.

15. http://www.ich.org/cache/compo/475-272-1.html#E6.

Chapter 4

1. James P. Womack, Daniel T. Jones, and Daniel Roos, *The Machine That Changed the World*, Simon & Schuster, New York, 2007.

2. Virtual pharma but not virtual responsibility, *Pharmaceutical Formulation and Quality*, Feb.–Mar. 2009, available at http://www.pharmaquality.com, search on article title.

3. L. F. Stead, R. Perera, C. Bullen, D. Mant, and T. Lancaster, *Cochrane Database Systems Review*, 1, 2008.

4. B. Hyrup, C. Andersen, L. V. Andreasen, B. Tandrup, and T. Christensen, *Expert Opinion Drug Delivery*, 5:927–933, 2005.

5. European patent, EP 1,825,589 and EP 1,523,242.

6. J. Jacobsen, L. L. Christrup, and N.-H. Jensen, *American Journal of Drug Delivery*, 2:75–88, 2004.

7. Fertin Pharma, unpublished results, 2010.

8. Ron Krawczyk, Blue Fin Consultants, http://www.consultbfg.com.

9. Prepared for the Kaiser Family Foundation by the Health Strategies Consultancy LLC, *Follow the Pill: Understanding the U.S. Commercial Supply Chain*, Mar. 2005, available at http://www.kff.org, accessed June 2007.

10. Importance of QbD in biotherapeutic development, presented at the BIA Committee Seminars, June 4, 2009.

11. Peter Rosholm, *BioProcess International*, 8(3):34–36, Mar. 2010.

12. Ernst and Young, *Beyond Borders Global Biotechnology Report*, 2009.

13. Regulation (EC) 1394/2007 on advanced therapy medicinal products.

14. CFR Title 21 Part 1271, Human Cells, Tissues and Cellular and Tissue-Based Products.

Chapter 5

1. Prepared for the Kaiser Family Foundation by the Health Strategies Consultancy LLC, *Follow the Pill: Understanding the U.S. Commercial Supply Chain*, Mar. 2005, available at http://www.kff.org, accessed June 2007.

2. APICS, The Association for Operations Management, details available at http://www.apics.org/.

Chapter 6

1. Mark Phillips, presentation at ManuPharma 2005.
2. M. E. Porter, *Competitive Advantage*, Free Press, New York, 1985, and *Competitive Strategy*, Free Press, New York, 1980.
3. Porter, *Competitive Advantage*, pp. 33–61.
4. Malcolm McDonald, http://www.malcolm-mcdonald.com/.
5. PricewaterhouseCoopers, *Pharma 2020, the Vision: Which Path Will You Take?* 2007.
6. J. Bank, *The Essence of Quality Management*, Prentice Hall, Upper Saddle River, NJ, 1992, p. 1/2.
7. James P. Womack, Daniel T. Jones, and Daniel Roos, *The Machine That Changed the World*, Simon & Schuster, New York, 2007.
8. *Biotech PharmaFlow Newsletter*, July–Aug. 2009.

Chapter 7

1. Jeffrey K. Liker, *The Toyota Way*, McGraw-Hill, New York, 2004, p. 7.
2. Details available at http://www.supply-chain.org/.
3. Martyn A. Ould, *Business Process Management: A Rigorous Approach*, BCS, Swindon, UK, 2005.
4. http://www.bptrends.com/.

Chapter 8

1. Eliyahu M. Goldratt, and J. Cox, *The Goal*, Gower, Aldershot, UK, 1989.

Chapter 9

1. Peter Kraljic, Purchasing must become supply management, *Harvard Business Review*, 61(5):109–117, 1983.
2. Paraphrased from an article in *Journal of Purchasing and Supply Management*, 11:141–155, 2005.
3. C. J. Marjolein Caniëls, and Cees J. Gelderman, *Purchasing Strategies in the Kraljic Matrix: A Power and Dependence Perspective*, Faculty of Management Sciences, Open University of the Netherlands, Heerlen, The Netherlands.
4. Chartered Institute of Purchasing and Supply, http://www.cips.org/professional resources/purchasingsupplymanagementmodel/strategicsourcinganalysis/defa ult.aspx, accessed Sept. 30, 2009.
5. Andrew Cox, Strategic outsourcing: avoiding the loss of critical assets and the problems of adverse selection and moral hazard, in *Business Briefing: Global Purchasing and Supply Strategies*, 2004, pp. 67–70.

6. *The McKinsey Quarterly*, Strategic Purchasing, 1991, 3 P25, Exhibit III, Procurement Development Model.

Chapter 10

1. http://www.wto.org/.
2. Can be contacted at http://www.barnesrichardson.com.
3. International Chamber of Commerce Publishing, *Incoterms 2010*, available at http://www.iccbooks.com.
4. Virtual pharma but not virtual responsibility, *Pharmaceutical Formulation and Quality*, Feb.–Mar. 2009, available at http://www.pharmaquality.com, search on article title.
5. http://www.wcoomd.org/home.htm.
6. http://publications.wcoomd.org/.
7. http://www.macmap.org.
8. http://www.bitd.org.
9. http://ec.europa.eu/enterprise/sectors/chemicals/reach/index_en.htm.
10. http://www.epa.gov/lawsregs/laws/tsca.html.
11. http://www.usda.gov/wps/portal/usdahome.
12. http://www.FDA.gov.
13. http://www.ema.europa.eu.
14. http://www.hta.gov.uk/.

Chapter 11

1. Michael Hammer and James Champy, Reengineering the corporation: a manifesto for business revolution, HarperCollins, Canada, 1993.
2. Elliot and Avison in 2005, Scoping the Discipline of Information Systems, http://media.wiley.com/product_data/excerpt/80/EHEP0008/EHEP000880.pdf.
3. Jan vom Brocke and Michael Rosemann, *Handbook on Business Process Management: Strategic Alignment, Governance, People and Culture*, Springer, 2010, http://www.bpm-handbook.com.
4. Details available at http://www.supply-chain.org/.
5. George Plossl, *The Best Investment—Control, Not Machinery*, Atlanta, Georgia, 1975, APICS, Material summarized with permission of the APICS.
6. http://www.pharmacovigilance.org.uk/legal-and-procedural/pharmacovigilance-definiton-and-glossary.
7. GAMP® is a Community of Practice within ISPE (www.ispe.org) and GAMP is a registered trademark of ISPE. Details of the main guide (GAMP 5) can be found at http://www.ispe.org/guidancedocs/operation_gxp, accessed Sept. 2010.
8. Contact Sylvia Collins at Nimbus Partners, http://www.nimbuspartners.com/.

Chapter 12

1. LERC (Lean Enterprise Research Centre), Annual Conference, Celtic Manor Resort, July 7, 2009, available at http://www.leanenterprise.org.uk.
2. Adam Smith, *The Wealth of Nations*, The University of Chicago Press, 1976.
3. A. Badiru (Ed.), *Handbook of Industrial and Systems Engineering*, CRC Press, Boca Raton, FL, 2005.
4. Lean Enterprise Institute, *Lean Lexicon: A Graphical Glossary for Lean Thinkers*, available at http://www.lean.org.
5. Elton Mayo, Hawthorne and the Western Electric Company, *The Social Problems of an industrial civilisation*, Routledge, London, 1949.
6. Douglas McGregor, *The Human Side of Enterprise*, McGraw-Hill, New York, 1960.
7. W. Edwards Deming, *The New Economics for Industry, Government, Education*, Second Edition, excerpt from pages 92–115.
8. W. Edwards Deming, *Out of the Crisis*, MIT Press, Cambridge, MA, 1986, pp. 23–24, available at http://mitpress.mit.edu/catalog.
9. *Lean Lexicon*, op. cit.
10. Eliyahu M. Goldratt and J. Cox, *The Goal*, Gower, Aldershot, UK, 1989.
11. Richard J. Schonberger, *World Class Manufacturing: The Lessons of Simplicity Applied*, Free Press, New York, 1986, pp. 201, 217–218.
12. James P. Womack, Daniel T. Jones, and Daniel Roos, *The Machine That Changed the World*, Simon & Schuster, New York, 2007.
13. *Lean Lexicon*, op. cit.
14. Ibid.
15. James P. Womack and Daniel T. Jones, *Lean Thinking*, Free Press, New York, 2003, p. 96.

Chapter 13

1. Contact David Cotterrell, managing director, Apex Healthcare Consulting, http://www.apex-consulting.co.uk.
2. Supply Chain Council, SCOR Framework and Reference Model, available at http://www.supply-chain.org, accessed Apr. 2010.
3. Mike Dales is Chairman of Insights, A Global Learning and Development Company, http://www.insights.com.

Chapter 14

1. U.S. FDA, http://www.fda.gov.
2. *Quieta non movere:* Don't move settled things, *or* don't rock the boat.
3. *Quinon proficit deficit:* He who does not advance goes backwards.

4. International conference on Harmonization, ICH Q6A Specifications: Test Procedures and Acceptance Criteria for New Drug Substances and New Drug Products: Chemical Substances, http://ema.europa.eu/docs/en-GB/document-Library-Scientific-guideline/2009/09/WC500002823.pdf.

5. *Quidquid latine dictum sit, altum videtur:* Anything said in Latin sounds profound.

6. http://www.fda.gov/cder/gmp/gmp2004/gmp_finalreport2004.htm.

7. Ibid.

8. http://www.ema.europa.eu/pdfs/human/ich/26514509en.pdf.

9. J. Woodcock (2005) Pharmaceutical quality in the 21st century: an integrated systems approach, presented at the AAPS Workshop on Pharmaceutical Quality Assessment: A Science and Risk-Based CMC Approach in the 21st Century.

10. U.S. Department of Health and Human Services, Food and Drug Administration, *PAT Guidance for Industry: A Framework for Innovative Pharmaceutical Development, Manufacturing and Quality Assurance*, FDA, Washington, DC, 2004.

11. International Conference on Harmonization, ICH Harmonized Tripartite Guideline: Q8(R1) Pharmaceutical Development, 2008, available at http://www.ich.org/LOB/media/MEDIA4986.pdf.

12. International Conference on Harmonization, ICH Harmonized Tripartite Guideline: Q9 Quality Risk Management, 2005, available at http://www.ich.org/LOB/media/MEDIA1957.pdf.

13. International Conference on Harmonization, ICH Harmonized Tripartite Guideline: Q10 Pharmaceutical Quality Systems, 2008, available at http://www.ich.org/LOB/media/MEDIA3917.pdf.

14. U.S. Food and Drug Administration, Submission of chemistry, manufacturing and controls information in a new drug application under the new pharmaceutical quality assessment system; notice of pilot program, *Federal Register*, 70(134):40719–40720, July 14, 2005.

15. U.S. Department of Health and Human Services, Food and Drug Administration, Notice of Pilot Program for Submission of Quality Information for Biotechnology Products in the Office of Biotechnology Products, Food and Drug Administration, Docket Number FDA-2008-N-03551, FDA, Washington, DC, 2008.

16. http://www.ema.europa.eu/pdfs/human/ich/16706804enfin.pdf.

17. U.S. Food and Drug Administration, *Guidance for Industry: CGMP For Phase 1 Investigational Drugs*, FDA, Washington, DC, July 2008.

18. U.S. Food and Drug Administration, *Guidance for Industry: For the Submission of Chemistry, Manufacturing and Controls Information for a Therapeutic Recombinant DNA-Derived Product or a Monoclonal Antibody Product for In Vivo Use*, Guidance for Industry 1-30, FDA, Washington, DC, 1996.

19. International Conference on Harmonization, ICH Topic Q8: Pharmaceutical Development: Note for Guidance on Pharmaceutical Development, European Medicines Agency, London, 2006, pp. 1–9.

20. International Conference on Harmonization, ICH Harmonized Tripartite Guideline: Q6B Specifications: Test Procedures and Acceptance Criteria for Biotechnological/Biological Products, 1999, available at http://www.ich.org/LOB/media/MEDIA432.pdf.

21. International Conference on Harmonization, ICH Topic Q10: Pharmaceutical Quality System: Note for Guidance on Pharmaceutical Quality Systems, European Medicines Agency, London, 2007, pp. 1–18.

22. S. Garcia-Munoz, J. F. MacGregor, and T. Kourti, Product transfer between sites using joint Y_PLS, *Chemometrics and Intelligent Laboratory Systems*, 79:101–114, 2005.

23. International Conference on Harmonization, ICH Harmonized Tripartite Guideline: Q5(E) Comparability of Biotechnological/Biological Products Subject to Changes in Their Manufacturing Process, 2004, available at http://www.ich.org/LOB/media/MEDIA1196.pdf.

24. U.S. Food and Drug Administration, *Guidance for Industry: Draft Guidance for Process Validation: General Principles and Practices*, FDA, Washington, DC, 2008, available at http://www.fda.gov/downloads/Drugs/GuidanceComplianceRegulatoryInformation/Guidances/UCM070336.pdf.

25. Guidance for Industry, PAT—A Framework for Innovative Pharmaceutical Development, Manufacturing, and Quality Assurance, http://www.fda.gov/downloads/Drugs/GuidanceComplianceRegulatoryInformation/Guidances/UCM070305.pdf, accessed Sept. 2010.

26. R. D. Snee, Quality by design: four years and three myths later, *Pharmaceutical Processing*, Feb. 2009, pp. 14–16.

27. International Conference on Harmonization, The Common Technical Document for the Registration of Pharmaceuticals for Human Use: Quality Overall Summary of Module 2; Module 3 Quality M4Q(RI), Sept. 2002, available at http://www.ich.org/LOB/media/MEDlA556.pdf.

28. Guideline on the Requirements to the Chemical and Pharmaceutical Quality Documentation Concerning Investigational Medicinal Products in Clinical Trials, CHMP/QWP/185401/2004 final, European Medicines Agency, London, Mar. 2006, available at http://www.emea.europa.eu/pdfs/human/qwp/18540104en.pdf.

Chapter 15

1. Nelson P. Repenning and John D. Sterman, Nobody ever gets credit for fixing problems that never happened: creating and sustaining process improvement, *California Management Review*, 43(4), Summer 2001.

2. Steven Spear, *Chasing the Rabbit*, McGraw-Hill, New York, 2009.

3. Thomas Kuhn, *The Structure of Scientific Revolutions*, Third Edition, University of Chicago Press, 1970.

4. Jeffrey K. Liker, *The Toyota Way*, McGraw-Hill, New York, 2004; Jeffrey K. Liker and David Meier, *Toyota Talent: Developing Your People the Toyota Way*,

McGraw-Hill, 2007; Jeffrey Liker and Michael Hoseus, *Toyota Culture: The Heart and Soul of the Toyota Way*, McGraw-Hill, 2008.

5. Emi Osono, *Extreme Toyota: Radical Contradictions That Drive Success at the World's Best Manufacturer*, Wiley, 2008.

6. P. Hines, P. Found, G. Griffiths, and R. Harrison, Staying lean: thriving, not just surviving, 2008, Published by Lean Enterprise Research Center, Cardiff University.

7. James P. Womack, Daniel T. Jones, and Daniel Roos, *The Machine That Changed the World*, Simon & Schuster UK Ltd., London, 2007.

8. J. Seddon, and B. O'Donovan, Rethinking lean service, presented at the LERC Conference, 2009, available at http://www.systemsthinking.co.uk, accessed Apr. 2010.

9. Spear, *Chasing the Rabbit*.

10. Based on book by Ian Glenday, *Breaking Through to Flow*, Lean Enterprise Academy, 2010.

11. P. M. Senge, *The Fifth Discipline: The Art and Practice of the Learning Organization*, Currency Doubleday, New York, 1990.

12.

13. Ibid., p. 2.

14. A. R. Kovner and K. Neuhauser, *Health Services Management: Readings, Cases, and Commentary*, 8th ed., Health Administration Press, Chicago, 2004.

15. L. V. Von Bertalanffy, *General Systems Theory: Foundations Development Applications*, George Braziller, New York, 1969.

16. Bridget Hutter, *Compliance: Regulation and Environment*, Clarendon Press, 1997.

17. Senges, *The Fifth Discipline*.

18. Ibid., p. 7.

19.

20. Senge, *The fifth discipline*.

21. L. C. Howard and J. B. McKinney, *Public Administration: Balancing Power and Accountability*, Praeger, Westport, CT, 1998.

Chapter 16

1. M. Williamson, *A Return to Love: Reflections on the Principles of "A Course in Miracles,"* HarperCollins, New York, 1992, Chap. 7, Sec. 3.

2. Dale Carnegie, *How to Win Friends and Influence People*, Simon & Schuster, New York, 1964.

3. Stephen Covey, *Seven Habits of Highly Effective People*, Simon & Schuster, 2004.

4. John J. Emerick, Jr., *Be the Person You Want to Be: Harnessing the Power of Neuro-Linguistic Programming to Reach Your Potential*, Prima Publishing, Rocklin, California, 1997.

5. Thomas Harris, *I'm OK, You're OK*, Arden Books Ltd., London, 1995.

6. Benjamin Hoff, *The Tao of Pooh*, Mandarin Paperbacks, 1989.

7. P. M. Senge, *The Fifth Discipline: The Art and Practice of the Learning Organization*, Currency Doubleday, New York, 1990.

8. W. Edwards Deming, *Out of the Crisis*, MIT Press, Combridge, MA, 1986, pp. 23–24.

9. Euromanagement, Welcome to the learning organization, presented at the Queen Elizabeth Conference Center, Jan. 30–31, 1995.

10. Abraham H. Maslow, *Towards a Psychology of Being*, Wiley, New York, 1998.

11. Frederick Hertzberg, *The Motivation to Work*,

12. Welsh Assembly Government Web site, http://wales.gov.uk/?skip=1&lang =en, accessed Apr. 2010.

13. Jeffrey K. Liker, *The Toyota Way*, McGraw-Hill, New York, 2004.

14. http://elisabethgoodman.wordpress.com.

15. Rob Goffee and Gareth Jones, *Clever: Leading Your Smartest, Most Creative People*, Harvard Business Press, Cambridge, MA, 2009.

16. Malcolm Gladwell, *Blink: The Power of Thinking Without Thinking*, Back Bay Books, New York, 2007.

17. Ben Goldacre, *Bad Science*, Harper Perennial, New York, 2009.

18. Edger H. Schein, *Organizational Culture and Leadership*, 3rd ed., Jossey-Bass, San Francisco, 2004.

19. Advisory, Conciliation and Arbitration Service (ACAS) UK, Best Practice in Industrial Relations, report compiled by Professor George Thomason, case study compiled by Brian Chaney, ACAS Head Office, 1993.

20. Steven M. R. Covey, *The Speed of Trust*, Free Press, New York, 2006.

21. E. Jaques, *Requisite Organization: Total System for Effective Managerial Organization and Managerial Leadership for the 21st Century*, Gower, Aldershot, UK, 1997.

22. D. Keuning and W. Opheij, Delayering organisations: how to beat bureaucracy and create a flexible and responsive organisation, in *Financial Times*, Pitman Publishing, London, 1993.

Chapter 17

1. P. Checkland, *Systems Thinking, Systems Practice*, Wiley, Hoboken, NJ, 1999.

2. Gareth Morgan, H. Lundbeck Eschews Outsourcing and Buys Elaiapharm, http://www.in-pharmatechnologist.com/content/search?SearchText= lundbeck+elaisapharm.

3. IMS Health, http://www.imshealth.com/portal/site/imshealth.

4. Michelle Hoffman, Editor, *Pharmaceutical Technology*, http://www.Pharma ceutical-technology.com.

5. Ram Balani, http://www.fdasmart.com.

INDEX